Women's Health

Editors

KAREN A. BLACKSTONE
ELIZABETH L. COBBS

CLINICS IN GERIATRIC MEDICINE

www.geriatric.theclinics.com

November 2021 • Volume 37 • Number 4

ELSEVIER

1600 John F. Kennedy Boulevard • Suite 1800 • Philadelphia, Pennsylvania, 19103-2899

http://www.theclinics.com

CLINICS IN GERIATRIC MEDICINE Volume 37, Number 4
November 2021 ISSN 0749-0690, ISBN-13: 978-0-323-83582-4

Editor: Katerina Heidhausen
Developmental Editor: Hannah Almira Lopez

Clinics in Geriatric Medicine (ISSN 0749-0690) is published quarterly by Elsevier Inc., 360 Park Avenue South, New York, NY 10010-1710. Months of issue are February, May, August, and November. Business and Editorial Offices: 1600 John F. Kennedy Blvd., Suite 1800, Philadelphia, PA 191023-2899. Periodicals postage paid at New York, NY, and additional mailing offices. Subscription prices are $295.00 per year (US individuals), $875.00 per year (US institutions), $100.00 per year (US & Canadian student/resident), $320.00 per year (Canadian individuals), $928.00 per year (Canadian institutions), $418.00 per year (international individuals), $928.00 per year (international institutions), and $195.00 per year (international student/resident). Foreign air speed delivery is included in all *Clinics* subscription prices. All prices are subject to change without notice. POSTMASTER: Send address changes to *Clinics in Geriatric Medicine,* Elsevier Health Sciences Division, Subscription Customer Service, 3251 Riverport Lane, Maryland Heights, MO 63043. **Telephone: 1-800-654-2452 (U.S. and Canada); 314-447-8871 (outside U.S. and Canada). Fax: 314-447-8029. E-mail:** journalscustomerservice-usa@elsevier.com **(for print support)** or journalsonlinesupport-usa@elsevier.com **(for online support).**

Reprints. For copies of 100 or more, of articles in this publication, please contact the Commercial Reprints Department, Elsevier Inc., 360 Park Avenue South, New York, New York 10010-1710. Tel.: 212-633-3874; Fax: 212-633-3820, E-mail: reprints@elsevier.com.

Clinics in Geriatric Medicine is covered in *MEDLINE/PubMed (Index Medicus), EMBASE/Excerpta Medica, Current Contents/Clinical Medicine (CC/CM),* and the *Cumulative Index to Nursing & Allied Health Literature.*

Printed in the United States of America.

Contributors

EDITORS

KAREN A. BLACKSTONE, MD, FAAHPM
Director, Hospice and Palliative Medicine Fellowship, The George Washington University, Director, Palliative Care Services, Washington DC Veterans Affairs Medical Center, Washington, DC, USA

ELIZABETH L. COBBS, MD, FACP, FAAHPM, AGSF
Geriatrics and Palliative Medicine, The George Washington University, Geriatrics, Extended Care and Palliative Care, Washington DC Veterans Affairs Medical Center, Washington, DC, USA

AUTHORS

ANITA AGGARWAL, DO, PhD
Professor of Medicine, The George Washington University School of Medicine and Health Sciences, Veterans Affairs Medical Center, Hematology/Oncology Section, Washington, DC; Adjunct Professor of Medicine, Uniformed Services University of the Health Sciences, Bethesda, Maryland, USA

WAHIDA AKBERZIE, MD
Sleep Fellow, Department of Neurology, The George Washington University School of Medicine and Health Sciences, Washington DC VA Medical Center, Washington, DC, USA

IVY AKID, MD
Clinical Instructor, Department of Medicine, Division of General Internal Medicine, Section of Palliative Medicine, Johns Hopkins School of Medicine, Johns Hopkins Hospital, Baltimore, Maryland, USA

TANIA ALCHALABI, MD
Assistant Professor of Medicine, Division of Geriatrics and Palliative Medicine, The George Washington University School of Medicine and Health Sciences, Washington, DC, USA

ESSRAA BAYOUMI, MD
Cardiovascular Disease Fellow, MedStar Washington Hospital Center, Georgetown University, VA Medical Center, Washington, DC, USA

MARIE A. BERNARD, MD
Chief Officer for Scientific Workforce Diversity, National Institutes of Health, Bethesda, Maryland, USA

SARAH T. CIGNA, MD, MS, FACOG
Assistant Professor, Department of Obstetrics and Gynecology, Alexandria, Virginia, USA

ELIZABETH CLARK, MD
Associate Professor of Clinical Medicine, Albert Einstein College of Medicine, Bronx, New York, New York, USA

PARTH DESAI, MD
Hematology and Oncology Fellow, National Heart, Lung and Blood Institute (NHLBI)/
National Institutes of Health (NIH), Bethesda, Maryland, USA

ANCA DINESCU, MD
Geriatrics and Palliative Care Department, Washington DC Veteran Administration
Medical Center, Assistant Professor, Internal Medicine, The George Washington
University, Washington, DC, USA

DANIELLE J. DOBERMAN, MD, MPH, HMDC
Assistant Professor, Department of Medicine, Division of General Internal Medicine,
Section of Palliative Medicine, Palliative Medicine Program, Johns Hopkins School of
Medicine, Johns Hopkins Hospital, Baltimore, Maryland, USA

MARISA DUNN, MD, MPH
Primary Care Physician, Jencare Senior Medical Center, Decatur, Georgia, USA

NANCY D. GABA, MD, FACOG
Professor and Chair, Department of Obstetrics and Gynecology, Washington, DC, USA

DEBRA L. GRAY, PT, DPT, DHS, MEd
Board Certified Geriatric Clinical Specialist, Certified Expert for the Aging Adult, Associate
Professor, University of St Augustine for Health Sciences, Practicing Physical Therapist,
Gray Therapy Education Consulting LLC, Jacksonville, Florida, USA

RENEE HICKSON, MD
Oak Street Healthcare, New Orleans, Louisiana; Department of Geriatrics and Palliative
Medicine, The George Washington University, Washington, DC, USA

CATHERINE G. HOEPPNER, MD, MS
Chief Resident, Department of Obstetrics and Gynecology, Washington, DC, USA

PATRICIA JONES, DrPH, MPH, MS, MBA
Office of Special Populations, National Institute on Aging, National Institutes of Health,
Bethesda, Maryland, USA

RACHAEL KANTOR, MD
Medical School of International Health, Faculty of Health Sciences, Ben-Gurion University
of the Negev, Be'er Sheva, Israel

PAMELA KARASIK, MD
Chief, Medical Service VA Medical Center, Professor of Medicine, The George
Washington University Medical Center, Washington, DC, USA

LYNN KATARIA, MD
Director, Sleep Laboratory, Clinical Assistant Professor, Department of Neurology, The
George Washington University School of Medicine and Health Sciences, Washington DC
VA Medical Center, Washington, DC, USA

FRED C. KO, MD
Associate Professor, Brookdale Department of Geriatrics and Palliative Medicine, Icahn
School of Medicine at Mount Sinai, New York, New York, USA; Geriatric Research
Education and Clinical Center, James J. Peters VA Medical Center, Bronx, New York,
USA

MOLLY LAFLIN, PhD, FSOAE
Professor Emeritus, Health Promotion, Bowling Green State University, Bowling Green, Ohio, USA

JOY A. LARAMIE, MSN, NP, ACHPN
Arlington, Virginia, USA

CAROLE B. LEWIS, PT, DPT, GCS, GTCCS, MPA, MSG, PhD, FSOAE, FAPTA
Editor-in-Chief, *Topics in Geriatric Rehabilitation*, President of Great Seminars and Books and Great Seminars Online, Practicing Physical Therapist, Adjunct Professor, The George Washington University School of Medicine and Health Sciences, Washington, DC, USA

SOPHIE LIN, MD
New York Medical College, Metropolitan Hospital Center, New York, New York, USA

TAHIRA I. LODHI, MD
Division of Geriatrics and Palliative Medicine, The George Washington University, Washington, DC, USA

JOANNE LYNN, MD, MA, MS
Policy Analyst, Center to Improve Eldercare, Altarum

MONICA PERNIA MARIN, MD
Department of Geriatrics and Palliative Medicine, The George Washington University, Washington, DC, USA

CATHERINE NAGY, MA
Office of Planning, Analysis, and Evaluation, National Institute on Aging, National Institutes of Health, Bethesda, Maryland, USA

CAROLINE PARK, MD, PhD
Geriatric Medicine Fellow, Section of Geriatrics, Division of Primary Care and Population Health, Stanford School of Medicine, Stanford Senior Care, Palo Alto, California, USA

JENNA PERKINS, MSN, WHNP-BC
Alexandria, Virginia, USA

CHRISTINA PRATHER, MD
Assistant Professor of Medicine, Division of Geriatrics and Palliative Medicine, Clinical-Director, GWU Institute for Brain Health and Dementia, The George Washington University School of Medicine and Health Sciences, Washington, DC, USA

LOUISA WHITESIDES, MD
Assistant Professor of Geriatrics and Palliative Medicine, The George Washington University Medical Faculty Associates, Washington, DC, USA

Contents

> Certain psychosocial elements, such as depression, anxiety, stress, lack of social support, and loneliness, should be considered as part of frailty. Women are more likely to be frail toward the end of life, because they live longer and are less likely to develop diseases with abrupt ends. Women are also more prone to develop psychosocial elements associated with frailty because of their lifetime stressors, poverty, and loneliness at the end of life. Clinicians should recognize this phenomenon and create early interventions to ensure women are able to live according to their preferences during the last part of their lives.

> Women's sexual health is a frequently ignored area of geriatric medicine. There are clearly defined criteria for sexual dysfunction that are organized by phase of sexual function, including desire, arousal, orgasm, and pain. The menopause transition and comorbid medical conditions (as well as their treatments) can contribute to alterations in sexual function. The partner must be included and involved in the evaluation and management to achieve a better intimate relationship in an established couple. A variety of effective and evidence-based treatments are available to women for sexual concerns in the geriatric population.

> Health care providers in all settings are likely to have the opportunity to care for lesbian, gay, bisexual, transgender, and/or queer (LGBTQ) persons. It is important to understand and respect the histories and experiences of these persons and the impacts in their later years. Attention must be paid to their unique psychological, social, and medical needs— not only the challenges but also the positive aspects that help develop resilience and establish a strong, if not traditional, community of care.

> Brain health and the health of the aging brain are topics of increased interest in recent years given the expected aging of the world's population. Many conditions associated with memory loss and other disorders of cognition have age as a risk factor. This article describes the healthy aging brain and theories about how to maintain brain health through later life. The role of gender in brain health and whether women are at increased risk of neurodegenerative disorders leading to dementia are discussed. Important factors that contribute to brain health, including nutrition, exercise, chronic disease management, and others, also are discussed.

The overall rate of advance care planning (ACP) in the general population remains low. ACP is a dynamic process that needs to be refined over time. ACP documentation includes the naming of a health care proxy, preferences regarding life-sustaining treatment interventions, and other, more disease-specific, interventions, such as chemotherapy, hemodialysis, and surgeries. The process should start early in someone's adult life, with a broad scope of defining what matters most for that person. Over time, the initial ACP could be refined to include more specific limitations of certain medical procedures. ACP documents achieved more standardization in the last several years.

Breast cancer is becoming increasingly prevalent in the women greater than 65 years of age. Most tumors are hormone receptor-positive in this group. Breast cancer screening recommendations for older women should be tailored based on life expectancy. Early stage breast cancer should be treated with conservative surgery followed by adjuvant endocrine therapy in HR+ patients. Primary endocrine therapy is a low-risk option for those with limited life expectancy. Adjuvant radiation therapy can be avoided in early stage, low-risk cancers. Evaluation should include comprehensive geriatric assessment. Treatment with less cytotoxic chemotherapy, HER-2 targeted therapies, and other biomarker-driven, molecularly targeted therapies should be sought whenever possible.

Frailty is an important clinical syndrome of age-related decline in physiologic reserve and increased vulnerability. In older adults, frailty leads to progressive multisystem decline and increased adverse clinical outcomes. The pathophysiology of frailty is hypothesized to be driven by dysregulation of neuroendocrine, inflammatory, and metabolic pathways. Sex-specific differences in the prevalence of frailty have been observed. Treatment interventions of geriatric care can be applied to the care of frail older women with these differences in mind. As additional evidence regarding sex-specific differences in frailty emerges, research efforts should encompass the development of screening tools and therapeutic interventions that optimize outcomes.

Exercise is associated with protective effects, yet most adult women in this country do not meet the physical activity recommendations set forth in the Physical Activity Guidelines for Americans. This article discusses how exercise affects disease and prevents functional decline. It also clarifies why exercise is not a generic cure-all but is instead a tool physicians can use with precision to affect a myriad of health issues. Specifics will be provided regarding physical fitness assessments and comprehensive treatments and how physicians can be more involved in using physical fitness to keep their older female patients healthy.

Cardiovascular disease is the major cause of death in women. Older women remain at risk for coronary artery disease/cardiovascular disease, but risk-modifying behavior can improve outcomes. Women have a different symptom profile and have been underdiagnosed and under-treated as compared with men. Although older women are underrepresented in trials, clinicians should be more attuned to the prevention, diagnosis, and treatment of cardiovascular disease in older women.

What are the effects of sleep disturbance and changes of sleep on aging women in the short and long term? Most research that has been done in recent years evaluates how sleep disorders and sleep disturbance may change mortality and outcomes of this population. Many confounding factors may be playing a role, including comorbid conditions. This article reviews sleep disorders including insomnia, circadian sleep-wake rhythm disorders, restless legs syndrome, disorders of hypersomnia, and sleep-disordered breathing in women aged 65 and older; prevalence of these disorders; and recommended treatment options.

The gold standard for diagnosis of osteoporosis is measurement of an individual's bone mineral density on dual-energy x-ray absorptiometry scan. If this value is less than or equal to 2.5 standard deviations less than that of an adult female reference population, a person is said to have osteoporosis, with this risk increasing as a person ages. Female gender is a large risk factor in developing osteoporosis, regardless of ethnic or racial group. Frailty is another key factor in determining likelihood to develop osteoporotic fractures. Bisphosphonates are the first line agents for treatment of osteoporosis.

CLINICS IN GERIATRIC MEDICINE

SERIES OF RELATED INTEREST

Medical Clinics
https://www.medical.theclinics.com/
Primary Care: Clinics in Office Practice
https://www.primarycare.theclinics.com/

THE CLINICS ARE AVAILABLE ONLINE!
Access your subscription at:
www.theclinics.com

Preface

Geriatrics Clinic in Women's Health

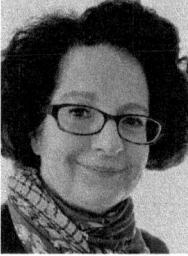

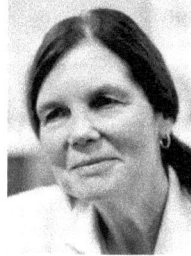

Karen A. Blackstone, MD, FAAHPM   Elizabeth L. Cobbs, MD, FACP, FAAHPM, AGSF
Editors

Older women comprise a diverse population of enormous complexity and opportunity. Recent discovery that many diseases, medications, and exposures affect women differently than men drives the current transformation in the research community to incorporate both female sex as a biological variable and female gender (culturally assigned attitudes, feelings, and behaviors) into all types of biomedical research from the laboratory bench to the patient's bedside to community-based health initiatives. A variety of contemporary health issues appear to be influenced by both sex and gender, including neurodegenerative diseases, hypertension, response to viral infection, chronic stress and depression, and the response to dietary fats and carbohydrates.[1]

As health care experts increasingly recognize nonbiological factors that influence older women's wellness, local, national, and international health care systems leaders have begun to address environmental and sociocultural concerns. The Age-Friendly Health System Initiative, formed through a collaboration between The John A. Hartford Foundation, the Institute for Healthcare Improvement, the American Hospital Association, and the Catholic Health Association of the United States, aims to improve health care outcomes for older adults, including women, through systematically applying evidence-based practices across health care systems and aligning with what matters to older adults and their family caregivers. To support international governments to develop age-friendly health and social policies, the World Health Organization (WHO) released a Policy Framework on Active Ageing in 2002. The Global Age-Friendly Cities Project developed out of WHO focuses on the environmental and social factors that influence healthy aging in urban settings. The aim of WHO Global Age-Friendly Cities is to engage cities around the world to make communities more age-friendly.

Our selection of topics for this issue reflects important and diverse issues influencing the health of older women. The list is by no means a comprehensive treatment of these

Clin Geriatr Med 37 (2021) xiii–xiv
https://doi.org/10.1016/j.cger.2021.06.002
0749-0690/21/© 2021 Published by Elsevier Inc.

issues. We hope to introduce key evidence in several important domains and spark further interest and discovery. Significant general subjects include the following: Aging and Health, the Science of Frailty, Frailty and Personal Care, Brain Health, Fitness, Sexuality, Sleep, and Advance Care Planning. Articles on special populations address Minority Women and LGBT wellness concerns. Articles on key medical syndromes affecting older women include the following: Bone Health, Diabetes, and Cancer.

We hope this collection of articles will inspire and inform you to learn more about the health of older women and how we can all contribute to successful aging for all women around the globe.

Karen A. Blackstone, MD, FAAHPM
Director, Hospice and Palliative Medicine Fellowship
The George Washington University
Director, Palliative Care Services
Washington DC Veterans Affairs Medical Center
Washington, DC, USA

Elizabeth L. Cobbs, MD, FACP, FAAHPM, AGSF
Geriatrics and Palliative Medicine
George Washington University
Geriatrics, Extended Care and Palliative Care
Washington DC Veterans Affairs Medical Center
Washington, DC, USA

E-mail addresses:
karen.blackstone@va.gov (K.A. Blackstone)
ecobbs@mfa.gwu.edu (E.L. Cobbs)

REFERENCE

1. Clayton JA. A path for better science and innovation, the 5th Annual Vivian W. Pinn Symposium to Highlight Benefits of Accounting for Sex and Gender in Biomedical Research. Available at: https://orwh.od.nih.gov/about/director/messages/path-better-science-and-innovation. Accessed May 3, 2021.

Diabetes Mellitus in Older Women

Tahira I. Lodhi, MD

KEYWORDS

- Diabetes mellitus • Older adults • Older women

KEY POINTS

- Gestational diabetes mellitus and prediabetes are 2 historical features that have research evidence for association with the development of diabetes in older women.
- Type 1 diabetes mellitus is characterized by the destruction of β cells of the endocrine pancreas, most likely through cell-mediated autoimmunity.
- Both basal and stimulated insulin levels in older adults are similar to those of insulin-sensitive young people, suggesting an inadequate adaptive response to insulin resistance in older subjects.
- Once a diagnosis of diabetes is established, a comprehensive geriatric assessment is performed to obtain a multiyear history of diabetes and identify multimorbidity.
- In an age-friendly health system, what matters most to a patient should determine the management goals, based on shared decision making between patient, caregiver, and health care provider.
- Nonpharmacologic management, oral hypoglycemic agents, and insulin are interventions for diabetes care.
- The critical step in developing a diabetes management plan for an older adult is establishing treatment goals for the short term and the long term. Managing comorbidities, including hypertension, hyperlipidemia, and cigarette smoking, also are part of the strategy.
- It is imperative to teach patients and caregivers to be able to recognize and treat hypoglycemia.
- Appropriate diabetes care for patients currently lacks quality standards and guidance on best clinical practices at the end of life.
- Dementia, including both Alzheimer and vascular type, is approximately twice as likely to occur in those with diabetes than age-matched nondiabetic control subjects.

Sharing hyperglycemia as a common phenotype, diabetes represents a heterogeneous group of disorders affecting multiple body systems. A large population-based prospective cohort study, consisting of women ages greater than 50 years old, has

Author Note: No grant funding or financial disclosures.
Division of Geriatrics and Palliative Medicine, George Washington University, 2300 M Street NW, Washington, DC 20037, USA
E-mail address: tlodhi@mfa.gwu.edu

shown evidence of a decreased risk of type 2 diabetes mellitus with moderate alcohol consumption in women.[1] Although the disease itself has no gender differences, coping strategies may be different.

DIAGNOSIS

Three methods can be used to determine a diagnosis of diabetes in all adults, regardless of age.[2,3] They are summarized in **Table 1**.

The American Diabetes Association (ADA) recommends screening all individuals older than age 45 years at 3-year intervals to detect prediabetes or diabetes using fasting plasma glucose (FPG) level, oral glucose tolerance test (OGTT), or glycosylated hemoglobin A_{1c} (HbA_{1c}) level, particularly those with a body mass index (BMI) greater than or equal to 25 kg/m^2. There is significant discordance in these 3 different criteria in diagnosing diabetes, especially in older adults. For example, if FPG is less than 126 mg/dL (7 mmol/L) but HbA_{1c} is greater than or equal to 6.5%, then HbA_{1c} should be repeated. If the repeat HbA_{1c} is greater than or equal to 6.5%, then the person is considered to have diabetes.

TYPES

Type 1 diabetes mellitus is characterized by the destruction of β cells of the endocrine pancreas, most likely through cell-mediated autoimmunity.[2,4] Markers of immune destruction, including pancreatic β-cell antibodies, other pancreatic cell–specific antibodies, and antibodies to insulin, have been found. Other patients may present with idiopathic type 1 diabetes mellitus, with no detectable autoimmunity. Older adults rarely present with new-onset type 1 diabetes mellitus. Due to an increase in longevity and improved cardiovascular mortality, patients with type 1 diabetes mellitus may live to old age. They become part of the spectrum of diabetes in the older adult population.

Approximately 90% of older adults have type 2 diabetes mellitus. Its exact etiology is unknown. Autoimmunity rarely is observed. It likely is multifactorial due to an interaction between genetics, lifestyle, and aging factors contributing to progressive insulin secretory defect and peripheral insulin resistance resulting in characteristic hyperglycemia.

Gestational diabetes mellitus (GDM) is defined as glucose metabolism first identified during pregnancy. It is not a part of the spectrum of diabetes in older adults. Still, an older woman with a history of GDM can present later in life with type 2 diabetes mellitus. In the United States, approximately 4% of all pregnancies are complicated by GDM. A reported 5% to 10% of women with GDM are found to have type 2 diabetes

Table 1 Laboratory diagnosis of diabetes			
Glycemic Status	Glycosylated Hemoglobin A_{1c}	Fasting Plasma Glucose	Oral Glucose Tolerance Test, 2 Hours
Normal	≤5.6%	<99 mg/dL (5.5 mmol/L)	<148 mg/dL (7.7 mmol/L)
Prediabetes	5.7%–6.4%	≥100–125 mg/dL (5.6–6.9 mmol/L)	149–199 mg/dL (7.8–11.0 mmol/L)
Diabetes	≥6.5%	≥126 mg/dL (7 mmol/L)	≥200 mg/dL (11.1 mmol/L)

FPG is glucose measurement after no caloric intake for at least 8 h. Any of these criteria should be confirmed on a separate day to establish the diagnosis of diabetes.

mellitus. These women have 20% to 50% chance of developing diabetes in the next 5 years to 10 years.[5] Polycystic ovary syndrome also is associated with insulin resistance, putting them at higher risk of developing diabetes.[6,7]

Rare but specific types of diabetes mellitus identified by the ADA include maturity-onset diabetes of youth, diseases of exocrine pancreas, excessive secretion of hormones, tumors, and medication-induced diabetes.

RISK FACTORS FOR DIABETES DEVELOPMENT

Box 1 summarizes the risk factors for diabetes development.

EPIDEMIOLOGY

The highest incidence of newly diagnosed diabetes is between the ages of 45 years to 64 years and 65 years to 79 years, with an estimated 12 new cases per 1000 people and 15 new patients per 1000 people in 2011, respectively. Prevalence is highest among patients older than 65 years, 27% compared with 18% in 45-year-old to 64-year-old age group (https://www.cdc.gov/nchs/hus/contents2018.htm#Table_014).

Per death certificate records, diabetes was the seventh leading cause of death in the United States from 1999 to 2019 (https://wonder.cdc.gov/controller/saved/D76/D99F205). Only 35% to 40% of people who died with diabetes had the diagnosis mentioned anywhere on their death certificate. Only 10% to 15% had it listed as a cause of death; 73% of deaths that occur among people ages 70 and older are attributable to diabetes.

AGING AND PATHOGENESIS OF TYPE 2 DIABETES MELLITUS

Fig. 1 depicts age-related changes resulting in hyperglycemia. People who do not meet the criteria for diabetes mellitus have an age-related increase in fasting glucose levels and a more slowing of return to normal glucose levels following an oral glucose challenge.[8,9]

Insulin Resistance

With aging, insulin resistance develops by several mechanisms, including decreased physical activity (PA), central adiposity, and age-related impairment of intracellular insulin signaling, reducing insulin-mediated mobilization of glucose transporters. These

---

Box 1
Diabetes risk factors

- BMI $\geq$25 kg/m^2
- Genetic predisposition: first-degree relative with diabetes
- Older women with a history of GDM
- History of hypertension
- History of dyslipidemia: in particular, elevated triglycerides, low high-density lipoprotein levels
- History of impaired fasting glucose
- History of impaired glucose tolerance
- History of previous HbA$_{1c}$ >5.7%
- Race: African American, Hispanic, Pacific Islander, Asian American, Native American

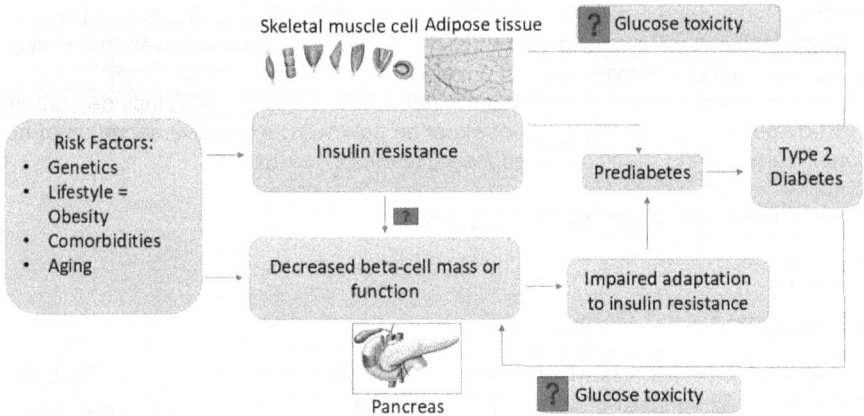

Fig. 1. Age-related changes resulting in hyperglycemia.

transporters are critical to glucose uptake and metabolism in insulin-dependent tissues, such as muscle and fat. Physiologically, in the presence of insulin resistance, a compensatory increase of insulin secretion, leading to increased circulating insulin levels, would be expected. Both basal and stimulated insulin levels in older adults, however, are similar to those of insulin-sensitive young people, suggesting an inadequate adaptive response to insulin resistance in older subjects. This maladaptive response leads to impaired insulin secretion and progression to impaired glucose tolerance and type 2 diabetes mellitus.[10] The resulting hyperglycemia contributes directly to insulin resistance and to impaired pancreatic β-cell function, thereby setting up a vicious cycle of maladaptive mechanisms.

There currently is little evidence for an age-related impairment of insulin effects on protein or fat metabolism.

Impaired Insulin Secretion

Multimorbidity, including hypertension, hyperlipidemia, and acute coexisting illness, are factors that affect both insulin sensitivity and insulin secretion in older adults. Furthermore, a critical illness can precipitate hyperglycemia because of the effects of stress hormones, the α-adrenergic effects of catecholamines released during stressful conditions lead to inhibition of insulin secretion. Many commonly used medications also contribute to hyperglycemia by causing insulin resistance in older people.

Genetics

The concordance rate for type 2 diabetes mellitus in identical twins approaches 100%, suggesting a strong genetic predisposition. The genetic alleles appear to affect the risk of type 2 diabetes mellitus primarily through impaired pancreatic β-cell function, reduced insulin action, or obesity risk.[11]

PRESENTATION

The most common presentation for type 2 diabetes mellitus in older adults is through routine laboratory work showing hyperglycemia. Few older people present with polyuria, polydipsia, and polyphagia. There may be gradual unexplained weight loss. Atypical symptoms of hyperglycemia like falls, urinary incontinence, fatigue, and confusion are common. Because type 2 diabetes mellitus can go undetected for years, some older adults with type 2 diabetes mellitus may present with a complication like retinopathy, nephropathy, or neuropathy as the presenting complaint.

Type 1 diabetes mellitus may have a more indolent course in an older adult. Diabetic ketoacidosis (DKA) might never occur because of early detection and treatment.

EVALUATION

Once a diagnosis of diabetes is established, a comprehensive geriatric assessment is performed to obtain a multiyear history of diabetes and identify multimorbidity. Medication and allergy histories are used to identify medications that could contribute to hyperglycemia or hypoglycemia and identify potential drug interactions. What matters to older adults can be elicited through social and family history, care goals, and advance directive discussions. Mentation can be elicited through formal neuropsychological testing for cognitive assessment. Mobility and life space assessments can be used to assess an older adult's functional status.

Physical examination should include a set of vital signs, including orthostatic blood pressure and baseline weight. Examination of eyes and cardiovascular, pulmonary, genitourinary, gastrointestinal, and neurologic systems should be done in detail, including skin examination.

A detailed neurologic examination should be done, including cranial nerve examination and monofilament test using a 10-g nylon for peripheral neuropathy; vibration sensation also should be tested with a tuning fork at the base of the big toe. This neuropathy evaluation should be carried out in conjunction with a careful foot examination to identify possible structural abnormalities.

A thorough evaluation of the cardiovascular system should be done given the cardiovascular disease (CVD) risk in older people with diabetes. Doppler evaluation should be made of carotids, extremity blood flow, and/or cardiovascular stress testing if there is any CVD suggestion. Silent myocardial infarction (MI) seems more common in patients with diabetes, so the stress testing threshold should be relatively low.

Diabetes knowledge should be evaluated using standardized diabetes knowledge tests by a diabetes educator or a suitably trained nurse.

Geriatric syndromes, including visual impairment, hearing impairment, urinary incontinence, and polypharmacy, affect self-care abilities and quality of life in older adults with diabetes. These should be assessed as part of a comprehensive geriatric assessment.

Laboratory evaluation should include, in addition to the diagnostic test for diabetes, a test for lipid panel, renal functions, and electrolytes, liver function tests and a spot qualitative urine test for the presence of protein in the urine. Any positive test should be repeated. A spot urine sample should be sent for quantitative measurement of urine protein and creatinine for a negative test. Microalbuminuria suggests early diabetic nephropathy. Such a test should be repeated twice in subsequent months for confirmation. If 2 or 3 of these tests are positive, intervention is warranted.

PREVENTION

Type 2 diabetes mellitus is a gradually progressive disorder of carbohydrate metabolism that may develop over 8 years to 10 years before a clinical diagnosis is made. Intensive lifestyle interventions, including weight loss and increased PA, can substantially reduce type 2 diabetes mellitus progression in high-risk people, for example, those with prediabetes. In the multicenter National Diabetes Prevention Program in the United States,[12,13] during the 3 years of active treatment, the program was more effective in people older than 60 than in younger people, reducing diabetes progression by more than 70% compared with the control group. Metformin also was used in the National Diabetes Prevention Program and was influential in slowing progression in younger adults but surprisingly was much less effective in older people above age 60 years. The benefit of lifestyle intervention appeared to be long-term among older adults as they had a reduced frequency of developing type 2 diabetes mellitus over the 10 years of follow-up.

MANAGEMENT
General Approach

In an age-friendly health system, what matters most to a patient should determine the management goals, based on shared decision making between patient, caregiver, and health care provider. A team's collaborative effort, including physicians, nurse practitioners, nurses, dietitians, pharmacists, and mental health professionals, who communicate with each other and involve the patient as an active participant, is vital to achieving care goals. A supportive social environment, adequate economic support, meal preparation, and availability also play a significant role in adherence to treatment regimens. It can be beneficial to have a social worker or other suitably trained personnel help with older diabetic patients' needs.

Establishing Goals

A critical step in developing a diabetes management plan for an older adult is establishing treatment goals for the short term and the long term. Short-term goals are to control hyperglycemia and glucose toxicity. Long-term goals are to prevent complications from long-standing diabetes based on life expectancy.[9] Managing comorbidities, including hypertension, hyperlipidemia, and cigarette smoking, also are part of the strategy.[14]

The ADA (Consensus Report, 2019) recommends the goals (listed in **Table 2**) for glycemia, blood pressure, and dyslipidemia in older adults.

Diabetes Self-Management Education

Diabetes self-management education is an ongoing, evidence-based process of facilitating the knowledge, and skills, necessary for diabetes self-care for an individual. It can be difficult to achieve.[15] Diabetes self-management education should be received at the time of diagnosis and as needed after that. It is associated with improved diabetes knowledge and self-care behavior, improved quality of life, lower HbA$_{1c}$, and lower costs. The Centers for Medicare & Medicaid Services reimburse the cost to beneficiaries if the diabetes self-management education is provided by a training program accredited by either the ADA or the American Association of Diabetes Educators. Despite Medicare reimbursement, only 55% of older adults 65 years to 74 years old and 47% of adults ages 75 years and older reported ever attending a diabetes self-management class.

Nonpharmacologic Treatment Options

Exercise
Exercise training can improve insulin sensitivity in people with decreased PA. Per the ADA, all adults with diabetes should perform at least 150 minutes per week of moderate-intensity aerobic PA, spread over at least 3 days a week, with no more than 2 consecutive days without exercise. As part of the exercise routine, resistance

Table 2
Diabetes management goals

Health Status	Rationale	Hemoglobin A_{1c}	Fasting Plasma Glucose (mg/dL)	Blood Pressure (mm Hg)	Lipids
Healthy	Longer life expectancy	<7.5%	90–130	<140/80	Statins unless contraindicated or not tolerated
Complex/ intermediate health	Intermediate life expectancy, high treatment burden, hypoglycemia vulnerability, fall risk	<8%	90–150	<140/80	Statins unless contraindicated or not tolerated
Very complex/ poor health	Limited remaining life expectancy makes benefit uncertain	<8.5%	100–180	<150/90	Consider benefit with statin (secondary prevention > primary)

training should be performed at least twice per week. More than 60% of adults with type 2 diabetes mellitus are not physically active. Only 12% of adults above age 75 years engage in 30 minutes of exercise 5 or more days per week and 65% report no leisure PA. Patients with low baseline PA are likely to experience more significant health benefits with a given increase in PA, especially with longer and more frequent exercise sessions. Each patient's exercise prescription should be individualized based on their ability to participate in an exercise program safely.

Diet
The ADA currently recommends medical nutrition therapy to be included in any diabetes care. The average American diet includes approximately 45% of calories from carbohydrates, 40% as fat and 15% protein, including with recommended quantities of vitamins and minerals. There is no convincing evidence for hyperglycemia control or diabetes complication prevention with the supplements.

Special considerations for older adults with diabetes mellitus include access to food due to functional disability, financial constraints, poor meal preparation skills, and lack of formal or informal support to obtain food. A decline in taste and smell appreciation and xerostomia can affect food intake as well. Ethnic food preferences, impaired cognition, and depression also can affect dietary intake.

A combination of caloric restriction and exercise is the best approach for an older adult with type 2 diabetes mellitus. BMI greater than 25 kg/m^2 is a marker of being overweight and an indication of reduced caloric prescription.[16] Because of an age-related decline in lean body mass, older individuals may have increased adiposity, especially central adiposity, without being overweight by usual BMI criteria. Documenting waist measurement is a better criterion in older adults for a prescription of caloric restriction rather than BMI.

Medications

Noninsulin glucose-lowering agents for the treatment of type 2 diabetes mellitus are shown in **Table 3**.

Table 3
Noninsulin glucose-lowering agents for the treatment of type 2 diabetes mellitus

Class	Route	Mechanism	Advantages	Disadvantages
Biguanide • Metformin	Oral • 500–1000 mg BID • Maximum 2500 mg/d	Decreased hepatic gluconeogenesis, possibly increased insulin-mediated uptake of glucose in muscles	No weight gain, minimal hypoglycemia, likely decreased microvascular and macrovascular events, extensive clinical experience	Gastrointestinal side effects (diarrhea and abdominal discomfort), lactic acidosis, contraindicated in the presence of progressive hepatic, renal, or cardiac failure
Sulfonylureas Glipizide Glyburide Glimepiride Gliclazide	Oral 2.5–10 mg BID 2.5–20 mg daily 1–4 mg daily 40 mg daily–160 mg BID	Increased insulin secretion from pancreatic β cells	Decreased microvascular events, extensive clinical experience	Hypoglycemia (especially with longer half-life: glyburide), weight gain, skin rash (including photosensitivity)
Meglitinides Repaglinide Nateglinide	Oral 0.5–4 mg QAC 60–120 mg QAC	Increased insulin secretion from pancreatic β cells	Decreased postprandial glucose excursions, dosing flexibility (before meals)	Hypoglycemia, weight gain, frequent dosing schedule
Thiazolidinediones Pioglitazone Rosiglitazone	Oral 15–45 mg daily 2–8 mg daily or BID	Increased insulin sensitivity	Minimal hypoglycemia, increase high-density lipoprotein cholesterol, decreased triglycerides (pioglitazone)	Weight gain, edema/heart failure, bone fractures, increase low-density lipoprotein cholesterol, ? increased myocardial infarction risk

Drug class	Dosing	Mechanism	Benefits	Side effects/cautions
DPP-4 inhibitors Sitagliptin Saxagliptin Vildagliptin Linagliptin Alogliptin	Oral 100 mg daily 2.5–5 mg daily 50 mg daily or BID 5 mg daily 25 mg daily	Increased insulin secretion (glucose-dependent), decreased glucagon secretion (glucose-dependent)	Minimal hypoglycemia, well tolerated, once-daily dosing	Urticaria/angioedema, ? increased risk of pancreatitis, ? increased heart failure hospitalization, high cost
GLP-1 receptor agonists Exenatide (Byetta) Exenatide extended-release Liraglutide Dulaglutide Albiglutide Lixisenatide	Injection 5–10 µg SC BID 2 mg SC weekly 0.6–1.8 mg SC daily 0.75 mg/0.5 mL SC weekly 30–50 mg SC weekly 10–20 µg SC daily	Increase insulin secretion (glucose-dependent), Decrease glucagon secretion (glucose-dependent), slows gastric emptying, increased satiety	Minimal hypoglycemia, weight reduction, Decreased postprandial glucose excursions	Gastrointestinal side effects (nausea, vomiting), increased heart rate, ? acute pancreatitis, C-cell hyperplasia/medullary thyroid tumors in animals
α-Glucosidase inhibitors Acarbose Miglitol	Oral 25–100 mg TID with meals 25–100 mg TID with meals	Slows intestinal carbohydrates digestion or absorption	Minimal hypoglycemia, decreased postprandial glucose excursions, ? decreased CVD events (STOP-NIDDM)	Generally modest HbA$_{1c}$ reduction, flatulence, abdominal discomfort, contraindicated in cirrhosis frequent dosing schedule (with meals)
Bile acid sequestrant Colesevelam	Oral 3750 mg daily (or 1875 mg BID) with meals	Unclear ? Decreased hepatic glucose production, ? increased incretin levels	Minimal hypoglycemia, decreased low-density lipoprotein cholesterol	Generally modest HbA$_{1c}$ reduction, constipation, increased triglycerides, reduced absorption of fat-soluble vitamins, high cost

(continued on next page)

Table 3
(continued)

Class	Route	Mechanism	Advantages	Disadvantages
Dopamine-2 agonist Bromocriptine, immediate-release form	Oral 1.6–4.8 mg QAM	Modulates hypothalamic regulation of metabolism, increased insulin sensitivity	Minimal hypoglycemia	Nausea, headache; orthostatic hypotension; potential exacerbation of psychosis; high cost
Amylin-like Pramlintide	Injection 60–120 µg SC QAC	Decreased glucagon secretion, slows gastric emptying, increased satiety	Reduced postprandial glucose excursions, weight reduction	Gastrointestinal side effects (nausea; vomiting), increased hypoglycemic risk of insulin, frequent dosing schedule, high cost
SGLT-2 inhibitors Canagliflozin Empagliflozin Dapagliflozin	Oral 100–300 mg daily 10–25 mg daily 5–10 mg daily	Decreased renal glucose reabsorption, increased urinary glucose excretion	Minimal hypoglycemia, weight reduction Decreased blood pressure useful at all stages of type 2 diabetes mellitus, once-daily dosing	Caution in renal insufficiency, genitourinary infections, genital yeast infections, polyuria, hyperkalemia, orthostatic hypotension, pancreatitis

Insulin agents lead to increased glucose disposal and decreased hepatic glucose production (**Table 4**). They are nearly universally responsive and likely lead to decreased microvascular risk.[17] Disadvantages are hypoglycemia risks, which vary based on the individual agent's dose and its course of action.

Combination of Insulin and Oral Agents

Insulin can be combined with using 1 or more oral agents, although there is little research on such regimens, specifically in older adults. Comparing several insulin regimens and oral therapy among people with type 2 diabetes mellitus with a mean age of 62 years found that fewer than 25% of patients achieve stringent HBA_{1c}.

MULTIMORBIDITY WITH DIABETES
Acute Complications: Hyperglycemia

The relationship between HbA_{1c} and mortality appears to be U-shaped rather than linear. Older patients with diabetes have a low risk of death or other complications at an HBA_{1c} between 6% and 9% but a higher risk with lower HbA_{1c} or higher HbA_{1c}. Adherence to diet, exercise, and oral hypoglycemic agents and insulin regimen maintains glycemic goals.

Diabetic ketoacidosis

DKA is uncommon in older people, but it can occur in older patients with type 1 diabetes mellitus when insulin is inappropriately discontinued or because of a significant underlying illness that interferes with a patient's self-care capability. As in younger people, the hallmarks of DKA are significant hyperglycemia, hyperosmolarity, and volume depletion. Systemic acidosis can be caused by marked elevation of ketoacids.

Table 4
Insulin for treatment of type 2 diabetes mellitus

Insulin Agents	Onset of Action	Peak Effect	Duration of Action
Long-acting	Approximately 2 h	No peak	20–24 h
Glargine 100	Approximately 2 h	3–9 h	6–24 h (dose-dependent;
Detemir			at $\geq$0.8 U/kg, mean duration of action is longer and less variable—22–23 h)
Ultra–long acting	Approximately 2 h	No peak	>40 h
Degludec	Approximately 6 h	No peak	28–36 h
Glargine 300			
Intermediate acting	Approximately 2 h	4–12 h	18–28 h
Human NPH	Approximately 2 h	6 h	15 h
Neutral protamine lispro			
Short acting	Approximately 30 min	2–4 h	5–8 h
Human regular			
Rapid acting	5–15 min	45–75 min	2–4 h
Lispro			
Aspart			
Glulisine			
Inhalation powder	5–15 min	50 min (wide variation)	2–3 h
Human insulin			

Treatment should focus on immediate insulin replacement to inhibit lipolysis and stop ketoacidosis, vigorous replacement of fluids, and a thorough evaluation to identify an underlying illness. Careful monitoring is required to ensure response and particularly to monitor the cardiovascular system for signs of failure.

Hyperosmolar nonketotic state

A hyperosmolar nonketotic state is characterized by hyperglycemia, hyperosmolarity, severe volume depletion, and associated renal insufficiency. The mortality rate is high because of associated underlying illnesses like pneumonia or CVA. Metabolic acidosis is not present, or, if present, it is caused by lactic acid rather than ketoacids. The reason for the failure to mobilize fatty acids despite severe insulin deficiency in these patients is unclear. Although insulin should be provided as part of initial therapy, the focus should be on volume and sodium replacement and on identification and intervention for major underlying illness. As volume status is corrected, in the presence of recovering renal function, glucose levels can fall precipitously. Therefore, attention must be paid to the avoidance of hypoglycemia.

Long-term complications

Several mechanisms may be at play to cause these complications in diabetic patients. One mechanism may be the interaction of chronic high glucose levels with cellular proteins, leading to the subsequent formation of advanced glycosylation end products.[11] When these products accumulate in slow turnover proteins, such as collagen, they potentially lead to tissue damage and injury.

Chronic hyperglycemia also can lead to the accumulation of the aldose reductase system's metabolic products, including nonmetabolized molecules, such as sorbitol. Such accumulation potentially can affect cellular energy metabolism and contribute to cell injury and death.

It may be speculated that an individual's genetic background may contribute directly to the risk of 1 or more long-term complications of diabetes, independent of the effects of hyperglycemia.

Interactions between diabetes and other comorbidities also may contribute to the manifestation and severity of diabetes-related complications. Diabetic patients with hypertension are at higher risk of nephropathy, retinopathy, and microvascular disease than are diabetic patients without hypertension.

Dementia, including both Alzheimer and vascular type, is approximately twice as likely to occur in those with diabetes than age-matched nondiabetic control subjects.[18] Approximately 20% of people enrolled in the Action to Control Cardiovascular Risk in Diabetes (ACCORD) trial, ages 40 years to 79 years, were found to have undiagnosed cognitive impairment at baseline. In the Health and Retirement Study of US people ages 53 years or older, more than 23% of those with diabetes and 20% of those with prediabetes had cognitive impairment. Cognitive impairment is associated with more inadequate glycemic control in clinical trials. It also is associated with a higher risk of severe hypoglycemia, which in turn is associated with a higher risk for dementia.

Elevated serum creatinine is a poor prognostic sign, suggesting that substantial kidney damage already has occurred. Angiotensin-converting enzyme inhibitors and angiotensin receptor blockers reduce the progression rate from microalbuminuria to overt proteinuria and diabetic nephropathy. Also, rigorous blood pressure control is essential for such individuals.

Growth factors, including vascular endothelial growth factor, growth hormone, and transforming growth factor β, have been postulated to develop diabetic retinopathy. Nonproliferative retinopathy is characterized by cotton wool spots, intraretinal hemorrhages, and microaneurysms. Proliferative retinopathy is characterized by new blood vessels forming on the retina's surface and can lead to vitreous. If proliferation continues, blindness can occur due to vitreous hemorrhage and traction retinal detachment. With no intervention, visual loss may occur. Laser photocoagulation and intraocular injection of inhibitors of vascular growth often prevent can it from progressing to blindness; therefore, close surveillance for the progression of retinopathy in patients with diabetes is crucial. Macular edema may occur at any stage of diabetic retinopathy, especially in older adults. It requires intervention because it is sometimes associated with rapid visual deterioration. Unfortunately, despite the evidence, only 50% of diabetic patients receive recommended screening retinopathy. This needs to be done by a trained ophthalmologist and not a primary care physician because, without a dilated eye examination, retinopathy cannot be visualized.

A diabetic patient exposed to a neurotoxic agent is more likely to get neuropathy. Peripheral neuropathy, present in 50% to 70% of all patients with diabetes, increases the risk of postural instability, balance problems, and muscle atrophy, limiting PA and increasing the risk of falls. The diabetic neuropathies encountered most frequently include distal symmetric polyneuropathy, autonomic neuropathy, thoracic and lumbar nerve root disease, polyradiculopathies, and individual cranial and peripheral nerve involvement, causing focal mononeuropathies affecting mostly the oculomotor nerve and the median nerve—asymmetric involvement of multiple powerful nerves resulting in mononeuropathy multiplex. Neuropathic dysfunction can involve organ systems and can be manifested by gastroparesis, constipation, diarrhea, bladder dysfunction, erectile dysfunction, exercise intolerance, resting tachycardia, silent ischemia, and even sudden death. There is no specific treatment. Primary management consists of controlling pain. The only medication that was shown to be effective for the treatment of diabetic neuropathy pain is pregabalin. Other agents that are probably effective include gabapentin, amitriptyline, duloxetine, venlafaxine, and tramadol. Lidocaine patches possibly are effective.

Women with diabetes have a higher risk of hip and proximal humerus fractures after adjusting for age, BMI, and bone density.

Individuals with diabetes have twice the odds of depression as those without diabetes. Older adults have a high mortality risk if they have both diabetes and depression.

Cardiovascular risk. Hyperglycemia, dyslipidemia, hypertension, and age-related cardiovascular system changes, including diminished vascular responsiveness, represent CVD risk factors in diabetic patients.[19] Obesity, insulin resistance, autonomic dysfunction, and inflammation are additional risk factors. Even in prediabetic individuals, a higher risk for coronary heart disease is present. Studies have not shown evidence, however, for CVD risk reduction with reduced hyperglycemia in older adults with diabetes. The ACCORD trial had to be terminated early due to a higher mortality rate in the intensively treated glycemic group.

The Collaborative Atorvastatin Diabetes Study included diabetic patients ages 40 years to 75 years.[20] It found that atorvastatin was associated with a 36% reduction in acute coronary events; cardiovascular prevention with statins as a significant secondary benefit emerges quickly, within 1 year to 2 years, suggesting that statins may be indicated in nearly all older adults with diabetes except those with end-stage disease and minimal life expectancy. The ACCORD lipid trial found no benefit to adding fenofibrate to statin therapy.

Lowering systolic blood pressure from very high levels to moderate targets, for example, from 170 mm Hg to 150 mm Hg, reduces cardiovascular risk in all the adults with diabetes. The ACCORD-BP trial[21] showed no benefit on major adverse cardiovascular events of systolic blood pressure targets less than 120 mm Hg compared with less than one 140 mm Hg but found a significant reduction in stroke. Low diastolic blood pressure, less than 70 mm Hg, may be a risk factor for older adults' mortality.

Aging and diabetes both are risk factors for cardiovascular events, and aspirin has known benefits for secondary prevention of CVD, dose range 75 mg to 162 mg. Primary prevention of CVD with aspirin use remains controversial in older adults because of the risk of bleeding.

Follow-up Care and Quality Indicators

- Self-monitoring of blood glucose individualized frequency
- HBA$_{1c}$ testing 2 times to 4 times a year
- Patient education and diabetes management annually
- Medical nutrition therapy annually
- Eye examination annually by an ophthalmologist
- Foot examination 1 time to 2 times a year by primary care physician and daily by the patient
- Screening for diabetic nephropathy annually
- Blood pressure measurement quarterly
- Lipid profile annually

Special issues

Hypoglycemia

Hypoglycemia can result from absolute therapeutic hyperinsulinemia, but, more commonly, it is the result of compromised physiologic and behavioral defenses against falling plasma glucose concentrations. The primary source of endogenous glucose is the liver. The liver contributes to recovery from hypoglycemia by increasing glucose production under the influence of counter-regulatory hormones, including cortisol, growth hormone, and epinephrine. Normally, there is a hierarchy of hypoglycemia responses with the release of counter-regulatory hormones, such as epinephrine and glucagon, occurring before a patient becomes symptomatic and aware of hypoglycemia. The initial symptoms include tachycardia, nervousness, and a sweating response, all of which can alert the patient to seek exogenous sources. Hunger often is a part of this response. Aging is associated with decreased β-adrenergic receptor function and reduced glucagon response to hypoglycemia.

A self-reported history of severe hypoglycemia (requiring another person's assistance)[22] predicts increased mortality 5 years later. Emergency department visit rates for hypoglycemia are 3-times higher among adults with diabetes ages 75 years or older compared with those ages 45 years to 64 years. It is imperative to teach patients and caregivers to be able to recognize and treat hypoglycemia,[23] as shown in **Fig. 2**.

LONG-TERM CARE FACILITIES

Approximately 22% of women in nursing homes have diabetes mellitus. Compared with those without diabetes, these patients are frailer, have a higher disease burden, have cognitive decline, and have increased risk of aspiration pneumonia and fecal incontinence. Based on several observational studies, residents in long-term care facilities have better survival if their HbA$_{1C}$ is higher, between 8% and 9%, consistent with ADA consensus panel recommendations.[24]

In nursing homes, various limitations need to be considered when administering medications[25–27]: staff level of training, staff-to-resident ratio, and understanding

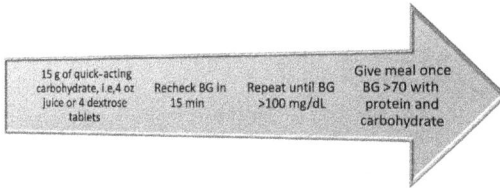

Fig. 2. In cases of hypoglycemia, give patients a quick-acting carbohydrate, which could be 4 oz fruit juice or 4 dextrose tablets. Recheck fingerstick blood sugar (FSBS) in 15 minutes. Repeat the cycle until FSBS is greater than 100 mg/dL. Give patients a meal with protein and carbohydrate once FSBS is greater than 70 mg/dL. (*Data from* Kasper D, Braunwald E. Harrison's Principles of Internal Medicine (16Th Edition). Blacklick, USA: McGraw-Hill Professional Publishing; 2005; and Asthana S, Halter J, High K et al. Hazzard's Geriatric Medicine And Gerontology, 7E. New York, N.Y.: McGraw-Hill Education LLC.; 2017.)

the risks associated with diabetes medications and insulin regimens. Their ability to provide meals timely and recognize and treat hypoglycemic symptoms rapidly is variable. Consistency of caloric intake is essential for a patient treated with insulin and may be challenging in a disabled nursing home resident.

Undernutrition is more of a problem in nursing homes than obesity. Diet therapy should focus on matching caloric intake to nutritional needs rather than restriction of calories. Weight loss in older adults is associated with an increased risk of death. A facility dietician can play a crucial role by educating facility aides and nurses on inappropriate consumption estimates.

PALLIATIVE CARE AND END-OF-LIFE CARE

Appropriate diabetes care for patients currently lacks quality standards and guidance on best clinical practices at the end of life. Diabetes UK commissioned a panel of professional groups and developed recommendations endorsed by the UK National Health Service.[28] The panel recognized no published evidence that justifies any glucose or HbA_{1C} target for end-of-life diabetes care management. They recommended glucose control target ranges between 108 mg/dL to 270 mg/dL. Hypoglycemic medications and monitoring still may be required to stay comfortable. Severe hyperglycemia, 350 mg/dL or higher, may impair comfort because it can lead to dehydration, infections, urinary incontinence, and falls. A more complicated glucose-lowering regimen that requires more monitoring may be appropriate if the prognosis is several months to a year, whereas minimizing glucose-lowering treatment and monitoring needs would be appropriate if a prognosis is days to weeks.

CLINICS CARE POINTS

- Diagnosis of diabetes can be done using an FPG level, OGTT, or HbA_{1C} values.
- Diet and exercise are the key first steps in the management of diabetes.
- A combination of caloric restriction and exercise is the best first approach for an older adult with type 2 diabetes mellitus.
- Oral glucose-lowering agents alone and insulin can be used to treat type 2 diabetes mellitus. Insulin is the mainstay of treatment in type 1 diabetes mellitus.
- Self-monitoring of blood glucose; HbA_{1C} testing; patient education; medical nutrition therapy; eye examination; foot examination; and screening for diabetic nephropathy, blood pressure measurement, and lipid profile are required at regular intervals.

REFERENCES

1. Beulens JWJ, et al. Alcohol consumption and risk of type 2 diabetes among older women. Diabetes Care 2005;28(12):2933–8.
2. American Diabetes Association. Diabetes care. J Clin Appl Res Educ 2019;42: 13–22.
3. Annual estimates of the resident population by sex, single year of age, race, and hispanic origin for the United States: April 1, 2010, to July 1, 2018, Population Division, US Census Bureau.
4. Hazzard's geriatric medicine and gerontology. 7th edition.
5. Feig DS, Zinman B, Wang X, et al. Risk of development of diabetes mellitus after diagnosis of gestational diabetes. CMAJ 2008;179(3):229–34.
6. Legro RS, Kunselman AR, Dodson WC, et al. Prevalence and predictors of risk for type 2 diabetes mellitus and impaired glucose tolerance in polycystic ovary syndrome: a prospective, controlled study in 254 affected women. J Clin Endocrinol Metab 1999;84(1):165–9.
7. Legro RS, Finegood D, Dunaif A. A fasting glucose to insulin ratio is a useful measure of insulin sensitivity in women with polycystic ovary syndrome. J Clin Endocrinol Metab 1998;83(8):2694–8.
8. Chang AM, Smith MJ, Galecki AT, et al. Impaired beta-cell function in human aging: response to nicotinic acid-induced insulin resistance. J Clin Endocrinol Metab 2006;91(9):3303–9.
9. Halter JB. Diabetes mellitus in an aging population: the challenge ahead. J Gerontol A Biol Sci Med Sci 2012;67(12):1297–9.
10. Mari A, Tura A, Natali A, et al, RISC Investigators. Impaired beta cell glucose sensitivity rather than inadequate compensation for insulin resistance is the dominant defect in glucose intolerance. Diabetologia 2010;53(4):749–56.
11. Harrison's Principles of internal medicine. 16th edition.
12. Center for Disease Control and Prevention. National diabetes prevention program 2019.
13. Center for Disease Control and Prevention. National diabetes statistics report, 2020. CDC > Diabetes home > Data and Statistics > National diabetes Statistics report.
14. Kirkman MS, et al. Diabetes in older adults: a consensus report. J Am Geriatr Soc 2012;60:2342–56.
15. Blaum C, Cigolle CT, Boyd C, et al. Clinical complexity in middle-aged and older adults with diabetes: the Health and Retirement Study. Med Care 2010;48: 327–34.
16. Rejeski WJ, Ip EH, Bertoni AG, et al, Look AHEAD Research Group. Lifestyle change and mobility in obese adults with type 2 diabetes. N Engl J Med 2012; 366(13):1209–17.
17. Holman RR, Paul SK, Bethel MA, et al. 10-year follow-up of intensive glucose control in type 2 diabetes. N Engl J Med 2008;359(15):1577–89.
18. Whitmer RA, Karter AJ, Yaffe K, et al. Hypoglycemic episodes and risk of dementia in older patients with type 2 diabetes mellitus. JAMA 2009;301(15):1565–72.
19. Cigolle CT, Blaum CS, Halter JB. Diabetes and cardiovascular disease prevention in older adults. Clin Geriatr Med 2009;25(4):607–41, vii-viii.
20. Colhoun HM. Effects of Atorvastatin on Kidney Outcomes and Cardiovascular Disease in Patients with Diabetes: An Analysis From the Collaborative Atorvastatin Diabetes Study (CARDS). American Journal of Kidney Diseases. 2009; 54: 810-9.

21. Buckley LF. Intensive Versus Standard Blood Pressure Control in SPRINT-Eligible Participants of ACCORD-BP. Diabetes Care 2017;40:1733–8.
22. Seaquist ER, Anderson J, Childs B, et al. Hypoglycemia and diabetes: a report of a workgroup of the American diabetes association and the endocrine society. Diabetes Care 2013;36(5):1384–95.
23. Punthakee Z, Miller ME, Launer LJ, et al, ACCORD Group of Investigators, ACCORD-MIND Investigators. Poor cognitive function and risk of severe hypoglycemia in type 2 diabetes: post hoc epidemiologic analysis of the ACCORD trial. Diabetes Care 2012;35(4):787–93.
24. Resnick HE, Heineman J, Stone R, et al. Diabetes in U.S. nursing homes, 2004. Diabetes Care 2008;31(2):287–8.
25. Munshi MN, Florez H, Huang ES, et al. Management of diabetes in long-term care and skilled nursing facilities: a position statement of the American diabetes association. Diabetes Care 2016;39(2):308–18.
26. National health and nutrition examination survey (NHANES) 2013–2016, National Center for Health Statistics, Centers for Disease Control and Prevention.
27. National health interview survey (NHIS) 2017–2018, National Center for Health Statistics, Centers for Disease Control and Prevention.
28. End of Life Diabetes Care. Clinical care recommendations. Commissioned by diabetes UK. 3rd edition 2018.

Coronavirus Disease 2019

Sophie Lin, MD[a], Rachael Kantor, MD[b], Elizabeth Clark, MD[c],*

KEYWORDS

- COVID-19 • Elderly • Nursing homes • Comorbidities • Telemedicine • Ageism
- Racism

KEY POINTS

- COVID-19 is highly pathogenic in older populations.
- Ageism and systemic racism have led to health care system failures, increase in risk of infection, and poor outcomes.
- Technology, maintenance of infection-control protocols, and home-based primary care can improve overall health care for older adults and better prepare for future disasters.

The novel coronavirus (COVID-19) outbreak in 2019 and subsequent pandemic have led to high morbidity and mortality rates, especially in the aging population, which accounts for 80% of all COVID deaths. Men have higher COVID-19 death rates, but women comprise the majority population older than 65 years, as well as the majority of caregivers.[1] Thus, COVID-19 is an urgent issue in older women's health.

In this article, the authors review manifestations of COVID-19 in older adults, normal physiologic changes and frequent comorbidities of aging that increase pathogenicity, factors contributing to overwhelming viral spread among seniors, negative effects on health and well-being resulting from measures to control the virus, and health-system improvements necessary to protect and care for this vulnerable population.

CASE 1

Mary Smith, age 63 years, is a Licensed Practical Nurse in an urban nursing home's (NH) dementia unit. COVID-19 struck in mid-March 2020, initially overwhelming infection-control protocols, personal protective equipment (PPE) supplies, testing capabilities, and staff rosters. Outbreak control was particularly difficult because cognitively impaired residents could not comply with mask wearing or physical distancing

The authors have nothing to disclose.
[a] New York Medical College, Metropolitan Hospital Center, 1901 First Avenue, New York, NY, 10029, USA; [b] Medical School of International Health, Faculty of Health Sciences, Ben-Gurion University of the Negev, Be'er Sheva, Israel; [c] Albert Einstein College of Medicine, Bronx, NY 10461, USA
* Corresponding author.
E-mail addresses: eliclark@montefiore.org; elizabethclarkmd@gmail.com

and frequently breached the isolation barrier. Two-thirds of the 43 unit's residents had confirmed COVID-19, 18 died, and ten survived. Others likely had asymptomatic, but unconfirmed, infections. Employees, including Ms Smith also became ill or needed to care for family members.

COVID-19 exacted a great emotional toll. Residents no longer recognized staff through PPE that blocked smiles and muffled voices, and recreational therapy was reduced to radios and coloring books. Certified nursing assistants (CNAs) and nurses curtailed nonessential tasks, resulting in depression and loneliness in many residents. Workdays were physically demanding and disheartening. A refrigerator truck in the parking lot served for months as the NH's morgue and a constant reminder of the virus's wrath. Ms Smith and colleagues mourned residents they had known for years.

Infection rates declined in late spring. By July, the refrigerator truck was gone, and the NH was COVID-19-free. Residents and staff are regularly tested. Employees are encouraged to work only at one facility. Infection-control protocols are followed, and adequate PPE dispensed. Recreation and other therapy services are at full capacity. There are even limited outdoor family visits.

Ms Smith feels the NH is better prepared for a second wave and is hopeful for the vaccine.

CASE 2

Sarah Jones and Miriam Brown, aged 86 and 85 years, respectively, are sisters whose families share a house—Sarah upstairs with her husband Abe; Miriam downstairs with husband Bob. Sarah is a breast cancer survivor. Both sisters have well-controlled hypertension and diabetes. They both function independently in the community, although Sarah's daughter Susan helps with transportation and shopping. Abe has advanced dementia and requires home-attendant services. Bob has mild cognitive impairment.

Through the first wave of the pandemic, the sisters kept the virus at bay. In November, one of Abe's home-attendants developed COVID-19. Abe became ill, was hospitalized, and died 3 days later. Sarah, Miriam, Bob, and Susan all tested positive but had mild symptoms. Susan is caring for the sisters and Bob. Everyone is sad, overwhelmed, and wishing people in the community had followed safety protocols more closely.

CASE 3

Carol Adams is a retired high school teacher who recently celebrated her 100th birthday. She never married but had several devoted former students including Dr Sanders, a physician, who became her health care proxy, and many dear friends in her building and church. Her medical problems include osteoporosis, arthritis, and unsteady gait. With increasing frailty, she needed a home-attendant for housekeeping and shopping, but she had no cognitive impairment. She managed her finances, medications, medical visits, and cooking independently. In January 2020, she had a mild respiratory infection but was clinically stable during a telemedicine visit in March.

In early April, her aide found Ms Adams with slurred speech and left-sided weakness. Afraid of COVID-19, Ms Adams refused to go to the emergency department (ED), and Dr Sanders supported that decision. Her home care hours were increased, and Ms Adams gradually recovered from her stroke. Seven of her closest friends, however, succumbed to COVID-19, as did several members of her congregation, all younger than she. Increased frailty and fear of infection now discourage Ms Adams from leaving her apartment. She feels fortunate to have enrolled in a program that provides primary care at home and is grateful for telephonic bereavement counseling and the support of surviving friends and former students. But the losses from the pandemic have left a hole in her heart that she doubts will ever heal.

INTRODUCTION

Beginning in late 2019, a cluster of infections by a novel coronavirus began in Wuhan, China, and quickly spread to other countries throughout the world. Severe acute respiratory syndrome coronavirus 2 (SARS-CoV-2) was the cause of the infection. In February 2020, the World Health Organization designated the disease as COVID-19, or coronavirus disease 2019.

Presentation

Most infected people experience mild to moderate respiratory illness and recover without special treatment. The elderly, and those with underlying comorbid conditions such as diabetes mellitus, hypertension, cardiovascular disease, respiratory illness, and chronic kidney disease, are more likely to develop serious disease. The case fatality rate in adults older than 80 years, which constitutes nearly half of NH residents, is approximately 15%.[2,3] Symptoms are nonspecific and vary tremendously.[2,4] Elderly patients can have present with milder or atypical symptoms, but nevertheless be more severely ill than younger patients.[5] A breakdown of symptoms of COVID-19 by severity and body system is presented in **Table 1**. Some people in all age-groups are asymptomatic. Presymptomatic and asymptomatic transmission of COVID-19 likely contributed to high infection rates in NHs.

Diagnosis

To date, there are two tests for active infection, molecular and antigen, and an antibody test for past infection. These tests are discussed in **Table 2**.

Common laboratory findings include lymphopenia, occasional thrombocytopenia, elevated C-reactive protein, and erythrocyte sedimentation rate. Specific organ damage may also be indicated in results because of the ability of COVID-19 to infect multiple organs; however, findings largely are nonspecific.[2] Radiographic findings can be highly variable, with typical ground-glass opacities and patchy infiltrates as seen in **Fig. 1** absent in roughly 33% of patients upon hospital admission.[2,14–16]

Pathophysiology

SARS-CoV-2 infects the host by binding to ciliated secretory cells in the nasal epithelium via angiotensin-converting enzyme (ACE-2). Host transmembrane protease serine type 2 (TMPRSS2) then primes the viral spike protein, allowing entry into the host cell.[17] Viral replication causes involvement of the remainder of the respiratory tract. Roughly 80% of patients clear the infection in 10 to 14 days with mild symptoms. However, as the disease progresses to the lower airways via the invasion of type II pneumocytes in the alveolar epithelium, where ACE-2 receptors are in high concentration, some people develop more serious symptoms. Release of inflammatory mediators including interleukin (IL)-1, IL-6, tumor necrosis factor α, and interferon λ, causes a cytokine storm. The immune system tries to limit lung destruction by sequestering the immune reaction and attempting to clear the virus as it continues to replicate and infect healthy lung tissue. The resulting cytotoxicity and destruction of both type I and II pneumocytes cause lung injury, acute respiratory distress syndrome, and respiratory failure.[17,18]

Table 1
Symptoms and clinical manifestations

System	Common Symptoms	Less Common or Severe Symptoms
Systemic[2,6]	Fever Fatigue Myalgia/arthralgia Pharyngitis Anorexia	Rhabdomyolysis Septic shock Multiorgan failure
Pulmonary[2,6]	Cough Dyspnea Chest tightness Tachypnea Sputum production	Hemoptysis Pneumonia ARDS
Cardiovascular[6,7]	Tachycardia Arrhythmia Acute myocardial injury with elevated troponin	Myocardial infarction Cardiomyopathy Pericarditis Myocarditis/heart failure Pulmonary embolism
Neurologic[8–11]	Anosmia/Ageusia Headache Dizziness Delirium Sleep disturbance Depression	Encephalitis Seizures Cerebral infarction Meningitis Guillain-Barré syndrome Miller Fisher syndrome Isolated cranial nerve palsies Acute hemorrhagic necrotizing encephalopathy Myelitis Autoimmune myopathy
Renal[6]	Acute renal failure	
Gastrointestinal[2,6,12]	Diarrhea Nausea/vomiting Hepatic injury	Gastrointestinal bleeding
Hematologic[6]	Lymphopenia Thrombosis	Disseminated intravascular coagulation

Dermatologic[13]	Acral lesions
	  (pseudo-chilblains,
	  "COVID hands
	  and toes")
	Rash (erythematous
	  or vesicular)
	Urticaria	

Abbreviation: ARDS, acute respiratory distress syndrome.
  Symptoms not specific to age. Elderly, and those with multiple comorbidities, more likely to have severe symptoms.

Through ACE-2 receptors, SARS-CoV-2 infects other host cells including enterocytes in the small intestine, arterial and venous endothelial cells, and cortical neurons and glia,[17] leading to the broad range of presenting symptoms and the potential for multiorgan failure (see **Table 1**).

One explanation for heightened susceptibility to severe disease among older adults is that ACE-2 receptor concentrations appear to increase with age. Older men have more ACE-2 receptors and TMPRSS2, possibly related to testosterone levels, while the number and function of innate immune cells are greater in older women. This

Table 2
Testing

	Molecular Test	Antigen Test	Antibody Test
Names	Gold standard test Diagnostic test NAAT RT-PCR	"Rapid" test Diagnostic test Protein/ Immunoglobulin test	Serologic test
Collection method	Nasopharyngeal, nasal, throat swab	Nasopharyngeal, nasal swab	Blood draw
When it is used	To determine active infection. To identify those who may be contagious or a risk to others.	To quickly determine active infection. To identify those who may be contagious or a risk to others. Less expensive than molecular tests.	To identify past infection and immune response. To identify those who might be able to donate convalescent plasma.
Results processing[a]	<48 h	<30 min	<48 h
Positive result indicates[b]	Active infection	Active infection	Past infection
Negative result indicates[b]	No active infection at time of sample collection	Viral proteins not detected. Does not rule out active infection. If concern for active infection, molecular test administration is recommended for confirmation.	No evidence of past infection. Does not rule out active infection.

Abbreviations NAAT, nucleic acid amplification test; RT-PCR, reverse transcriptase polymerase chain reaction.
[a] Times vary by manufacturer institution and test load burden.
[b] Sensitivity and specificity of test vary by manufacturer and trial data between 61.7% and 93.3% and 84.2% to 100%, respectively. Results affected by administration method.
Data from Weissleder R. et al. Covid-19 Diagnostics in Context (V1.50 ed., Rep.). MGH Center for Systems Biology. https://csb.mgh.harvard.edu/covid. Accessed November 19, 2020; and Wiersinga WJ, Rhodes A, Cheng AC, et al. Pathophysiology, Transmission, Diagnosis, and Treatment of Coronavirus Disease 2019 (COVID-19): A Review. *JAMA*. 2020;324(8):782-793.

may contribute to the higher morbidity and mortality among older men than older women, as noted in a European study.[1] There also appear to be gender differences in the effect of COVID-19 treatments. For instance, women have increased risk of QT interval prolongation on electrocardiogram and *torsades de pointes*.[1,17]

Comorbidities and Frailty

The presence of multiple comorbidities in older people increases both morbidity and mortality from COVID-19. **Table 3**, adapted from Ejaz and colleagues,[19] depicts the mechanisms by which SARS-CoV-2 causes symptoms in people with various comorbidities. Physical and cognitive functions, which are included in frailty indices, also contribute to outcomes from COVID-19 infection. One study found a direct correlation between higher Clinical Frailty Score and mortality.[20]

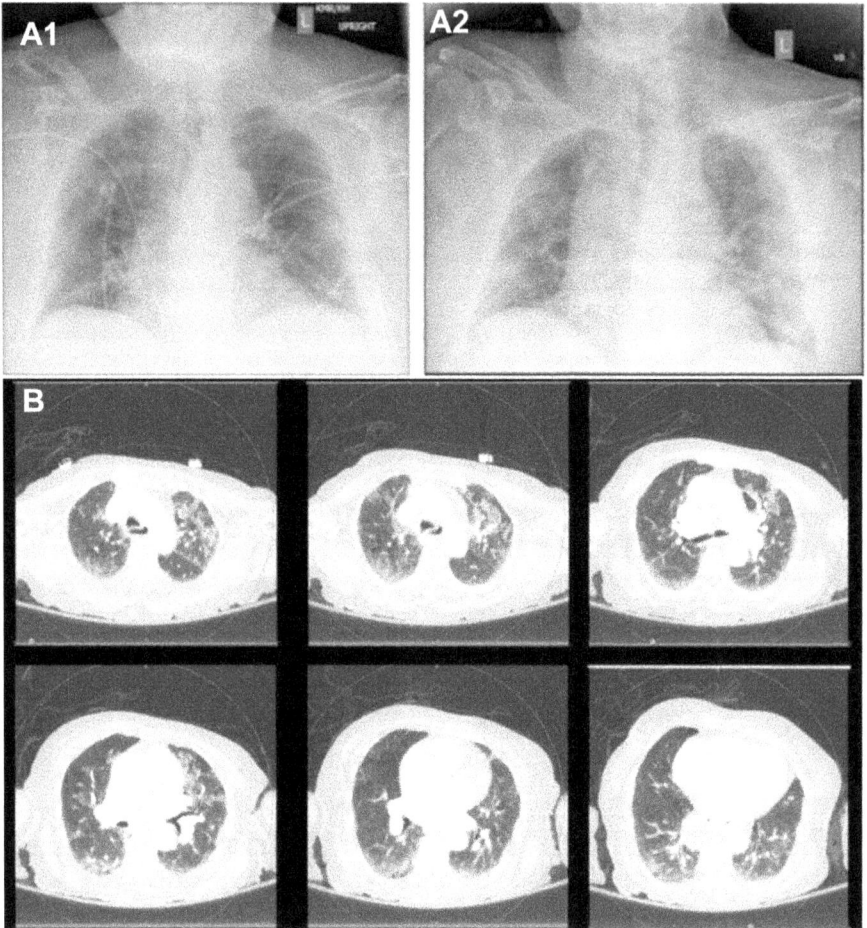

Fig. 1. Radiological Identification. (*A*) [1] CXR at admission, and [2] at 36 hours, shows progression of pulmonary findings. (*B*) CT scan demonstrates mild-moderate ground-glass opacities favoring the periphery. (*Modified from* Shea H, Holinski J, Benedetti R, et al. Mechanical Ventilation for COVID-19. https://courses.edx.org/courses/course-v1:HarvardX+COV19x+1T2020/course/. Published April 13, 2020. Accessed November 30, 2020.)

Health System and Societal Factors

Socioeconomic factors, including race and ethnicity, influence risk and severity of COVID-19. Blacks, Hispanic/Latinx, and Native Americans have been disproportionately impacted by COVID-19. The CDC reported Blacks are 1.4 times more likely to contract COVID-19 than their White counterparts but make up only 13% of the United States (US) population. Hispanic/Latinx and Native Americans are both 1.7 and 1.8 times more likely to contract the disease. **Fig. 2** represents a direct correlation of race and age to incidence of COVID-19 infection, hospitalizations, and mortality.[21]

Societal factors have also contributed to gender differences in infection rates and disease severity. In many countries, men are more likely to smoke and drink alcohol, both risk factors for comorbidities. Women are more likely to be caregivers, including frontline and essential workers.[1] In the US, a disproportionate number of people whose livelihoods place them at higher risk for COVID-19 exposure are Black and

Table 3
Comorbidities, mechanism, and symptoms

Comorbidity	Mechanism/Pathophysiology	Symptoms
Hypertension	Upregulation of ACE-2 expression	Severe hypertension Pneumonia-like symptoms
Cardiovascular disease	Impaired immune system	Myocardial injury/infarction
Chronic obstructive pulmonary disease	Upregulation of ACE-2	Hypoxemia
Asthma	Delayed innate immune response	Chronic respiratory diseases Pneumonia-like symptoms
Diabetes	Increased ACE-2 expression Impaired T-cell function	Pneumonia-like symptoms
Obesity	High levels of cytokines, adipokines, interferons	Chronic low-grade abdominal inflammation extending to lungs.
Human Immunodeficiency Virus	Antiretroviral therapy and impaired immune system increased ACE-2 expression	Pneumonia-like symptoms Jaundice
Malignancy	Impaired immune system	ARDS
Liver disease	Increased hepatic ACE-2 expression	Elevated serum aminotransferases
Renal disease	Increased renal ACE-2 expression	Acute kidney injury
Advancing age	Weakening immune system Mechanism of comorbidities	Reflects comorbidities

Adapted from Ejaz H, Alsrhani A, Zafar A, et al. COVID-19 and comorbidities: Deleterious impact on infected patients. *J Infect Public Health.* 2020;13(12):1833-1839.; with permission.

Hispanic/Latinx women.[21] Generally, women have less access to health care and are at greater risk of losing financial stability because of the pandemic. They are also more likely to experience domestic abuse and depression stemming from social isolation.[22]

The devastating impact of COVID-19 on older adults requiring long-term care—in the community and residential facilities such as NHs—cannot be explained solely by physiologic changes of aging, multiple comorbidities, or even increased exposure during personal care. The health care system failed to keep the virus out of NHs, to contain its spread once inside, and to provide appropriate care for those who became ill. Proximate causes include lack of effective infection control protocols and inadequate PPE, screening, and testing.[23] At a more basic level, this "perfect storm", as described by Ouslander and Grabowski, stems from society's wanton disregard for its older citizens and those who care for them.[24] Long-term care has too long been undervalued, underfunded, and highly segregated. Low pay and limited sick leave, especially for CNAs and home aides, result in employees' having multiple jobs and increasing risk of interfacility viral spread.[25] The pandemic has heightened racial and economic disparities in care.[22,26] NHs with greater crowding and caring for predominantly Medicaid or racial and ethnic minority residents had higher infection rates, while those with higher nurse staffing ratios and better quality ratings provided potential for better outbreak control.[27,28]

COLLATERAL DAMAGE

Besides direct mortality and morbidity, the COVID-19 pandemic has had many indirect effects including delayed diagnosis and treatment of life-threatening conditions,

A COVID-19 Cases, Hospitalization, Deaths in Minority groups compared to White Counterpart

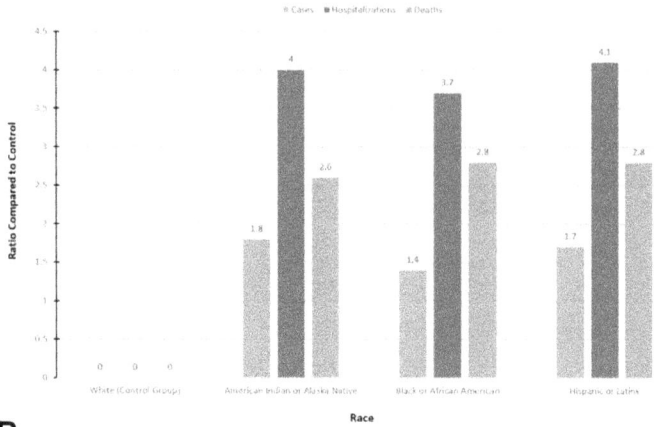

B COVID-19 Hospitalizations and Death rates by age when compared to 18-29 year olds

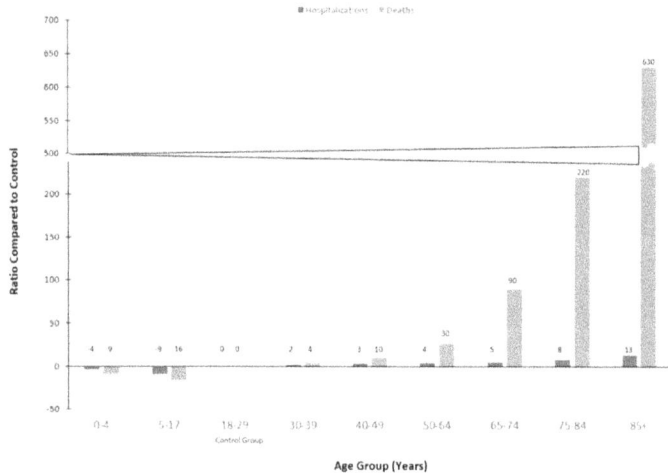

Fig. 2. Effects of COVID-19 on Minority and Different Age Groups. Numbers above the horizontal axis represent raw data as of 11/30/20. Ex. (A) 1.8 times more cases of COVID-19 in American Indian/Alaskan Natives than White counterparts. (B) 0- to 4-year-olds are 4 times less likely to be hospitalized than 18- to 29-year-old counterparts. (Data from Special Populations Data in the U.S. CDC and Prevention. https://www.cdc.gov/coronavirus/2019-ncov/cases-updates/special-populations/index.html. Accessed November 10, 2020.)

delayed health screenings, problems with medication management, increased elder abuse rates, decreased cognitive function, worsening depression, and decreased physical function and mobility.

Delayed Treatment and Screenings

Fear of infection kept many patients from timely hospital treatments and routine medical care. The decrease in ED visits for stroke, myocardial infarction, and appendicitis during the pandemic's peak was followed by an increase in presentations much later in the illness trajectory, when medical intervention is palliative rather than curative.[29] Cancer treatments have been interrupted. Critical decisions about surgery, radiotherapy, and chemotherapy must consider risks of frequent office visits and hospital admission. Advance directives also need to be discussed with patients to assess treatment goals. The International Society for Geriatric Oncology advocates using geriatric assessment to aid in decision-making in older adults.[30]

Medication Management

In the authors' clinical experience, medication management during the pandemic has been particularly challenging. Prolonged closings of many pharmacies and clinics interrupted renewal and dispensing of prescriptions, follow-up appointments, and regular laboratory tests needed to manage chronic conditions including diabetes, long-term anticoagulation, and hypertension.[31] Telemedicine became and remains a lifeline for medication renewal and follow-up of medical conditions.[32] Home-lab services are one solution, although not all insurances provide coverage. Strategies to minimize pharmacy trips include 90-day prescriptions and the use of mail-order pharmacies or home delivery from local pharmacies.

Similarly, patients who are regularly followed up by home-care nurses for medication administration may have this care delayed. Medication reconciliation may be even more challenging during care transitions. Medication adherence will also likely decline for many patients during the pandemic, possibly leading to poor health outcomes.[31]

Elder Abuse

Before the pandemic, approximately 1 in 10 people older than 60 years suffered from abuse or financial exploitation.[33] This has increased tenfold since the pandemic started.[22] Elder abuse is the "intentional act or failure to act by a caregiver or another person in a relationship involving an expectation of trust that causes or creates a serious risk of harm to an older adult."[34] Risk of abuse increases with level of dependence. Quarantine has increased both dependence and the time older adults spend with potential abusers. Financial and emotional stresses as well as social isolation may instigate elder neglect or abuse.[33] Providers must be vigilant for signs of elder abuse and advocate for this vulnerable population.

Cognitive Function and Mental Health

In one British study, frail older adults with COVID-19 were more likely to present with delirium than nonfrail adults of the same age with odds ratios of 3.22 in the hospitalized and 2.29 in the community-based cohort.[35] Disease-related factors that increase delirium risk include hypoxia, electrolyte imbalances, and forced isolation for long periods away from family. Hospital-related factors include minimal direct patient care and the use of PPE, which disproportionately affects the hearing impaired.[30]

Older adults with dementia face special challenges during the pandemic. They have difficulty accessing public health information. Many cannot remember to self-quarantine or to wear masks. Isolation may exacerbate behavioral problems in dementia patients, and the common need for outside caregivers increases risk of infection.[36]

The pandemic has affected older adults' mental health. Social isolation can worsen symptoms in those previously diagnosed with depression. Worries about the pandemic and loss of social connections have increased the incidence of new-onset depression and anxiety. The preponderance of mortality among older adults, and the derailment of usual end-of-life, funeral, burial, and mourning processes, increases the risk of complicated grief.[37] Bereavement in communities of color has been heightened by disproportionate distribution of COVID-19 deaths.[38]

Access to mental health care and bereavement services has been limited. Even with the transition to virtual therapy, current resources have not kept up with demand. Many older adults have difficulty using these alternative services. Monitoring medications via telemedicine presents an additional challenge.[39]

Physical Function and Mobility

Home isolation, leading to decline in daily physical activity, increases the risk of sarcopenia, multimorbidity, and mortality.[40] Increasing exercise can reverse these negative physical effects and improve mental well-being. Physicians recommend prescribing home-based resistance exercise for all older adults, with at least 150 minutes of moderate-intensity aerobic activity or 75 minutes of vigorous-intensity aerobic activity per week.[41]

Interruption of subcutaneous antiresorptive injections for osteoporosis could accelerate the rate of bone loss. A recent study found that even a 4-month delay in denosumab administration significantly increased vertebral fracture risk.[42] If patients cannot self-administer the injection or arrange an in-person visit to receive it, plans should be made to switch to an oral bisphosphonate.[43]

Osteoporotic fractures are an example of increased indirect risks of COVID-19 for older adults. Deconditioning during the pandemic leads to increased falls and fractures. The risk of falling and potential mortality is increased further if older adults become infected with COVID-19. Prompt surgical treatment is essential to preserve ambulation and independence. This might be delayed because patients may refuse necessary hospitalization for fear of contracting the virus, or patients medically optimized for surgery may have procedures postponed for active infection or awaiting COVID-19 test results.[43] Fall-prevention strategies during the pandemic are essential to decrease fragility fractures, as are protocols for surgery in patients with COVID-19.

WHAT MATTERS MOST: LESSONS LEARNED FROM COVID-19
Ethical Considerations

As the numbers of COVID-19 hospitalizations increase, the health care system may be overwhelmed, leading to the rationing of limited resources. Age has been reportedly used as a cutoff for denying admission to intensive care and mechanical ventilation, prioritizing this life-saving equipment for younger patients.[44] Advance-care planning should be addressed and documented properly. Care must be taken to distribute resources ethically and not exclude people from receiving potentially life-saving procedures solely based on age or predicted life expectancy.[45] Racial and ethnic minorities are particularly at risk for not receiving resources.[21] Active efforts need to be made to ensure truly equitable distribution of all resources.

Ageism or "stereotyping, prejudice, and discrimination toward people by age,"[46] is not a new sentiment. At the peak of the pandemic, mainstream media coverage discussed the risk of COVID-19 to the elderly, changing the narrative of the virus to a *disease of the old*. Social media also perpetuated negative attitudes toward the aging population, frequently referring to the virus as the #*BoomerRemover* accompanied by ageist memes. Facebook posts or tweets implied that the lives of the elderly were less valuable than those of the younger population.[47] The overall tone toward this at-risk population was unsympathetic. Ageism has increased since the pandemic, as reflected by views that older people should be sacrificed for the good of society, and there have been reports of increased hate crimes against older adults.[33,48]

Hope for the Future

The pandemic has expanded the use of telemedicine, increasing access to care for the geriatric population and allowing many geriatric syndromes to be identified, discussed, and managed remotely. Challenges in telemedicine include patients' lack of internet access or proficiency. The high prevalence of age-related hearing loss and cognitive impairment in this population makes working with these technologies even more difficult.[32] Benefits of this new communication modality include enhanced observation and greater receptiveness to counseling. Practitioners can observe patients in their own environment instead of a health care facility, providing valuable information. Does the patient appear well-kept and healthy? Does the environment look safe? Are caregivers present and attentive? There should be a systematic approach to assessing these factors within the remote geriatric assessment. In addition, patients and caregivers may feel more comfortable addressing difficult topics in their home environment and can be counseled simultaneously.[33] Telemedicine should not replace but serve as an adjunct to the in-person visit, highlighting the need for expanded house call programs.

In December 2020, administration of two COVID-19 vaccines began in the US, bringing hope for the pandemic's end.[49] However, widespread vaccination may not be completed until late 2021. Thus, continued vigilance in maintaining infection control in health care facilities and in the community is essential to protect everyone, especially the vulnerable elderly population until herd immunity is achieved.

SUMMARY

SARS-CoV-2 has had a devastating impact on older adults. Many older survivors suffered prolonged effects on health, function, and independence. While the virus's unequal effect on the elderly can be attributed to intrinsic physiologic and health factors associated with aging, the pandemic has uncovered numerous fault lines in our health care system. Ageism and systemic racism play an outsized role in poor COVID-19 outcomes, and the pandemic has brought many health-system deficiencies, especially in NHs, into focus. Older adults have suffered disproportionately from interruptions in routine health care; social and physical isolation; increased incidence of elder abuse; difficulties obtaining food, medication, and help at home; and grief. Along with regular implementation of telemedicine visits, pharmacy medication deliveries and the resurrection of the physician house call should be considered. Now is the time to start creating better mass casualty, infection, and pandemic protocols to improve care for all of our citizens, especially the most vulnerable.

CLINICS CARE POINTS

- When considering a diagnosis of COVID-19, be aware of both typical and atypical clinical presentations.
- In order to decrease exposure to COVID-19, consider prescribing to pharmacies that deliver to patients and writing 90-day prescriptions.
- The pandemic has highlighted the need for house call programs, which would significantly benefit seniors. Physicians should advocate for expansion of such services.
- Be able to help seniors access community resources for food, finances, and social support.
- Telemedicine is a valuable adjunct tool for the evaluation and management of geriatric patients that provides a window into home environments.

- Be aware of ageist and racist biases that may place older patients at risk for being unable to access necessary medical care and other resources.

REFERENCES

1. Gebhard C, Regitz-Zagrosek V, Neuhauser HK, et al. Impact of sex and gender on COVID-19 outcomes in Europe. Biol Sex Differences 2020;11(1):29.
2. Neumann-Podczaska A, Al-Saad SR, Karbowski LM, et al. Covid 19 - clinical picture in the elderly population: a qualitative systematic review. Aging Dis 2020; 11(4):988–1008.
3. Zheng Z, Peng F, Xu B, et al. Risk factors of critical & mortal COVID-19 cases: a systematic literature review and meta-analysis. J Infect 2020;81(2):e16–25.
4. Baj J, Karakuła-Juchnowicz H, Teresiński G, et al. COVID-19: specific and non-specific clinical manifestations and symptoms: the current state of knowledge. J Clin Med 2020;9(6):1753.
5. Lauretani F, Ravazzoni G, Roberti MF, et al. Assessment and treatment of older individuals with COVID 19 multi-system disease: clinical and ethical implications. Acta Biomed 2020;91(2):150–68.
6. Hussain A, Kaler J, Tabrez E, et al. Novel COVID-19: a comprehensive review of transmission, manifestation, and pathogenesis. Cureus 2020;12(5):e8184.
7. Su YB, Kuo MJ, Lin TY, et al. Cardiovascular manifestation and treatment in COVID-19. J Chin Med Assoc 2020;83(8):704–9.
8. Garg RK. Spectrum of Neurological manifestations in covid-19: a review. Neurol India 2020;68(3):560–72.
9. O'Hanlon S, Inouye SK. Delirium: a missing piece in the COVID-19 pandemic puzzle. Age Ageing 2020;49(4):497–8.
10. Paliwal VK, Garg RK, Gupta A, et al. Neuromuscular presentations in patients with COVID-19. Neurol Sci 2020;41(11):3039–56.
11. Brouwer MC, Ascione T, Pagliano P. Neurologic aspects of covid-19: a concise review. Infez Med 2020;28(suppl 1):42–5.
12. Portincasa P, Krawczyk M, Machill A, et al. Hepatic consequences of COVID-19 infection. Lapping or biting? Eur J Intern Med 2020;77:18–24.
13. Daneshgaran G, Dubin DP, Gould DJ. Cutaneous manifestations of COVID-19: an evidence-based review. Am J Clin Dermatol 2020;21(5):627–39.
14. Weissleder R, Lee H, Pittet MJ. Covid-19 diagnostics in context (V1.50 ed., Rep.). MGH center for systems biology. Available at: https://csb.mgh.harvard.edu/covid. Accessed November 19, 2020.
15. Wiersinga WJ, Rhodes A, Cheng AC, et al. Pathophysiology, transmission, diagnosis, and treatment of coronavirus disease 2019 (COVID-19): a review. JAMA 2020;324(8):782–93.
16. Shea H, Holinski J, Benedetti R, et al. Mechanical ventilation for COVID-19 2020. Available at: https://courses.edx.org/courses/course-v1:HarvardX+COV19x+1T2020/course/. Accessed November 30, 2020.
17. Yuki K, Fujiogi M, Koutsogiannaki S. COVID-19 pathophysiology: a review. Clin Immunol 2020;215:108427.
18. Parasher A. COVID-19: current understanding of its pathophysiology, clinical presentation and treatment [published online ahead of print, 2020 Sep 25]. Postgrad Med J 2020;97(1147):312–20.
19. Ejaz H, Alsrhani A, Zafar A, et al. COVID-19 and comorbidities: Deleterious impact on infected patients. J Infect Public Health 2020;13(12):1833–9.

20. Hewitt J, Carter B, Vilches-Moraga A, et al. The effect of frailty on survival in patients with COVID-19 (COPE): a multicentre, European, observational cohort study. Lancet Public Health 2020;5(8):e444–51.

21. Special populations data in the U.S. CDC and prevention. Available at: https://www.cdc.gov/coronavirus/2019-ncov/cases-updates/special-populations/index.html. Accessed November 10, 2020.

22. D'cruz M, Banerjee D. 'An invisible human rights crisis': the marginalization of older adults during the COVID-19 pandemic - an advocacy review. Psychiatry Res 2020;292:113369.

23. Fallon A, Dukelow T, Kennelly SP, et al. COVID-19 in nursing homes. QJM 2020; 113(6):391–2.

24. Ouslander JG, Grabowski DC. COVID-19 in nursing homes: calming the perfect storm. J Am Geriatr Soc 2020;68(10):2153–62.

25. VanHoutven CH, DePasquale N, Coe NB. Essential long-term care workers commonly hold second jobs and double-or triple-duty caregiving roles. J Am Geriatr Soc 2020;68(8):1657–60.

26. Shippee TP, Akosionu O, Ng W, et al. COVID-19 pandemic: exacerbating racial/ethnic disparities in long-term services and supports. J Aging Soc Policy 2020; 32(4–5):323–33.

27. Brown KA, Jones A, Daneman N, et al. Association between nursing home crowding and COVID-19 infection and mortality in Ontario, Canada. JAMA Intern Med 2020;181(2):229–36.

28. Li Y, Temkin-Greener H, Shan G, et al. COVID-19 infections and deaths among Connecticut nursing home residents: facility correlates. J Am Geriatr Soc 2020; 68(9):1899–906.

29. Feral-Pierssens AL, Claret PG, Chouihed T. Collateral damage of the COVID-19 outbreak: expression of concern. Eur J Emerg Med 2020;27(4):233–4.

30. Battisti NML, Mislang AR, Cooper L, et al. Adapting care for older cancer patients during the COVID-19 pandemic: recommendations from the international society of geriatric Oncology (SIOG) COVID-19 working group. J Geriatr Oncol 2020; 11(8):1190–8.

31. Brandt N, Chou J. Optimizing medication management during the COVID-19 pandemic: it takes a village. J Gerontol Nurs 2020;46(7):3–8.

32. Nieman CL, Oh ES. Connecting with older adults via telemedicine. Ann Intern Med 2020;173(10):831–2.

33. Makaroun LK, Bachrach RL, Rosland AM. Elder abuse in the time of COVID-19-increased risks for older adults and their caregivers. Am J Geriatr Psychiatry 2020;28(8):876–80.

34. Elder Abuse|Violence Prevention|Injury Center|CDC. Centers for disease control and prevention. 2020. Available at: https://www.cdc.gov/violenceprevention/elderabuse/index.html. Accessed November 11, 2020.

35. Bunders MJ, Altfeld M. Implications of sex differences in immunity for SARS-CoV-2 pathogenesis and design of therapeutic interventions. Immunity 2020;53(3):487–95.

36. Mok VCT, Pendlebury S, Wong A, et al. Tackling challenges in care of Alzheimer's disease and other dementias amid the COVID-19 pandemic, now and in the future. Alzheimers Dement 2020;16(11):1571–81.

37. Goveas JS, Shear K. Grief and the COVID-19 pandemic in older adults. Am J Ger Psych 2020;28(10):1119–25.

38. Cooper LA, Williams DR. Excess death from COVID-19, community bereavement, and restorative justice for communities of color. JAMA Netw 2020;324(15): 1491–2.

39. Bojdani E, Rajagopalan A, Chen A, et al. COVID-19 Pandemic: impact on psychiatric care in the United States. Psychiatry Res 2020;289:113069.

40. Roschel H, Artioli GG, Gualano B. Risk of increased physical inactivity during COVID-19 outbreak in older people: a call for Actions. J Am Geriatr Soc 2020; 68(6):1126–8.

41. Füzéki E, Groneberg DA, Banzer W. Physical activity during COVID-19 induced lockdown: recommendations. J Occup Med Toxicol 2020;15:25.

42. Lyu H, Yoshida K, Zhao SS, et al. Delayed denosumab injections and fracture risk among patients with osteoporosis : a population-based cohort study. Ann Intern Med 2020;173(7):516–26.

43. Upadhyaya GK, Iyengar K, Jain VK, et al. Challenges and strategies in management of osteoporosis and fragility fracture care during COVID-19 pandemic. J Orthop 2020;21:287–90.

44. Rosenbaum L. Facing covid-19 in Italy - ethics, logistics, and therapeutics on the epidemic's front line. N Engl J Med 2020;382(20):1873–5.

45. Farrell TW, Francis L, Brown T, et al. Rationing limited healthcare resources in the COVID-19 era and beyond: ethical considerations regarding older adults. J Am Geriatr Soc 2020;68(6):1143–9.

46. Ageing and Health. World health organization. Available at: https://www.who.int/ ageing/ageism/en/. Accessed November 11, 2020.

47. Jimenez-Sotomayor MR, Gomez-Moreno C, Soto-Perez-de-Celis E, et al. An evaluation of tweets about older adults and COVID-19. J Am Geriatr Soc 2020;68(8): 1661–5.

48. Han SD, Mosqueda L. Elder abuse in the COVID-19 era. J Am Geriatr Soc 2020; 68(7):1386–7.

49. CDC. COVID Data Tracker. Available at: https://covid.cdc.gov/covid-data-tracker/#vaccinations. Accessed December 26, 2020.

Minority Women

Renee Hickson, MD[a],*, Monica Pernia Marin, MD[b],
Marisa Dunn, MD, MPH[c]

KEYWORDS

• Hispanics • Latinx • The 5 M's • Geriatric assessment • Black women

KEY POINTS

- Variables such as BMI, diabetes, smoking status, renal function, and psychiatric affect are modifiable predictors of frailty in older Black and Hispanic/Latinx women.
- Performance-based application of assessment tools and measures used to determine cognitive and functional status should be administered with language and cultural sensitivity.
- Psychosocial factors such as educational attainment, socioeconomic living conditions, extent of community involvement, and social networking positively affect cognition in older Black and Hispanic/Latinx women.
- Comprehensive coverage health plans that include broader prescription drug coverage can reduce the clinical, economic, and social morbidity that disproportionately affects our most vulnerable seniors.
- Health goals for older Black and Hispanic/Latinx women are directed toward the preservation of functional independence to engage in social, occupational, and spiritual activities and maintenance of societal roles, and less likely to be disease-focused.

INTRODUCTION

The World Health Organization defines health as a state of physical, mental, and social well-being, not merely the absence of disease and infirmity.[1] Long before we need medical care, our foundation for health begins in our homes, schools, neighborhoods, and societal institutions.[2] Cultural characteristics have a strong influence in the way we perceive ourselves, others, and the world. Experiences shared from old to new generations over time can also shape the way a particular population finds its place in society. Ultimately, these experiences influence how people interpret illness, pain, and death.

A quick look back into history is sufficient to put in perspective how older Black and Hispanic American women have experienced health care systems fraught with disparities toward minority groups. Racism as well as cultural and gender biases have

[a] Oak Street Healthcare, 4800 Chef Menteur Highway, New Orleans, LA 70126, USA;
[b] Department of Geriatrics and Palliative Medicine, The George Washington University, 2150 Pennsylvania Avenue Northwest, Washington, DC 20037, USA; [c] Jencare Senior Medical Center, 2124 Candler Road, Decatur, GA 30032, USA
* Corresponding author.
E-mail address: drHicky3@gmail.com

Clin Geriatr Med 37 (2021) 523–532
https://doi.org/10.1016/j.cger.2021.05.013
0749-0690/21/© 2021 Elsevier Inc. All rights reserved.

engendered lack of trust and cause barriers for these women to receive optimal health care. Sadly, disparities have widened. It is imperative that providers seek to understand and consider specific needs, expectations, and circumstances that are germane to minority women.

The proportion of older Hispanic/Latinx adults in the United States is expected to double by 2050, becoming the largest group of older ethnic minorities.[3,4] There is vast evidence of significantly higher cardiovascular risk among Hispanics when compared with non-Hispanic whites,[5] and heart disease accounted for more than 40% of the mortality rate among older Black women.[6] A recent systematic review of studies of aging with multiple conditions found older people, women, and people who were socioeconomically deprived to be affected by multiple morbidities with increasing disability and functional decline, worse quality of life, and higher health costs.[7]

Given this context, this article is written in the framework of the 5 M's. The 4 M's being promoted by the Center for Medicare & Medicaid Services (CMS) are Mobility, Mentation, Medications, and What Matters.[8–10] The 5th M is for Multicomplexity, which refers to the presence of multiple chronic health conditions treated in one individual while considering all the components comprising a person's global health status.[11] We hope this concise literature review, as it relates specifically to older Black and Hispanic/Latinx women, serves to educate providers and prompt them to address disparities in our health care systems to promote healthy aging for these patients.

MOBILITY AND MULTICOMPLEXITY

It is estimated that almost 40% of community-dwelling older Americans report some limitation in daily activities due to chronic conditions.[12] Older Black Americans have higher rates of chronic conditions and increased risk of prolonged functional disability and impairment,[13] and studies confirmed higher incidence of disability in activities of daily living (ADLs) and higher fear of falling among elderly Hispanic adults.[14,15] Although many studies have demonstrated the association between falls and impairment of mobility and balance,[16,17] a broader view of how mobility relates to the multicomplexity of older Black and Hispanic women, and the factors that potentially affect the development of frailty, is warranted.

Body mass index (BMI), muscle strength, range of motion, and activity level are potentially modifiable conditions that contribute to balance and mobility. Galanos and colleagues reported that either a high or low BMI is associated with a greater risk of falling, even in situations where the activity level is low and muscle strength is less.[18] Compared to older white women, these factors simply lead older Black women to avoid situations or activities that put them at risk for falling.[19] A study of older adults reported hazard ratios for disability that doubled the hazard ratios for mortality among individuals with a BMI over 30 kg/m^2.[20] The importance of variables such as BMI, diabetes, smoking status, and negative affect, as predictors of frailty among Mexican-American older adults, represent modifiable characteristics or behaviors not previously identified as risk factors for frailty among non-Hispanic white or minority populations.[21]

Medical histories that include multiple comorbidities including chronic kidney disease have been associated with poor physical performance, cognitive impairment, and frailty,[20–23] and estimated glomerular filtration rate was associated with decline in basic and instrumental ADLs.[24] However, merely inquiring about these activities may be insufficient to assess the real social and psychological impact of reduced function. More recent research introducing concepts such as life-space mobility reflects a broader view of physical ability and participation in society for older Black patients and may provide important prognostic information about morbidity and incident functional impairment.[25] A validated tool such as the Life-Space Assessment (LSA) developed by investigators at the University of Alabama at Birmingham (UAB), in which higher composite scores represent greater mobility, has prognostic utility, as those with scores lower than 30 were reported to be 10 times more likely to die within 4 years.[25,26]

As studies such as the African-American Health point out, the appropriate use and application of tools that identify older Black (and Hispanic) patients at risk of disability and mortality are needed so that interventions can be developed.[27] For example, the FRAIL scale exhibits strong predictive validity for new disability and mortality and includes a comorbidity measure which may prove valuable.[28] Data from the Hispanic Established Population for Epidemiologic Studies of the Elderly revealed that performance-based measures are better predictors of mortality than self-assessments in elderly Mexican-Americans.[29] Hispanic/Latinx adults who have poor English proficiency show a higher incidence of disability in ADLs and a higher fear of falling.[14,15] The language of the interview may influence the association between the performance-based measure and the self-report because it serves as a proxy for very different, culturally based, cognitive conceptions of illness.[30,31]

The correlation between physical performance and cognition has been well-established[32,33] and executive functioning is deemed essential to preserved functional status.[34,35] In Black women, one study confirmed that executive functioning is significantly associated with physical performance.[35] The addition of executive functioning measures such as the Stroop effect, would improve assessment of disability risk, especially in older Black women whose declines in physical performance are an early indicator of disability.[36–38] Utilization of appropriate assessment tools will allow providers to perform an accurate evaluation of functional status in older Black and Hispanic women.

MENTATION

Cognitive impairment and dementia often lead to disability and care dependence, with the impact of dementia seeming to vary depending on ethnic and racial differences. Black and Hispanic/Latinx adults have a higher rate of cardiovascular disease including diabetes and hypertension, both associated with an elevated risk of dementia.[5] Black Americans have shorter life expectancy than Hispanics[4]; therefore, Hispanic women are more likely to live longer with some degree of cognitive impairment. Specifically, there is higher reported cognition, slower cognitive decline, and later presentation of impairment in foreign-born Hispanics when compared with those born in the United States.[39]

Bangen and collaborators reported worse cognitive performance on all cognitive domains including memory, language, and visuospatial abilities among diabetics in an ethnically diverse group of older adults when compared with nondiabetics.[40] Cognitive impairment may be reflected on neuroimaging studies[41,42] highlighting the frontal subcortical region, which is particularly sensitive to the effects of cardiovascular risk factors and vascular burden.[43,44] Perhaps dementia should be conceptualized as a product of both biological and cultural factors because genetics and cardiovascular disease may help explain disparities in the incidence and prevalence of Alzheimer disease, and race-specific cultural factors may impact diagnosis and treatment.[45]

The potential impact of the study of contextual variables shows that neighborhood homogeneity and socioeconomic context are relevant to cognitive decline among older Mexican Americans and important for cognitive health.[46] Psychosocial factors such as educational attainment, social networking, and mentally stimulating activities protect against dementia.[47,48] Larger social networks seem to have a protective influence on cognitive function among elderly women.[49]

The effect of education on cognitive impairment is more pronounced among ethnic minorities. Not only does higher education extend life in good cognitive health, but it also shortens the period of cognitive impairment.[48] This protective effect of high education is observed to be even stronger among older Black patients.[50] More education did not protect individuals from developing neurodegenerative and vascular neuropathology by the time they died but it mitigated the impact of pathology on the clinical expression of dementia before death.[50–52] Conversely, a low education level may also limit an accurate assessment of cognition in older adults,[48] and the addition of a language barrier among older Hispanic/Latinx adults makes assessments even more challenging.

There is an enormous need to optimize cognitive assessment tools that can be tailored to the patient's education level and preferred language. The additional implication of racial biases inherent in cognitive screening tools could potentially be reduced by controlling for literacy level or using savings scores in psychometric analyses.[45] Cognitive test scores are influenced by many factors, so equating lower test scores with presence of disease effects ignore the other sometimes more substantial contributions of nondisease variables.[48,53]

Policies to improve the social and economic environments for older adults in diverse populations could potentially delay the onset of dementia.[54] Education and prevention strategies to decrease cerebrovascular risk factors should be emphasized on a national scale and directed particularly to growing minority populations.

MEDICATIONS

Black and Hispanic elderly women live longer with cognitive impairment and cardiovascular comorbidities; often making careful and calculated choices regarding the use of prescription medications, complementary and alternative medications (CAMs), and the practice of self-medicating. Basic economic principles apply in that low income and high out-of-pocket drug costs play an important role in medication adherence. Other factors include interethnic differences in attitudes and behaviors toward medical decisions, reflecting different experiences in the health care system.[55–57]

Many low-income older adults may be forced to choose between their medications and food, clothing or other goods and services.[58] Increases in age-related health expenses, coupled with reduced access to adequate medical and pharmaceutical assistance also leads to the habit of self-medication.[59] In one systematic review, the mean prevalence of older adults taking nonprescription drugs was approximately 40%.[60] In addition, the elderly in ethnic groups and cultures use CAM as part of healing systems.[61] Among elderly Mexican-American women, there is a dual system of health care (allopathic and CAM) operating in a complementary way.[62] CAM modalities used by Hispanic/Latinx older adults mostly are dietary supplements, home remedies, and curanderos—herbalist/folk medicine practitioners. Although ethnic older adults consult a physician for medical problems, most CAM users (62%) did not inform their physician they were using it.[61] The Hispanic Health and Nutrition Examination Survey (HHANES 1982–1984) found that among folk healer users, only 4.7% were older than 65 years, were more apt to perceive their health as fair to poor, and were dissatisfied with medical care received.[62] Lack of medical insurance was more frequently noted among Hispanic CAM users, resulting in lower utilization of formal services and higher self-treatment due to lack of access.[61]

Physicians should be alert to the possibility of medication restriction among their older patients who are underinsured or have no coverage. A more comprehensive coverage plan, and policies that limit medication costs, may help reduce medication restriction and with it the clinical, economic, and social morbidity that disproportionately affects our most vulnerable seniors.[63,64]

WHAT MATTERS

For an older Black woman and her caregivers, the ability to remain independent and to care for herself is perhaps more important than any specific disease or diagnosis. To describe what really matters to older Black and Hispanic/Latinx women in America is merely an attempt to portray only some of their motivations, goals, and views toward chronic illness and well-being. We hope this helps clinicians and health care workers to expand their perspectives beyond the examination room and build trust within minority communities.

Older Black women suffer from chronic disease for longer periods and develop cardiovascular disease risk factors earlier than age 65 years.[65] One might consider evaluating for the degree of cumulative psychosocial stress that results from acute negative life events along with chronic stressors derived from family, and interpersonal relationships, work environment, discrimination, and safety. These factors may explain in part why cardiovascular health is significantly lower among Black American women when compared with whites.[65,66] Poor cardiovascular health translates into unexpected cardiovascular events, which eventually compromise function and independence ultimately leading to social isolation. However, for these women, health goals are not always oriented to disease-specific targets (adequate blood pressure, and blood glucose, etc.). In many instances, health goals are directed toward preservation of functional independence sufficient to engage in social activities. Even when viewed as debilitated, older Black women are more likely to make efforts to maintain control over health as committed practitioners of self-care, rather than making behavioral or environmental changes such as diet or exercise (disease-oriented goals).[67,68]

It appears that the roles Black women play in society may also have a part in their cardiovascular health. Janssen and colleagues (2011) investigated the effect of multiple roles (spouse, parent, employee, and caregiver) on the progression of coronary artery calcification in Black and white women during a follow-up period of 2 years. Stress and reward levels were assessed during this time. Results showed that higher role rewards among Black women were associated with lower progression of coronary artery calcification leading to some cardiovascular benefit.[69] Health care providers should acknowledge the relevance of these roles for older Black women because their ability to continue in these roles seems to be the main motivation for maintaining personal autonomy (including control over medical decisions) while preventing overburdening of family members at the end of their lives.[70]

There are several interrelated dimensions that serve as the foundations of inner strength in older Hispanic women with chronic illness. These dimensions include drawing strength from the past, focusing on possibilities, being supported by others, knowing one's purpose, and nurturing the spirit.[71] Spirituality should be located as a point of connection with older women to create safe spaces for open communication.[72,73] Understanding the belief that God controls the timing and nature of death shapes perceptions of quality of life as well as certain decisions regarding life-sustaining treatments and end-of-life care.[74] Locating one's personal perspective on suffering, mortality, and the process of dying should also be included for consideration. The role of the health care provider is to serve as God's instrument of healing.[75]

Early and active engagement of caregivers and family members should be encouraged as it offers valuable information about the family principles, dynamics, faith, and cultural background, which can guide providers to facilitate goals of care conversations and decisions regarding health.[76] Other aspects that appear relevant during goals of care discussions include feelings of fulfillment, hopefulness and acceptance, and acknowledgment of barriers to accessing care or general mistrust in the health care system. At the end of life, a more personalized health care conversation is best.

SUMMARY

The relationship between health, illness, life, and death is determined in part by culture, tradition, personal experiences, and psychological factors. Moreover, tradition, education, and socioeconomic factors play a role in the way people live and their approach to health care. Diversity is increasing, and the health care system must evolve accordingly. Known disparities in the health and care of older Black and Hispanic/Latinx women can be reduced by recognition of cultural and biological factors of diseases that affect them. Education is key, as providers should work to reduce the gap in communication between older minority women and the research needed to address and improve their care. Improving education and resources in high-risk ethnic communities with physical, social, and cognitively stimulating interventions would certainly improve the quality of life for all concerned.

CLINICS CARE POINTS

- Performance-based tools provide more accurate assessment than self-reporting
- Accuracy of cognitive tests is increased when administered with language and cultural specificity.
- Adherence to prescribed therapies is dependent on patient and provider awareness of insurance coverage constraints and affordability of medication.
- BMI and renal function should be assessed in frailty and disability determinations
- Helping older Black and Hispanic/Latinx women maintain their societal roles is a key component of attaining health goals.
- Consider socioeconomic living conditions and community/social networks when assessing mood and cognition in older minority women.

DISCLOSURE

The authors have nothing to disclose.

REFERENCES

1. World Health Organization. 2018.
2. Robert Wood Johnson Foundation. 2018.
3. Passel JS, Cohn D, U.S. Pew Research Center. Washington, DC: Population projections: 2005-2050 2008.
4. Available at: https://www.census.gov/data/tables/2014/demo/popproj/2014-summary-tables.html. Accessed April 10, 2020.

5. Balfour PC Jr, Ruiz JM, Talavera GA, et al. Cardiovascular disease in hispanics/latinos in the United States. J Lat Psychol 2016;4(2):98–113.
6. Satcher D. Eliminating racial and ethnic disparities in health: the role of the ten leading health indicators. J Natl Med Assoc 2000;92(6):315–318.2.
7. King DE, Xiang J, Pilkerton CS. Multimorbidity trends in the U.S. adults. 1988-2014. J Am Board Fam Med 2018;31:503–13.
8. Center for Medicaid & Medicare services. Available at: www.cms.gov. Accessed April 10, 2020.
9. Hartford foundation for public giving. Available at: www.hfpg.org. Accessed May 10, 2020.
10. Improving health & healthcare worldwide. Available at: www.ihi.org. Accessed June 10, 2020.
11. Suls J, Green PA, Boyd CM. Multimorbidity: implications and directions for health psychology and behavioral medicine. Health Psychol 2019;38(9):772–82.
12. National Center for Health Statistics. Health, United States, 2018. Hyattsville (MD): US Department of Health and Human Services, Public Health Service, Centers for Disease Control, National Center for Health Statistics; 2018.
13. Bulutaoand RA, Anderson NB. In: Understanding racial and ethnic differences in health in late life: a research agenda. Washington, DC: National Academies Press; 2004. for the Committee on Population, Division of Behavioral and Social Sciences and Education, National Research Council.
14. Song J, Chang HJ, Tirodkar M, et al. Racial/ethnic differences in activities of daily living disability in older adults with Arthritis: a longitudinal study. Arthritis Rheumatol 2007;57(6):1058–66.
15. James EG, Conatser P, Karabulut M, et al. Mobility limitations and fear of falling in non-English speaking older Mexican-Americans. Ethn Health 2017;22(5):480–9.
16. Graafmans WC, Ooms ME, Hofstee HMA, et al. Falls in the elderly: a prospective study of risk factors and risk profiles. Am J Epidemiol 1996;143:1129–36.
17. Lord SR, Ward JA, Williams P, et al. Physiological factors associated with falls in older community-dwelling women. J Am Geriatr Soc 1994;42:1110–7.
18. Galanos AN, Pieper CF, Cornoni-Huntley JC, et al. Nutrition and function: is there a relationship between body mass index and the functional capabilities of community-dwelling elderly? J Am Geriatr Soc 1994;42:368–73.
19. Means KM, Rodell DE, O'Sullivan PS, et al. Comparison of a functional obstacle course with an index of clinical gait and balance and postural sway. J Gerontol A Biol Sci Med Sci 1998;53:M331–5.
20. Al Snih S, Ottenbacher KJ, Markides KS, et al. The effect of obesity on disability vs mortality in older Americans. Arch Intern Med 2007;167(8):774–80.
21. Ottenbacher KJ, Graham JE, Al Snih S, et al. Mexican Americans and frailty: findings from the Hispanic established populations epidemiologic studies of the elderly. Am J Public Health 2009;99(4):673–9.
22. Odden MC, Chertow GM, Fried LF, et al. Cystatin C and measures of physical function in elderly adults: the health, aging, and body composition (HABC) study. Am J Epidemiol 2006;164:1180–9.
23. Wilhelm-Leen ER, Hall YN, Tamura MK, et al. Frailty and chronic kidney disease: the third national health and nutrition evaluation Survey. Am J Med 2009;122:664–671 e662.
24. Bowling CB, Sawyer P, Campbell RC, et al. Impact of chronic kidney disease on activities of daily living in community-dwelling older adults. J Gerontol A Biol Sci Med Sci 2011;66:689–94.

25. Brown CJ, Roth DL, Allman RM, et al. Trajectories of life-space mobility after hospitalization. Ann Intern Med 2009;150:372–8.
26. Sawyer Baker P, Allman RM. Resilience in mobility in the context of chronic disease and aging: cross-sectional and prospective findings from the UAB study of aging. New York: Cambridge University Press; 2010.
27. Miller DK, Wolinsky FD, Malmstrom TK, et al. Inner city, middle-aged African Americans have excess frank and subclinical disability. J Gerontol A Biol Sci Med Sci 2005;60A:207–12.
28. Malmstrom T, Miller D, Morley J. A comparison of four frailty models. J Am Geriatr Soc (Jags) 2014;62(4):721–6.
29. Angel R, Ostir GV, Frisco ML, et al. Comparison of a self-reported and a performance-based assessment of mobility in the hispanic established population for epidemiological studies of the elderly. Res Aging 2000;22(6):715–37.
30. Angel R, Thoits P. The impact of culture on the cognitive structure of illness. Cult Med Psychiatry 1987;11(4):465–94.
31. Angel R, Williams K. Chapter 3: cultural models of health and illness. In: Paniagua FA, Yamada A-M, editors. Handbook of multicultural mental health (second edition): assessment and treatment of diverse populations. Academic Press; 2013. p. 49–68.
32. Sawyer Baker P, Allman RM. Resilience in mobility in the context of chronic disease and aging: cross-sectional and prospective findings from the UAB study of aging. New York: Cambridge University Press; 2010.
33. Yochim BP, Lequerica A, MacNeill SE, et al. Cognitive initiation and depression as predictors of future instrumental activities of daily living among older medical rehabilitation patients. J Clin Exp Neuropsychol 2008;(30):236–44.
34. Johnson JK, Lui LY, Yaffe K. Executive function, more than global cognition, predicts functional decline and mortality in elderly women. J Gerontol A Biol Sci Med Sci 2007;62(10):1134–41.
35. Lewis MS, Miller LS. Executive control functioning and functional ability in older adults. Clin Neuropsychol 2007;21(2):274–85.
36. Atkinson HH, Rosano C, Simonsick EM, et al. Cognitive function, gait speed decline, and comorbidities: the health, aging and body composition study. J Gerontol A Biol Sci Med Sci 2007;62:844–50.
37. Miller DK, Wolinsky FD, Malmstrom TK, et al. Inner city, middle-aged African Americans have excess frank and subclinical disability. J Gerontol A Biol Sci Med Sci 2005;60A:207–12.
38. Malmstrom TK, Miller DK, Morley JE. A comparison of four frailty models. J Am Geriatr Soc 2014;62(4):721–6.
39. Garcia MA, Saenz JL, Downer B, et al. Age of migration differentials in life expectancy with cognitive impairment: 20-year findings from the hispanic-EPESE. Gerontologist 2018;58(5):894–903 [published correction appears in Gerontologist. 2017 Oct 1;57(5):1008].
40. Bangen KJ, Gu Y, Gross AL, et al. Relationship between type 2 diabetes mellitus and cognitive change in a multiethnic elderly cohort. J Am Geriatr Soc 2015; 63(6):1075–83.
41. Dufouil C, De Kersaint-Gilly A, Besancon V, et al. Longitudinal study of blood pressure and white matter hyperdensities: the EVA MRI cohort. Neurology 2001;56(7):921–6.
42. Ylikoski A, Erkinjuntti T, Raininko R, et al. White matter hyperdensities on MRI in the neurologically nondiseased elderly: analysis of cohorts of consecutive subjects aged 55-85 years living at home. Stroke 1995;26(7):1171–7.

43. Cahn-Weiner DA, Boyle PA, Malloy PF. Tests of executive function predict instrumental activities of daily living in community-dwelling older individuals. Appl Neuropsychol 2002;9(3):187–91.

44. Carlson JE, Ostir GV, Black SA, et al. Disability in older adults 2: physical activity as prevention. Behav Medicin 1999;24(4):157–68.

45. Chin AL, Negash S, Hamilton R. Diversity and disparity in dementia: the impact of ethnoracial differences in Alzheimer disease. Alzheimer Dis Assoc Disord 2011; 25(3):187–95.

46. Sheffield KM, Peek KM. Neighborhood context and cognitive decline in older Mexican Americans: results from the hispanic established populations for epidemiologic studies of the elderly. Am J Epidemiol 2009;169(9):1092–101.

47. Qiu C, De Ronchi D, Fratiglioni L. The epidemiology of the dementias: an update. Curr Opin Psychiatry 2007;20(4):380–5.

48. Gross AL, Mungas DM, Crane PK, et al. Effects of education and race on cognitive decline: an integrative study of generalizability versus study-specific results. Psychol Aging 2015;30(4):863–80.

49. Crooks VC, Lubben J, Petitti DB, et al. Social network, cognitive function, and dementia incidence among elderly women. Am J Public Health 2008;98(7):1221–7. https://doi.org/10.2105/AJPH.2007.115923.

50. Reuser M, Willekens FJ, Bonneux L. Higher education delays and shortens cognitive impairment: a multistate life table analysis of the US Health and Retirement Study. Eur J Epidemiol 2011;26(5):395–403.

51. Fratiglioni L, Rocca W. Epidemiology of dementia. In: Boller F, Cappa SF, editors. Handbook of neuropsychology: aging and dementia. Elsevier Sc Publ Amsterdam; 2001. p. 193–215.

52. Fratiglioni W. Prevention of Alzheimer's disease and dementia. Major findings from the Kungsholmen Project. Physiol Behav 2007;92(1):98–104.

53. Early DR, Widaman KF, Harvey D, et al. Demographic predictors of cognitive change in ethnically diverse older persons. Psychol Aging 2013;28(3):633–45.

54. Garcia MA, Downer B, Chiu CT, et al. Racial/ethnic and nativity differences in cognitive life expectancies among older adults in the United States. Gerontologist 2019;59(2):281–9.

55. Hopp FP, Duffy SA. Racial variations in end-of-life care. J Am Geriatr Soc 2000; 48:658–63.

56. McKinley ED, Garrett JM, Evans AT, et al. Differences in end-of-life decision making among Black and white ambulatory cancer patients. J Gen Intern Med 1996; 11:651–6.

57. Escarce JJ, Epstein KR, Colby DC, et al. Racial differences in the elderly's use of medical procedures and diagnostic tests. Am J Public Health 1993;83:948–54.

58. Lagnado L. The uncovered; drug costs can leave elderly a grim choice: pills or other needs; when a trip to the pharmacy costs $400, and Medicare doesn't pay for any of it; buying medicines on credit. Wall Street J 1998;A1(E).

59. Barros e SAM, Barros JAC, Olivera SAMPB. Self-medication in the elderly of the city of Salgueiro, state of penambuco. Rev Bras Epidemiol 2007;10:75–85.

60. Jerez-Roig J, Mederios L, Silva V, et al. Prevalence of self-medication and associated factors in an elderly population: a systematic review. Drugs Aging 2014; 31(12):p883–96.

61. Najm W, Reinsch S, Hoehler F, et al. Use of complementary and alternative medicine among the ethnic elderly. Altern Ther Health Med 2003;9(3):50–7.

62. Drug Utilization Research Group, Latin America. Multicenter study on self-medication and self-prescription in six Latin American countries. Clin Pharmacol Ther 1997;61:488–93.

63. Mayers RS. Use of folk medicine by elderly Mexican-American women. J Drug Issues 1989;10:283–95.

64. Soumerai SB, Ross-Degnan D. Inadequate prescription-drug coverage for Medicare enrollees – a call to action. N Engl J Med 1999;340:722–8 (published erratum appears in N Engl J Med 1999;340:976).

65. Malek A, Cushman M, Lackland D, et al. Secondhand Smoke exposure and Stroke: the reasons for geographic and racial differences in Stroke (REGARDS) study. Am J Prev Med 2015;49(6):e89–97.

66. Burroughs Pena M, Mbassa R, Slopen N, et al. Cumulative psychosocial stress and ideal cardiovascular health in older women: data by race/ethnicity. Circulation 2019;139(17):2012–21.

67. Golden M. The wide circumference of love. New York: Arcade; 2017.

68. Turner C, Battle J. Old enough to know: the impact of health values on self-care among elderly Black men and women. West J Black Stud 2010;34(1):1–12.

69. Janssen I, Powell LH, Jasielec MS, et al. Progression of coronary artery calcification in Black and white women: do the stresses and rewards of multiple roles matter? Ann Behav Med 2012;43(1):39–49.

70. Nath SB, Kirschman KB, Lewis B, et al. Place called LIFE: exploring the advance care planning of African-American PACE enrollees. Soc Work Health Care 2008; 47(3):277–92.

71. Dingley C, Roux G. Inner strength in older Hispanic women with chronic illness. J Cult Divers 2003;10(1):11–22. PMID: 12776543.

72. Pesut B, Reimer-Kirkham S. Situated clinical encounters in the negotiation of religious and spiritual plurality: a critical ethnography. Int J Nurs Stud 2010;47(7): 815–25.

73. Rao AS, Desphande OM, Jomoona C, et al. Elderly Indo-Caribbean Hindus and end-of-life care: a community-based exploratory study. J Am Geriatr Soc 2008; 56(6):1129–33.

74. Carr D. Racial differences in end-of-life planning: why don't Blacks and latinos prepare for the inevitable? Omega J Death Dying 2011;63(1):1–20.

75. Johnson KS, Elbert-Avila KI, Tulsky JA. The influence of spiritual beliefs and practices on the treatment preferences of African-Americans: a review of the literature. J Am Geriatr Soc 2005;53(4):711.

76. Brown E, Patel R, Kaur J, et al. The interface between South Asian culture and palliative care for children, young people, and families- a discussion paper. Issues Compr Pediatr Nurs 2013;36(1/2):120–43.

Aging and Women's Health
An Update from the National Institute on Aging

Catherine Nagy, MA*, Patricia Jones, DrPH, MPH, MS, MBA,
Marie A. Bernard, MD

KEYWORDS

- Aging • Clinical care • Women's health

KEY POINTS

- Older women outnumber older men in the United States, and the proportion of the population that is female increases with age.
- Older women may experience a range of physical, cognitive, social, and emotional challenges.
- Women of color and members of other marginalized groups often have unique concerns that may not be immediately apparent to clinicians.
- The National Institute on Aging of the National Institutes of Health supports a vibrant program of aging research with many immediately implementable findings for the busy clinician.

INTRODUCTION

Mrs J, a 76-year-old black woman, presents to her primary care provider for a periodic visit. She has no complaints beyond mild knee discomfort with prolonged sitting. She has known hypertension. She has several questions about how to optimize her health:

- She states that she wants to live as long as possible without being a burden to her children and has heard that metformin can prolong life and health in older adults. Should she take it?
- She has also read that a daily aspirin will help her prevent heart problems. Should she take aspirin?
- She expresses deep concern over eventually developing Alzheimer disease (AD). What steps can she take to prevent it?

Older women outnumber older men in the United States, and the proportion of the population that is female increases with age. In 2019, women accounted for

The authors report no conflicts or disclosures.
National Institute on Aging, National Institutes of Health, Bethesda, MD 20892, USA
* Corresponding author.
E-mail address: nagyk@nia.nih.gov

approximately 54% of Americans ages 65 and older and nearly 65% of Americans ages 85 and older.[1] Despite living longer, however, older women are more likely than older men to report depressive symptoms or limitations in physical function, for reasons that are not entirely clear.[2] Data suggest that older women are also more likely to live alone (a potential indicator or risk factor for isolation, lack of care-givers, or lack of support) and live in poverty at a disproportionately high rate.[2]

As introduced in earlier chapters of this *Geriatric Clinics* volume, the "Geriatric 5 Ms" provide a useful lens through which we can examine Mrs J's unique case, and through her, other clinical concerns common among older women.

DISCUSSION
Multicomplexity

Overall, Mrs J is in excellent physical health, suffering from one diagnosed chronic condition, hypertension, and probably suffering from osteoarthritis given her age and the description of symptoms (**Box 1**). Although multimorbidity is common among older men and women,[3] as many as 45% of adults 65 to 74 have limited comorbidities.[4] Multimorbidity increases steeply with older age, has different patterns in men and women, and varies by race/ethnicity. For example, a recent study found dyads and triads of diseases including cancer were more common among older men, while dyads and triads that included arthritis and osteoporosis were more common among women. In addition, multimorbidity was most common among Black persons, followed by Whites and then Asian Americans.[3]

Although she asks whether she should take aspirin to prevent heart disease, the answer, surprisingly, is no. The Aspirin in Reducing Events in the Elderly (ASPREE) trial found that for adults 75 and older, daily aspirin had no effect on the incidence of myocardial infarction or stroke, physical disability, or dementia. It was, however, associated with a significantly increased risk of serious bleeding.[5–7] Further analysis has shown that the initiation of aspirin may accelerate cancer progression.[8] Notably, the ASPREE results do not address whether older adults who initiated aspirin use at a younger age should discontinue its use.[8]

Mrs J can safeguard her health by achieving optimal control of her blood pressure. The groundbreaking SPRINT trial demonstrated that targeting a systolic blood pressure of less than 120 mm Hg, compared with less than 140 mm Hg, in patients at high risk for cardiovascular events but without diabetes resulted in lower rates of fatal and nonfatal major cardiovascular events and death from any cause.[9] Mrs J's systolic

---

Box 1
Mrs J's history and physical exam

PMH: G2P2, no other hospitalizations.

Meds: Hctz 25 mg Qd; Tylenol prn.

FH: Both parents had hypertension, with mother dying with AD and father with vascular dementia; 1 sister A & W with obesity, hypertension, hypercholesterolemia.

SH: retired school administrator, volunteering 20 h/wk in the school system, and had been exercising with a mall walking group until the COVID pandemic.

ROS: negative.

VS: BP = 138/88 (home readings consistent) Ht = 5'4" Wt = 140 lbs BMI = 24.

PE—unremarkable with the exception of mild crepitance on knee flexion and extension.

blood pressure, while not dangerously high, is still significantly higher than the SPRINT investigators recommend, and the feasibility and desirability of intervening through either lifestyle or medication should be discussed.

Mrs J's history does not reflect prior hyperlipidemia. However, given her age, family history, and hypertension, a lipid panel should be considered. If hyperlipidemia is identified, and should lifestyle interventions fail, the risks and benefits of statins should be discussed. Evidence supporting the use of statins for primary prevention of atherosclerotic cardiovascular disease in adults 75 and older is lacking. Statin use may be associated with muscle weakness and pain, cognitive symptoms, and incident diabetes mellitus, and these risks may or may not be acceptable to an older patient who, like Mrs J, prioritizes independence and a high quality of life.[10] The ongoing Pragmatic Evaluation of Events and Benefits of Lipid-Lowering in Older Adults (PREVENTABLE) trial, supported by the National Institute on Aging (NIA) and the National Heart, Lung, and Blood Institute, will provide needed clarity around the question of statin use among the "oldest old."

Should Mrs J be prescribed metformin specifically to extend healthy life span? Metformin is one of a number of interventions including dietary manipulations, mTOR (mechanistic target of rapamycin) inhibitors, and senolytics (compounds targeting cellular senescence) being studied for their potential to enhance the duration of health and independence, or health span, by targeting fundamental aging processes rather than specific disease mechanisms.[11] Although some interventions have shown promise in animal studies, large-scale clinical trials have yet to demonstrate efficacy in human subjects. Mrs J should not take metformin in the hope that it will help her remain healthy for longer—but she and her physician should keep an eye on the emerging research.

Mind

Mrs J expresses worry about developing AD. This is not an unreasonable concern given her family history and her hypertension. In addition, African Americans, like Mrs J, are 4 times more likely to develop AD than their White counterparts and may differ in risk factors and disease manifestation.[12] For example, some studies have suggested that African Americans may experience an earlier age of onset and present with more severe clinical symptoms of disease,[13] possibly because compared with non-Hispanic Whites, minority patients are less likely to seek medical advice until they are further along in the disease course.[14] Genetic factors that predispose to AD may also differ between African Americans and non-Hispanic Whites.[15,16]

Moreover, sex and gender differences have been noted in the prevalence, manifestation, disease course, and prognosis of AD between men and women. For example, neurodegeneration and clinical symptoms appear more rapidly in women once a diagnosis of AD has been proposed, with the rapid progression potentially due to neurobiological vulnerabilities in the female brain post menopause.[17] Furthermore, sex mediates at least some forms of genetic risk; carrying 1 or 2 copies of the APOE ε4 allele increases AD risk in both men and women, but the effect is stronger in women.[18] Men and women also differ in the types of dementia with which they are most likely to be diagnosed, with women more likely to be diagnosed with AD and men with vascular, Lewy body, or mixed dementia.[17]

The USPTF has stated that "although there is insufficient evidence to recommend for or against screening for cognitive impairment, there may be important reasons to identify cognitive impairment early. [...] Clinicians should remain alert to early signs or symptoms of cognitive impairment (eg, problems with memory or language) and evaluate the individual as appropriate."[19] The NIA provides access to a variety of screening tools that may be employed within the clinic, are reliable and valid, and can be administered in 10 minutes or less.

Results from the recent SPRINT-MIND study underscore the importance of blood pressure control in Mrs J's particular case. In this study, intensive blood pressure control (goal of SBP<120 mm Hg), compared with standard control (SBP<140 mm Hg), resulted in a 19% reduction in the rate of developing mild cognitive impairment (MCI) and a 15% reduction in the rate of composite MCI and probable dementia.[20]

Mrs J may also be a candidate for a prevention trial, particularly if she resides near an NIA-supported Alzheimer's Disease Research Center. Currently, NIA supports over 200 prevention and intervention trials for AD and related forms of dementia. The Alzheimer's Disease Education and Referral Center and the alzheimers.gov Web site, both sponsored by the NIA, are excellent resources for patients, caregivers, and clinicians.

In addition to AD, screening for mental health and social history is an important task. As noted, older women are more likely than men to report depressive symptoms or limitations in physical function and are more likely to live alone (a potential indicator or risk factor for isolation, lack of caregivers, or lack of support).[2] With the onset of the COVID-19 pandemic, data show that persons 65 and older, particularly women, and older persons with household incomes less than $25,000 reported higher rates of anxiety and depression.[21]

Mobility

Until recently, Mrs J has enjoyed a physically active lifestyle. Unfortunately, her mall walking group stopped walking because of the COVID pandemic, but she should be encouraged to walk outdoors if it is safe for her to do so and to incorporate exercise into her daily life.

Research has shown that a "healthy lifestyle" that includes regular physical activity, never smoking, moderate alcohol intake, and a robust social network compresses the period of late-life disability.[22] The Lifestyle Interventions and Independence for Elders study demonstrated that an exercise intervention encompassing walking, resistance training, balance exercises, and stretching decreased disability by 18% in participants who were age 70 to 89.[23] Exercise and physical activity may also help reduce the risk of falls: a recent meta-analysis found that among well-controlled studies, the rate of falls was 23% lower among the participants in exercise groups than among those in the control groups.[24] The effect was most pronounced among exercise programs involving balance or functional exercise. Evidence for regimens involving other types of exercise (walking, dance, and so forth) is less robust.

Another issue related to mobility is driving. While older adults engage in safer driving behaviors than other age groups, including more frequently wearing seat belts, driving when conditions are safest, and not drinking and driving, older persons, including those aged 75 and older, have higher crash death rates than middle-aged drivers (aged 35–54), largely because they are more vulnerable to severe injury.[25,26]

The decision to discontinue driving can be challenging, given that it may sharply curtail independence and ability to maintain social ties, particularly for individuals who live in rural settings or in places where walking is unsafe. Furthermore, women are more likely to self-regulate driving activities and stop driving when they perceive it to no longer be safe, potentially contributing further to isolation.[27] In this instance, Mrs J may be appropriately questioned about her driving activity and about vision and cognitive changes that may make driving unsafe.

Recognizing the limitations some older women may experience due to changes in daily routines due to the pandemic, including anxiety and depression related to social isolation, clinicians may consider implementing a shared decision-making model with their female patients to identify creative strategies and substantive plans to promote physical activity while physically distancing. In addition, maintaining nutritional health may require additional support if patients like Mrs J are no longer driving and depend on others to deliver groceries or prepared meals or to provide transportation.

Medications

Polypharmacy remains a widespread issue for older adults. Studies have shown that 10% of the US population, and 30% of older adults, take 5 or more medications concurrently.[28] This increases the risk of adverse effects of individual drugs and drug combinations. In 1 study, the strongest predictor of a potentially harmful medication in an older cohort was number of medications taken.[29] The US Deprescribing Research Network, established by the NIA, is currently conducting studies of the benefits, risks, and effects of reducing prescriptions in older adults.

Mrs J reports regularly using just 2 medications—hydrochlorothiazide and acetaminophen, compounds between which adverse interactions have not been widely reported. However, she should be cautioned that switching from acetaminophen to a nonsteroidal anti-inflammatory drug may be associated with an increase in systolic blood pressure[30] and should only be attempted under a physician's supervision. Additional history should be obtained regarding the use of other over-the-counter medications, herbal preparations, and dietary supplements, as there is the potential for interactions with prescribed drugs.

Mrs J does not report use of menopausal hormone therapy (MHT), which remains an option for some women with menopause-related symptoms. The NIA funded Study of Women's Health Across the Nation demonstrated that menopausal vasomotor symptoms persist for years and vary based on racial origin—with average duration of symptoms ranging from a few years to up to a decade. African American women, such as Mrs J, suffered the longest average duration of 10 years.[31] There are a variety of nonmedicinal and medication approaches to controlling vasomotor instability. Research has demonstrated that certain selective serotonin reuptake inhibitors may relieve vasomotor symptoms.[32,33] However, women with severe persistent symptoms may be candidates for MHT, still the most effective means of treating menopausal symptoms. The risks of MHT for women over age 60 are well documented and include increased risk of coronary heart disease, venous thromboembolism, and dementia. These women should be closely followed and should be fully apprised of the risks and benefits of treatment.[34]

What Matters Most

Shared decision-making between health care providers and patients facilitates open and transparent communication with providers, improves patient satisfaction, reflects the patient's goals, supports adherence to treatment plans, and in some instances may reduce health care costs.[35,36] One such paradigm is goal-oriented patient care, which focuses on health and functional goals specific to the individual.[37] In particular, patient priority-directed care (PPC), an approach developed by multiple advisory groups representing patients, caregivers, clinicians, health system experts, and health technology leaders, facilitates the integration of care across specialties to help meet patients' specific, actionable, and achievable health outcome goals within the context of their care preferences.[38] Adoption of PPC has been shown to be feasible in the clinical setting.[39]

It is apparent that one thing that "matters most" to Mrs J is her independence, as signaled by her statement that she "doesn't want to be a burden for her children." Maintaining independence, including remaining in the home and managing activities of daily living, may become increasingly challenging to older adults, particularly those with functional or cognitive limitations. In a recent study, the top 3 variables that serve as barriers to independent living for older adults include memory/cognitive loss, wandering or running away, and the need for assistance with medications.[40] Concerns about mobility and managing a specific medical condition were also frequently mentioned.

Emerging technologies, such as health monitoring devices, accident detection, socially assistive robots, and "smart home" systems, may help older adults, including those with dementia, maintain health and independence for a longer period. For persons with dementia, apps and other technologies may provide reminders, aid autobiographical memory, or provide sequential instruction for wayfinding as well as diverse tasks.[41] Barriers to using technology may include lack of knowledge about and confidence in the ability to use new technological devices; lack of appropriate instruction; health barriers; and cost.[42] A recent study indicated that US Internet users ages 65 and older are less confident than their younger counterparts when using new electronic devices, and a majority require assistance when learning to use a new device. Of note, only a third of disabled older adults had home broadband Internet, which could impinge on their ability to use several technologies for which Internet access is required or desirable.[43]

For those with access, a number of new technologies are currently either available or in development.[44] Technologies such as smart phones with GPS and map features can assist older persons who are active but require direction assistance. Resources such as Amazon Alexa or Echo can aid memory. There are also resources to enhance physical activity and promote social interaction as well as tools such as Tile Mates Bluetooth tracking to aid with locating misplaced items.

SUMMARY

While many older women such as Mrs J enjoy overall good health, healthy aging is a process. Furthermore, older patients are not a monolith but rather a heterogeneous group with unique needs. In the context of major social shifts such as the COVID-19 pandemic as well as (in many cases) ongoing stressors such as racial disparities, it is important for providers to see themselves as members of a health service team and recognize the importance of engaging the expertise of other social support and health care providers. The strategies outlined above may help clinicians partner with women like Mrs J to proactively address and maintain their specific health needs.[45] Going forward, clinicians can foster additional discovery to enhance aging by referring patients for aging clinical trials—including AD studies. Information can be found at Clinical Trials | National Institute on Aging.

CLINICS CARE POINTS

- Tight control of blood pressure benefits both physical and cognitive health in older individuals.
- Evidence does not support use of aspirin for primary prevention of heart disease.
- Screening for mental health and social history, including driving ability, is crucial in this population.

REFERENCES

1. Annual estimates of the resident population by sex, age, race alone or in combination, and hispanic origin for the United States: April 1, 2010 to July 1,

2019 (NC-EST2019-ASR5H). US Census Bureau Population Division; 2020. Available at: https://www.census.gov/newsroom/press-kits/2020/population-estimates-detailed.html. Accessed January 1, 2021.

2. Federal Interagency Forum on Aging-Related Statistics. Older Americans 2016: key indicators of well-being. Available at: https://agingstats.gov/docs/LatestReport/Older-Americans-2016-Key-Indicators-of-WellBeing.pdf. Accessed January 1, 2021.

3. Rocca WA, Boyd CM, Grossardt BR, et al. Prevalence of multimorbidity in a geographically-defined American population: patterns by age, sex, and race/ethnicity. Mayo Clin Proc 2014;89(10):1336–49.

4. Forman DE, Maurer MS, Boyd C, et al. Multimorbidity in older adults with cardiovascular disease. J Am Coll Cardiol 2018;71(19):2149–61.

5. McNeil JJ, Woods RL, Nelson MR, et al. Effect of aspirin on disability-free survival in the healthy elderly. N Engl J Med 2018;379(16):1499–508.

6. McNeil JJ, Wolfe R, Woods RL, et al. Effect of aspirin on cardiovascular events and bleeding in the healthy elderly. N Engl J Med 2018;379(16):1509–18.

7. McNeil JJ, Nelson MR, Woods RL, et al. Effect of aspirin on all-cause mortality in the healthy elderly. N Engl J Med 2018;379(16):1519–28.

8. McNeil JJ, Gibbs P, Orchard SG, et al. Effect of aspirin on cancer incidence and mortality in older adults. J Natl Cancer Inst 2020;113(3):258–65.

9. SPRINT Research Group. A randomized trial of intensive versus standard blood-pressure control. N Engl J Med 2015;373(22):2103–16.

10. Leya M, Stone NJ. Statin prescribing in the elderly: special considerations. Curr Atheroscler Rep 2017;19(11):47.

11. Tchkonia T, Palmer AK, Kirkland JL. New horizons: novel approaches to enhance healthspan through targeting cellular senescence and related aging mechanisms. J Clin Endocrinol Metab 2020;106(3):e1481–7.

12. Barnes LL, Bennett DA. "Alzheimer's disease in African Americans: risk factors and challenges for the future. Health Aff (Millwood) 2014;33(4):580–6.

13. Manly JJ, Jacobs D, Mayeux R. Alzheimer's disease among different ethnic and racial groups. In: Terry RD, Katzman R, Bick KL, et al, editors. Alzheimer's disease. 2. Philadelphia: Lippincott Williams and Wilkins; 1999. p. 117–31.

14. Chui HC, Gatz M. Cultural diversity in Alzheimer disease: the interface between biology, belief, and behavior. Alzheimer Dis Assoc Disord 2005;19(4):250–5.

15. Evans DA, Bennett DA, Wilson RS, et al. Incidence of Alzheimer disease in a biracial urban community: relation to apolipoprotein E allele status. Arch Neurol 2003; 60(2):185–9.

16. Reitz C, Jun G, Naj A, et al. Variants in the ATP-binding cassette transporter (ABCA7), apolipoprotein E e4 and the risk of late-onset Alzheimer disease in African Americans. JAMA 2013;309(14):1483–92.

17. Podcasy JL, Epperson CN. "Considering sex and gender in Alzheimer's disease and other dementias. Dialogues Clin Neurosci 2016;18(4):437–46.

18. Altmann A, Tian L, Henderson VW, et al. Sex modifies the APOE-related risk of developing Alzheimer's disease. Ann Neurol 2014;75(4):563–73.

19. US Preventive Services Task Force. Screening for cognitive impairment in older adults: US Preventive Services Task Force recommendation statement. JAMA 2020;323(8):757–63.

20. SPRINT MIND Investigators for the SPRINT Study Group. Effect of standard vs. intensive blood pressure control on probable dementia. JAMA 2019;521(6):553–61.

21. Koma W, True S, Biniek JF, et al. One in four older adults report anxiety or depression amid the COVID-19 pandemic. KFF; 2020. Available at: https://www.kff.org/medicare/issue-brief/one-in-four-older-adults-report-anxiety-or-depression-amid-the-covid-19-pandemic/. Accessed January 1, 2021.

22. Jacob ME, Yee LM, Diehr PH, et al. Can a healthy lifestyle compress the disabled period in older adults? J Am Geriatr Soc 2016;64(10):1952–61.

23. Pahor M, Guralnik JM, Ambrosius WT, et al. Effect of structured physical activity on prevention of major mobility disability in older adults: the LIFE study randomized clinical trial. JAMA 2014;311(23):2387–96.

24. Sherrington C, Fairhall NJ, Wallbank GK, et al. Exercise for preventing falls in older people living in the community. Cochrane Database Syst Rev 2019;1(1): CD012424.

25. Older adult drivers. Centers for disease control and prevention. 2020. Available at: https://www.cdc.gov/transportationsafety/older_adult_drivers/index.html. Accessed January 1, 2021.

26. Cicchino JB. Why have fatality rates among older drivers declined? The relative contributions of changes in survivability and crash involvement. Accid Anal Prev 2015;83:67–73.

27. Bergen G, West BA, Luo F, et al. How do older adult drivers self-regulate? Characteristics of self-regulation classes defined by latent class analysis. J Saf Res. 2017;61:205–10.

28. Quinn KJ, Shah N. A dataset quantifying polypharmacy in the United States. Sci Data 2017;4:170167.

29. Jirón M, Pate V, Hanson LC, et al. Trends in prevalence and determinants of potentially inappropriate prescribing in the United States: 2007 to 2012. J Am Geriatr Soc 2016;64(4):788–97.

30. Pavlicević I, Kuzmanić M, Rumboldt M, et al. Interaction between antihypertensives and NSAIDs in primary care: a controlled trial. Can J Clin Pharmacol 2008;15(3):e372–82.

31. Avis NE, Crawford SL, Greendale G, et al. Duration of menopausal vasomotor symptoms over the menopause transition. JAMA Int Med 2015;175(4):531–9.

32. Yoon SH, Lee JY, Lee C, et al. Gabapentin for the treatment of hot flushes in menopause: a meta-analysis. Menopause 2020;27(4):485–93.

33. Drewe, J., Bucher, K. A., & Zahner, C. (2015). A systematic review of non-hormonal treatments of vasomotor symptoms in climacteric and cancer patients. SpringerPlus, 4, 65. https://doi.org/10.1186/s40064-015-0808-y.

34. North American Menopause Society. The 2017 hormone therapy position statement of the North American Menopause Society. Menopause 2017;24(7):728–53.

35. National Learning Consortium. Shared decision making: Fact sheet. Health IT.gov. 2013. Available at: https://www.healthit.gov/sites/default/files/nlc_shared_decision_making_fact_sheet.pdf. Accessed January 1, 2021.

36. The consumer benefits of patient shared decision making. In: ALTARUM healthcare value hub research brief 37. 2019. Available at: https://www.healthcarevaluehub.org/advocate-resources/publications/consumer-benefits-patient-shared-decision-making. Accessed January 1, 2021.

37. Reuben DB, Tinetti ME. "Goal-oriented patient care – an alternative health outcomes paradigm. N Engl J Med 2012;366(9):777–9.

38. Tinetti ME, Esterson J, Ferris R, et al. Patient priority-directed decision making and care for older adults with multiple chronic conditions. Clin Geriatr Med 2016;32(2):261–75.

39. Blaum CS, Rosen J, Naik AD, et al. Feasibility of implementing patient priority care for older adults with multiple chronic conditions. J Am Geriatr Soc 2018; 66(10):2009–16.
40. DiGennaro Reed FD, Strouse MC, Jenkins SR, et al. Barriers to independent living for individuals with disabilities and seniors. Behav Anal Pract 2014;7(2):70–7.
41. Koo BM, Vizer LM. Examining mobile technologies to support older adults with dementia through the lens of personhood and human needs: scoping review. JMIR Mhealth and Uhealth 2019;7(11):e15122.
42. Vaportzis E, Clausen MG, Gow AJ. Older adults perceptions of technology and barriers to interacting with tablet computers: a focus group study. Front Psychol 2017;8:687.
43. Anderson M, Perrin A. Tech adoption climbs among older adults. Pew Research Foundation; 2017. Available at: https://www.pewresearch.org/internet/2017/05/17/tech-adoption-climbs-among-older-adults/. Accessed January 1, 2021.
44. Astell AJ, Bouranis N, Hoey J, et al. Technology and dementia: the future is now. Dement Geriatr Cogn Disord 2019;47:131–9.
45. Hartgerink, J. M., Cramm, J. M., Bakker, T. J., van Eijsden, A. M., Mackenbach, J. P., & Nieboer, A. P. (2014). The importance of multidisciplinary teamwork and team climate for relational coordination among teams delivering care to older patients. Journal of advanced nursing, 70(4), 791–799. https://doi.org/10.1111/jan.12233.

The Psychosocial Effects of Frailty on Women

Louisa Whitesides, MD[a],*, Joanne Lynn, MD, MA, MS[b]

KEYWORDS

- Frailty • Psychosocial • Gender differences • Elder orphan • Late life singlehood

KEY POINTS

- Depression, anxiety, lifetime stressors, lack of social support, and loneliness are part of frailty.
- Frailty disproportionately affects women, as they live longer and are less likely to have diseases that lead to abrupt ends.
- Additional lifetime obligations make women more prone to the psychosocial concomitants of frailty.
- Clinicians should recognize the psychological and social elements of frailty as part of the syndrome in women, recognize the signs of prefrailty, and create comprehensive care plans for those becoming frail.

INTRODUCTION

This article highlights the important psychosocial components of frailty, the ways in which they may disproportionately affect older women, and the possible strategies that might reduce the adverse effects. Depression, anxiety, stress, decrease in quality of life, lack of resilience, and lack of social and financial support are all part of frailty. They can predispose individuals to the condition, accelerate its onset, and add to its challenges. Once someone is frail, these psychosocial elements increase vulnerability, and thus increase risk of suffering, hospital admissions, and death. The authors of this article are not exempt, nor are any other women who might live into an old age.

Women's lives follow various courses, but many feature familial caregiver roles that make them more prone to exhaustion, depression, and anxiety. Often alone in their last years, women face declining strength, energy, and capabilities. With limited financial resources, support, and companionship, women must navigate the medical and supportive care systems on their own. Given this common life course, women are at higher risk of developing psychological and social limitations along with and

[a] George Washington University Medical Faculty Associates, 2300 M St. NW, Third floor, Washington, DC 20037, USA; [b] Center for Eldercare Improvement, Altarum, 2000 M St, NW, Suite 400, Washington, DC 20036, USA
* Corresponding author.
E-mail address: lwhitesides@mfa.gwu.edu

Clin Geriatr Med 37 (2021) 543–552
https://doi.org/10.1016/j.cger.2021.05.003
0749-0690/21/© 2021 Elsevier Inc. All rights reserved.

because of frailty. When viewing psychosocial and physical health as parts of a bigger picture, one can better understand why more women are frail and what clinicians can do to mitigate the effects.

DEFINITION: THE CONCEPT OF FRAILTY

As Ko and Park illustrate in their article in this volume, some view frailty as meeting certain phenotypic criteria; others see it as an accumulation of deficits. At the center of both philosophies is the concept of increased vulnerability to adverse outcomes—disability, health care utilization, and death—due to decreased reserve. Frail adults recover more slowly or not at all from physical stresses, such as illness or injury. Their bodily homeostasis is in a precarious balance.[1] All of the definitions point to reduced capability to manage daily needs, and most include sarcopenia and reduced mobility. Regardless of the definition, frailty correlates with advanced years, disabilities, and with dying in old age.

In operationalizing the concept of frailty in research, most investigators focus on the subjects' physical changes or functional decline. Although clinicians can readily document these changes, frailty encompasses more than failing organ systems and thus requires a more integrative approach.[2] Based on literature review and expert opinion, Gobbens and colleagues[3] present a more holistic model of the condition. This model incorporates relationships and psychological well-being. Including these elements in the concept of frailty may enable diagnosing and treating affected individuals in newly targeted and effective ways.[3]

CURRENT EVIDENCE: THE PSYCHOSOCIAL ELEMENTS ASSOCIATED WITH FRAILTY

Psychological and social health play roles in the aging process. Some seem to protect against the development of frailty. Others seem to go hand in hand with frailty and may come to be considered as part of the condition. The causal relationship among frailty, declining health, and mood is not entirely clear. Most studies simply show correlations between a definition of frailty and another defined condition, such as depression, disability, or weight loss. These correlations are important, but they leave considerable uncertainty as to whether 1 condition causes or precedes the other. Rigorous intervention studies should yield understanding as to what elements can be mitigated in order to improve the experience of patients. For example, patients with positive attitudes are likely to be healthy, mobile, and robust, while patients with negative attitudes may be more likely to be ill, immobile, and frail. But whether one's attitude is a cause, or an effect, is unclear. In becoming frail, an individual could lose her confidence and command and adopt a destructive attitude. Alternatively, a person with a negative outlook could forgo exercise and nutrition and lack a sense of purpose and thereby more readily develop the signs of frailty.

Researchers have tested the correlation of frailty and positive features of psychological health, including emotional vitality, sense of meaning or purpose, and perceived quality of life, and some may have protective effects. An observational analysis saw that emotional vitality correlated with a slower decline among disabled older women.[4] Another showed that greater purpose was positively associated with psychological well-being and reported good health.[5] Layte and colleagues[6] demonstrated in their Irish cohort study that quality of life can increase with age, as long as the person continues to have reasonable health, strong relationships, and social interaction. In this study, even as people developed physical disabilities, their quality of life remained high.

Frailty correlates with depression, although which comes first is difficult to determine. For example, many frail individuals lack energy (as part of the Fried definition of the syndrome), which is also a common feature of depression. Multiple studies have shown that depressed older adults who are not yet frail, whether on antidepressants or not, are at higher risk of developing prefrailty or frailty.[7] This observation makes it plausible that depression could be a cause of frailty; however, they both could arise from the same source, and depression simply be the earlier manifestation.

Fillit and Butler coined the term "frailty identity crisis" in 2009 to describe the maladaptive psychological processes that can occur in older adults and caregivers as an individual moves from fitness to frailty. This transition can be a period of great vulnerability. A person becoming more frail can take an adaptive and accepting approach, which could be termed responsible dependency. Others, in contrast, develop feelings of denial, anger, and depression. This latter coping mechanism can lead to a miserable existence and increased medical costs because of frequent admissions and polypharmacy as elders seek treatments for their accumulating ailments.[8,9]

Social health also correlates with frailty in similar ways. Simply having social relationships correlates with lower risk of mortality in older adults.[10] Connections to others provide a sense of purpose, as described previously, and a means of obtaining supportive services when needed (ie, potential caregivers or advocates). On the other hand, individuals who feel lonely have a 1.85 times higher risk of becoming frail.[11] In fact, loneliness and social isolation are correlated with various comorbidities, including sleep problems, poor cardiovascular health, depression, and cognitive decline.[12(p133)]

Sociodemographic factors may play a role in the development of the frailty syndrome. Older individuals with lower income are more likely to develop frailty,[13] as are those with lower education levels.[14–16] Others have shown that specific medical diagnoses related to lower socioeconomic status, such as obesity and diabetes, go hand in hand with frailty.[17] One study suggests that neighborhoods with homogenous groups of people have fewer frail residents,[18] perhaps because of more available neighborly supports. All of these associations speak to the relationship between frailty and social determinants of health.[19] These findings illustrate how the environment in which one lives can strongly affect the timing and course of functional decline.

CONCERNS: THE PSYCHOSOCIAL EFFECTS ON WOMEN

More women become frail than men, and these psychosocial variables likely play a large role in the development of frailty.[1,20] First and foremost, women live longer than men, for various reasons.[21] Many women escape the fatal conditions, like myocardial infarctions or accidental injuries, that kill men, and instead live into advanced age with arthritis, sarcopenia, and cognitive decline that, together, add up to frailty.[22] With living longer comes a host of social obligations and transitions, including caregiving for spouses or loved ones, death of family members and friends, singlehood, and isolation. Support systems may break down with these life changes and leave women with depleted financial resources and a tattered psyche. Thus, many women find themselves alone, poor, and depressed toward the end of their lives, and especially vulnerable to frailty.

Before the onset of frailty, many women serve as caregiver to one or more family members—a role that is, both stressful and rewarding. The most recent AARP (American Association of Retired Persons) caregiver report estimates that 3 in every 5 women take on caregiving to an adult at some point. Although caregivers often report that their role gives them a sense of meaning or purpose, many also must cope with emotional, financial, and physical stresses.[23] Interestingly, research suggests that male caregivers find more purpose when serving in this role.[24] Some postulate that the task-oriented nature of caregiving is more appealing to men. As well, most men do not perform household tasks in earlier years of life, so it is possible that they find the novelty of this work more invigorating.[12(p144)] Regardless, women are more likely to perform this largely thankless, time-consuming role as a volunteer caregiver.

On top of these emotional burdens, women suffer financial hardships by taking on caregiving. Currently, 1 in 4 caregivers reports that it is extremely to moderately difficult to access affordable community services such as meals, transportation, and in-home aides and request financial help for their care recipient.[23] As well, 62% of caregivers report needing more education and/or training in caring for their recipient and themselves.[23] Because few services support them, caregivers frequently need to work outside of the home in order to make ends meet. At the same time, caregivers cannot put in the hours necessary at work because of their duties at home. As hourly wage earners, these realities mean lower income and job insecurity. Although income falls, household expenses increase because of the needs of the disabled care recipient. Any saved money—often meant for the caregiver's retirement security—may be spent. One AARP study quotes nearly $300,000 lost in retirement savings and income for a full-time family caregiver.[25] The care recipient's death is the end to a social partnership and brings with it a series of financial losses for the surviving partner. Aside from the $300,000 lost to the caregiver, whatever retirement benefits that came into the household from the aged spouse cease. At this point, women not only suffer the psychological distress of losing a loved one and being alone, but also the drastic loss of income.[12]

Finally, the caregiving role can be physically demanding. As frail family members decline, they may require assistance in activities of daily living, such as bathing, toileting, and transferring. Caregivers risk injury by helping a frail family member with these tasks.[23] The physical aspects of caregiving are often particularly difficult for women. First, women, especially aging women, have less muscle strength than men, thus making heavy lifting more challenging. Second, women are more prone to musculoskeletal diseases such as arthritis. Stiff joints make it harder to lift, twist, and maneuver disabled family members.[12(p143)]

These strains can take their toll on the caregiver. According to the AARP, 1 in 4 caregivers report either that they were unable to care for themselves or that their own health got worse when they cared for their family member.[23] Many may also turn to destructive habits, such as smoking, alcohol, or comfort food, in order to cope with ongoing stress[12] Spousal caregivers who are themselves considered prefrail are at high risk of decline into frailty.[26] In the process of providing this service, women face worsening emotional, financial, and physical health, only to be left alone after caregiving ends.

The transition to solitude—often called late life singlehood—can be a particularly vulnerable time. The bereft former caregiver mourns the loss of loved ones without contemporaries to turn to, since the former caregiver may be the last surviving member of her cohort, and caregiving itself may well have created severe isolation. Women who care for a spouse until the spouse dies are particularly exposed to accumulating ailments of their own for several reasons (eg, because they neglected their own health, and because they deeply appreciated the companionship of their spouse). In comparison, lifelong single women actually fare quite well in later life.[12] Those women who do have other relationships to bolster them fare better at this transition, as would be expected.[27] Although some women are able to experience mental, spiritual, and emotional growth during late life singlehood, others may develop depression, alcohol abuse, and further decline in health.[28]

Many women in late life singlehood find themselves without an identifiable volunteer caregiver, and often not even a family member or friend to help make decisions and manage affairs. These un-befriended elders face difficulties in coordinating medical care and in assuring supportive services. Some predict that as many as 1 in 4 baby boomers will become elder orphans, without a family member to care for them as they age.[29] Women in these situations are more likely to end up in a nursing home, rather than cared for in their own homes. The impoverishment associated with caregiving and widowhood makes many women unable to pay for the services needed to live comfortably.[30] Women find ourselves in situations where they must rely on public services such as Medicaid nursing homes, where they cannot maintain our desired sense of self-respect and control over the course of their lives.

The world does not look kindly on aging women either. Media have long portrayed older women in a negative light. From the age of 35, women are perceived as past their prime. Younger women dread wrinkles and gray hair. Media are in part to blame for these stigmas placed on women. Aging women are frequently not included on prime-time television,[31] although this situation now may be better than previous generations. Ageism is instilled in children at a young age as well. Even old female Disney characters are witch-like or wicked.[32] Rather than recognizing and understanding older women's possibilities and needs, women's frailty becomes grotesque to most of the population.

When women reach the end of life, they often have no one to advocate for their existence. By that point, women no longer have substantial responsibilities to families and careers; they often have lost their financial resources, and they have lost at least some physical abilities. Women may have been living alone in a nursing home slowly declining for some time before coming to the end of life. The SUPPORT study aptly illustrates this lack of advocacy among aging men versus women. In this study, older women did not receive the same vigor in medical treatments, such as dialysis and mechanical ventilation, toward the end of life as their male counterparts.[33–35] This split shows the differences in the way men and women are generally perceived at the end of their lives. Although men remain important—because they have financial assets and family members advocating for them—women often become obsolete.

FUTURE DIRECTIONS

This outline provides a bleak picture of the way women decline toward the end of life. Women live longer, and their lifetime stressors and social situation as death approaches make them particularly prone to depression, loneliness, isolation, poverty, and, in turn, frailty. As a consequence, many women will live their last days confined to a mediocre nursing home and die without a fight. At the same time, this picture is full of opportunity for improvement. The authors call on all clinicians for wide-ranging reform in order to reduce the incidence and impact of frailty and thereby improve the lives of aging women.

First, all clinicians must be able to address women's mental health concerns appropriately. Prior to old age, women experience large amounts of stress to care for families, then must cope with the transition to solitude. These life events make women particularly susceptible to depression and anxiety. Multiple articles highlight the fact that women's life events and societal opinions of aged women leave them vulnerable to severe mental health conditions.[36,37] Psychiatric conditions like depression, anxiety, substance use, and compulsions are not part of normal aging. As well, cognitive decline may act as a guise for some of these underlying psychiatric issues. Taking dementia at face value is not enough.[38] In fact, distinguishing between dementia, delirium, and depression can be important, although challenging.

To date, however, few steps have been taken to recognize, appreciate, and treat these frequently debilitating mental health conditions in older women. Budding physicians must be educated in geriatric care, since, regardless of the field they choose, the care of older adults will likely be a part of it. Current internal medicine residents now must receive just 4 weeks of geriatric training, a recent increase from 2 as of last year.[39] This lack of training is clearly evident when one looks at the trends of psychiatric medication prescribing in frail elders. The table, courtesy of Nils Franco at Altarum using data from CareJourney, illustrates the ranges of some critical outcomes that affect the care of dependent older adults in 721 large US counties. According to these data, on average, 17% of these elders were using benzodiazepines, and 10% were on psychotropic medications, both of which should be prescribed rarely (**Table 1**). Clinicians should come to know the performance of their local eldercare system and act to improve shortcomings.

Second, clinicians must be able to identify the signs of prefrailty. Physicians should be counseling explicitly and specifically on exercise, social support, and sleep, and recognizing women's life stressors prior to old age. One place to start is to screen for caregiving, a major emotional, financial, and physical stressor that many women experience. Currently, caregivers are not receiving the financial or educational resources they need to carry out their role successfully. Clinicians can help by attempting to make caregivers lives easier in simple ways. Clinicians should know community resources—social workers, pastors, assisted transportation and meal delivery services-and be able to connect patients with needed services. Clinicians should find places to clearly list caregivers' names in the electronic medical record system. Clinicians should make caregivers visible by stressing the value of their involvement to fellow clinicians.

Clinicians can also advocate on the policy level. Although increasing the wages of aides would be a simple fix, families or organizations—like Medicare or Medicaid—would need to pay these wages, and both parties are already under financial constraints.[40] Clinicians must first ask why Medicare does not have the dollars to assist with this crucial piece to health care for older adults. Although Medicare spends

---

Table 1
The range of eldercare performance by counties in the United States for Medicare beneficiaries with Parts A and B and evidence of having 2 or more activities of daily living dependencies on an OASIS (home care) or MDS (nursing home care) assessment in 2018, for counties with greater than 1000 such patients (N = 721 counties)

The Performance Issue	The Performance Range	The Mean
Proportion using benzodiazepines	4.2%–39.3%	17.6%
Proportion using psychotropics	4.6%–32.3%	9.9%
Proportion having stage 3–4 or unstageable pressure ulcers	1.7%–13.8%	5.6%
Proportion spending down into Medicaid in the year	1.4%–32.3%	8.7%
Cost to Medicare, per person per month	$2012-$5165	$3294
Cost to Medicare in last month of life, per person	$8567-$34,135	$15,715

Data provided by Nils Franco and CareJourney, 12/13/2020.

millions of dollars a year for patients to receive advanced cancer therapies, it does not subsidize in-home supportive services.[41]

Dollars aside, one should also think about ways to come up with more creative solutions to address future caregiving needs. Japan, for example, has taken a total community approach to care of dementia patients, largely based on volunteers to assist with behavioral disturbances related to dementia.[42] Others look into use of technology, like robots, to assist with caregiving; however, at this point, it is unclear whether technology will be available only to those with economic means. Although interesting, these solutions are limited in scope. Reducing the burden of caregiving will require a multipronged approach that addresses the health of the caregiver and the needs of the recipient.[43]

Third, clinicians should develop comprehensive care plans with their aging female patients to ensure that women are able to live and socialize in the ways they choose. These care plans should include preferences on where women would like to live, how they would like to live, and where and how they would like to die. If a woman would like to age in place, clinicians should be able to assist her in carrying out this plan. Senior services and centers should be available to all those in need of them[44] and more widespread through diverse sociodemographic areas. As well, if a woman needs medical care in the home, clinicians should direct her to home-based practices in the area.[45]

As women move farther into activities of daily living (ADL) dependency, clinicians also need to understand how to care for these patients in more effective ways, preferably in the home or assisted living. Currently, frail elders often receive care that does not address their needs, but which have high costs. As illustrated in CareJourney's data set, Medicare patients (both men and women) who are dependent in 2 or more ADLS as reported through MDS and OASIS are not getting the care they need, and, despite this, are under financial constraints. Far too many develop deep pressure ulcers, a largely avoidable and terribly onerous experience. Up to 8.7% spend down to Medicaid within the first year of being ADL dependent. Despite this, they are spending, on average $3294 Medicare dollars per month (see **Table 1**). The authors contend that this money is often not being spent in ways that align with the preferences and maximum well-being of the patients.

Comprehensive care plans may address some of the more important aspects of care for any given woman while decreasing the amount of unnecessary spending. Although the term often connotes advanced care planning—often associated with DNR (do not resuscitate)/DNI orders and goals of care—a comprehensive plan should encompass so much more. Clinicians should know what women would want toward the end of life.[46] Women should be clear about what matters most (eg, for example, what foods they would want to eat or what music they would like to hear).

Finally, clinicians should be strong participants in changing the views of aging women on a societal level. Ageism leads to women's marginalization in society. Women's own social views push them to the outskirts of society toward the end of life. Older women are doomed to become supernumerary beings if society continues to value youth and conventional productivity to its current degree. In all facets of life, aging has become undesirable. In the same way women speak out against discrimination in the workforce, they must speak out against discrimination in old age.

SUMMARY

In summary, clinicians should recognize the psychological and social elements of frailty as part of the syndrome. Depression, anxiety, lifetime stressors, lack of social support, and loneliness likely all play roles in its development. Frailty disproportionately affects women, as they live longer and are less likely to have diseases that lead to abrupt ends. Their additional lifetime obligations make them more prone to the psychosocial conditions of frailty. Women too often spend their last days alone, disabled and financially drained, with little physical or emotional support. Clinicians should appreciate this phenomenon and provide resources to women in order to enhance the experience of old age. Clinicians should educate themselves about geriatric syndromes in order to understand the differences between depression, delirium, and dementia; aggressively treat prefrailty and screen for caregiving; create comprehensive care plans for their frail elders so that, despite disability, their preferences are met; and advocate for these patients on a societal level. By changing clinicians' opinions of aged women, women's lives in the last part of life can be so much better.

CLINICS CARE POINTS

- Depression, anxiety, lifetime stressors, lack of social support, and loneliness are part of frailty.
- Frailty disproportionately affects women, as they live longer and are less likely to have diseases that lead to abrupt ends.
- Additional lifetime obligations make women more prone to the psychosocial concomitants of frailty.
- Clinicians should recognize the psychological and social elements of frailty as part of the syndrome in women, recognize the signs of prefrailty, and create comprehensive care plans for those becoming frail.

DISCLOSURE

The authors have nothing to disclose.

REFERENCES

1. Albert SM. The dynamics of frailty among older adults. JAMA Netw Open 2019; 2(8):e198438.
2. Bergman H, Ferrucci L, Guralnik J, et al. Frailty: an emerging research and clinical paradigm—issues and controversies. J Gerontol A Biol Sci Med Sci 2007; 62(7):731–7.
3. Gobbens RJJ, Luijkx KG, Wijnen-Sponselee MT, et al. Towards an integral conceptual model of frailty. J Nutr Health Aging 2010;14(3):175–81.
4. Penninx BW, Guralnik JM, Bandeen-Roche K, et al. The protective effect of emotional vitality on adverse health outcomes in disabled older women. J Am Geriatr Soc 2000;48(11):1359–66.
5. Irving JD, Davis S, Collier A. Aging with purpose: systematic search and review of literature pertaining to older adults and purpose. Int J Aging Hum Dev 2017; 85(4):403–37.
6. Layte R, Sexton E, Savva G. Quality of life in older age: evidence from an Irish cohort study. J Am Geriatr Soc 2013;61:S299–305.
7. Buigues C, Padilla-Sanchez C, Fernandez Garrido J, et al. The relationship between depression and frailty syndrome: a systematic review. Aging Ment Health 2015;19(9):762–72.
8. Fillit H, Butler RN. The frailty identity crisis. J Am Geriatr Soc 2009;57(2):348–52.

9. Andrew MK, Fisk JD, Rockwood K. Psychological well-being in relation to frailty: a frailty identity crisis? Int Psychogeriatrics 2012;24(8):1347–53.
10. Holt-Lunstad J, Smith TB, Layton JB. Social relationships and mortality risk: a meta-analytic review. PLoS Med 2010;7(7):e1000316.
11. Gale CR, Westbury L, Cooper C. Social isolation and loneliness as risk factors for the progression of frailty: the English Longitudinal Study of Ageing. Age and Ageing 2018;47(3):392–7.
12. Carr D. Golden years?: social inequality in later life. New York: Russell Sage Foundation; 2018.
13. Myers V, Drory Y, Goldbourt U, et al. Multilevel socioeconomic status and incidence of frailty post myocardial infarction. Int J Cardiol 2014;170(3):338–43.
14. Etman A, Kamphuis CBM, Van Der Cammen TJM, et al. Do lifestyle, health and social participation mediate educational inequalities in frailty worsening? Eur J Public Health 2015;25(2):345–50.
15. Hoogendijk EO, van Hout HP, Heymans MW, et al. Explaining the association between educational level and frailty in older adults: results from a 13-year longitudinal study in The Netherlands. Ann Epidemiol 2014;24(7):538–44.e2.
16. Feng Z, Lugtenberg M, Franse C, et al. Risk factors and protective factors associated with incident or increase of frailty among community-dwelling older adults: a systematic review of longitudinal studies. PLoS One 2017;12(6):e0178383.
17. Fugate Woods N, Lacroix AZ, Gray SL, et al. Frailty: emergence and consequences in women aged 65 and older in the women's health initiative observational study. J Am Geriatr Soc 2005;53(8):1321–30.
18. Aranda MP, Ray LA, Snih SA, et al. The protective effect of neighborhood composition on increasing frailty among older Mexican Americans. J Aging Health 2011;23(7):1189–217.
19. De Labra C, Maseda A, Lorenzo-López L, et al. Social factors and quality of life aspects on frailty syndrome in community-dwelling older adults: the VERISAÚDE study. BMC Geriatr 2018;18(1):66.
20. Ofori-Asenso R, Chin KL, Mazidi M, et al. Global incidence of frailty and prefrailty among community-dwelling older adults. JAMA Netw Open 2019;2(8):e198398.
21. Collard RM, Boter H, Schoevers RA, et al. Prevalence of frailty in community-dwelling older persons: a systematic review. J Am Geriatr Soc 2012;60(8):1487–92.
22. Mauvais-Jarvis F, Bairey Merz N, Barnes PJ, et al. Sex and gender: modifiers of health, disease, and medicine. Lancet 2020;396(10250):565–82.
23. 2020 report. Caregiving in the US. NAC and AARP. Available at: https://www.aarp.org/content/dam/aarp/ppi/2020/05/full-report-caregiving-in-the-united-states. Accessed December 1, 2020.
24. Lin IF, Fee HR, Wu H-S. Negative and positive caregiving experiences: a closer look at the intersection of gender and relationship. Fam Relations 2012;61(2):343–58.
25. The Metlife study of caregiving costs to working caregivers: double jeopardy for baby boomers caring for their patients. Metlife Mature Market Institute; 2011. Available at: https://www.caregiving.org/wp-content/uploads/2011/06/mmi-caregiving-costs-working-caregivers.pdf. Accessed December 1, 2020.
26. Potier F, Degryse J-M, Bihin B, et al. Health and frailty among older spousal caregivers: an observational cohort study in Belgium. BMC Geriatr 2018;18(1):291.
27. Kinsel B. Resilience as adaptation in older women. J Women Aging 2005;17(3):23–39.
28. Bogunovic O. Women and aging. Harv Rev Psychiatry 2011;19(6):321–4.

29. Carney MT, Fujiwara J, Emmert BE, et al. Elder orphans hiding in plain sight: a growing vulnerable population. Curr Gerontol Geriatr Res 2016;2016:1–11.
30. Houser A. Women and long-term care. AARP Public Policy Institute. Fact Sheet Web site. 2007. Accessed December 21, 2020. Available at: https://www.aarp.org/content/dam/aarp/ppi/2017-01/women-and-long-term-services-and-supports.pdf.
31. Vernon JA, Phillips T, Wilson J. Media stereotyping: a comparison of the way elderly women and men are portrayed on prime-time television. J Women Aging 1990;2(4):54–68.
32. Robinson TCM, Magoffin D, Moore J. The portrayal of older characters in Disney animated films. J Aging Stud 2007;21:203–13.
33. Bird CE, Shugarman LR, Lynn J. Age and gender differences in health care utilization and spending for Medicare beneficiaries in their last years of life. J Palliat Med 2002;5(5):705–12.
34. Shugarman LR, Bird CE, Schuster CR, et al. Age and gender differences in Medicare expenditures and service utilization at the end of life for lung cancer decedents. Womens Health Issues 2008;18(3):199–209.
35. Shugarman LR, Bird CE, Schuster CR, et al. Age and gender differences in Medicare expenditures at the end of life for colorectal cancer decedents. J Womens Health (Larchmt) 2007;16(2):214–27.
36. Weissman J, Levine SR. Anxiety disorders and older women. J Women Aging 2007;19(1–2):79–101.
37. Goldstein RD, Gruenberg AM. Major depressive disorder in the older adult: implications for women. J Women Aging 2007;19(1–2):63–77.
38. Rodeheaver D, Datan N. The challenge of double jeopardy. Toward a mental health agenda for aging women. Am Psychol 1988;43(8):648–54.
39. ACGME Program Requirements for Graduate Medical Education in Internal Medicine. 2020 Accreditation Council for graduate medical education (ACGME) 2020. Available at: https://acgme.org/Portals/0/PFAssets/ProgramRequirements/140_InternalMedicine_2020.pdf?ver=2020-06-29-161610-040. Accessed December 21, 2020.
40. Weller CAB, Cohen M, Stone R. Making care work pay: how paying at least a living wage to direct care workers could benefit care recipients, workers, and communities. Leading age LTSS Center; 2020. Available at: https://www.ltsscenter.org/wp-content/uploads/2020/09/Making-Care-Work-Pay-Report-FINAL.pdf. Accessed December 21, 2020.
41. Medicare.gov: the official US government site for Medicare. 2020. Available at: medicare.gov; https://www.medicare.gov/coverage. Accessed December 21, 2020.
42. McCurry J. "Dementia towns": how Japan is evolving for its ageing population. London: The Guardian; 2018.
43. Smith A, Anderson M. Automation in everyday life. Washington DC: Pew Research Center; 2017.
44. Kadowaki L, Mahmood A. Senior centres in Canada and the United States: a scoping review. Can J Aging 2018;37(4):420–41.
45. Rotenberg J, Kinosian B, Boling P, et al. Home-based primary care: beyond extension of the independence at home demonstration. J Am Geriatr Soc 2018;66(4):812–7.
46. Tip sheet: the 5Ms of geriatrics. 2020. Available at: healthinaging.org; https://www.healthinaging.org/tools-and-tips/tip-sheet-5ms-geriatrics. Accessed December 21, 2020.

Sexual Health

Catherine G. Hoeppner, MD, MS*, Sarah T. Cigna, MD, MS,
Jenna Perkins, MSN, WHNP-BC, Nancy D. Gaba, MD

KEYWORDS

- Sexual health • Menopause • Couplepause • Dyspareunia

KEY POINTS

- Sexual health is an important measure of quality of life in the geriatric population.
- Although many symptoms of sexual dysfunction can be tied to changes in hormones, others are related to comorbid medical conditions and partner-related issues.
- There are a variety of safe and effective treatments for sexual concerns in older adults.

BACKGROUND

Women's sexual health is a frequently ignored area of geriatric medicine, encompassing desire, arousal, lubrication, orgasm, and pain.[1] Most patients are willing to discuss sexual health concerns if providers initiate the conversation[2,3]; however, many older adults feel that providers are not forthcoming with information.[4] Female sexual health and function is multifactorial, and physiologic and psychosocial influences must be considered when providing comprehensive care.

It is difficult to know the true prevalence of female sexual dysfunction (FSD) given the variations in classification and changes in diagnostic criteria.[1] As women age, sexual problems increase; however, distress decreases, making the prevalence of FSD stable over the life span.[2] Sexual dysfunction is characterized into desire, arousal, orgasm, and pain. Historically, sexual dysfunction was attributed to the psychological realm. For this reason, many health care practitioners were, and continue to be, guided by the *Diagnostic and Statistical Manual of Mental Health Disorders* (DSM). In the fifth edition of the DSM (DSM-V), 3 categories of FSD are described: female sexual interest and arousal disorder, female orgasm disorder, and genitopelvic pain or penetration disorder. The classification by the International Society for the Study of Women's Sexual Health is preferred because it allows for a more precise diagnosis and addresses areas omitted by DSM-V.[1] The DSM-V diagnostic criteria are viewed as more stringent among sexual health experts.[1] **Table 1** outlines the

The George Washington University School of Medicine and Health Sciences, 2150 Pennsylvania Avenue Northwest, Suite 6A-427, Washington, DC 20037, USA
* Corresponding author.
E-mail address: cghoeppner@gmail.com

Clin Geriatr Med 37 (2021) 553–577
https://doi.org/10.1016/j.cger.2021.05.004
0749-0690/21/© 2021 Elsevier Inc. All rights reserved.

Table 1
DSM-V versus International Society for the Study of Women's Sexual Health nomenclature

Nomenclature	Definition (Present for ≥6 mo and causes significant distress)	Considerations in the Elderly
DSM-V		
Female sexual interest and arousal disorder (FSIAD)	Lack of, or significantly decreased, sexual interest/arousal, as manifested by at least 3 of the following: 1. Absent/decreased interest in sexual activity. 2. Absent/decreased sexual/erotic thoughts or fantasies. 3. No/decreased initiation of sexual activity, and typically unreceptive to a partner's attempts to initiate. 4. Absent/decreased sexual excitement/ pleasure during sexual activity in almost all or all (approximately 75%–100%) sexual encounters (in identified situational contexts or, if generalized, in all contexts). 5. Absent/decreased sexual interest/ arousal in response to any internal or external sexual/erotic cues (eg, written, verbal, visual). 6. Absent/decreased genital or nongenital sensations during sexual activity in almost all or all (approximately 75%–100%) sexual encounters (in identified situational contexts or, if generalized, in all contexts).	There is a natural decrease in vaginal dryness depending on a woman's age and menopausal status Polypharmacy in the elderly may explain lack of sexual desire or arousal Another medical condition in the elderly (ie, diabetes, arthritis) may better explain the sexual dysfunction
Female orgasm disorder	Presence of one of the following in almost all or all (approximately 75%–100%) occasions of sexual activity: 1. Marked delay in, marked frequency of or absence of orgasm 2. Markedly decreased intensity of orgasm in	Menopausal status is inconsistently linked to orgasm dysfunction More likely in women with vulvovaginal atrophy
Genitopelvic pain or penetration disorder	Persistent or recurrent difficulties with one (or more) of the following: 1. Vaginal penetration during intercourse. 2. Marked vulvovaginal or pelvic pain during vaginal intercourse or penetration attempts. 3. Marked fear or anxiety about vulvovaginal or pelvic pain in anticipation of, during, or as a result of vaginal penetration. 4. Marked tensing or tightening of the pelvic floor muscles during attempted vaginal penetration.	Seen in women with lichen sclerosis or vulvovaginal atrophy Consider difficulties with male partner as well, such as erectile dysfunction

Nomenclature	Definition (Present for $\geq$6 mo)	Considerations in Elderly
International Society for the Study of Women's Sexual Health		

Hypoactive sexual desire disorder	Manifests as any of the following:
	1. Lack of motivation for sexual activity by
	  a. Decreased or absent spontaneous desire (sexual thoughts/fantasies)
	  b. Decreased or absent desire to erotic cues or stimulation or inability to maintain desire or interest
	2. Loss of desire to initiate or participate in sexual activity, including behavioral responses such as avoidance of sexual activity, that is, not secondary to sexual pain disorders and is combined with clinically significant personal distress that includes frustration, grief, incompetence, loss, sadness, sorrow, or worry
		Vasomotor symptoms of menopause may interfere with desire
		Pain arising from genitourinary syndrome of menopause or pelvic floor dysfunction may inhibit desire
		Depression can affect sexual desire and vice versa
		Drugs that act on the serotonergic, dopaminergic, and prolactin systems may affect desire

Female genital arousal disorder	Inability to develop or maintain adequate genital response, including: 1. Vulvovaginal lubrication 2. Engorgement of genitalia 3. Sensitivity of genitalia	Chronic medical problems such as cardiovascular disease, diabetes, hypertension, are risk factors for arousal disorder Substance use disorder may affect arousal Patients with previous pelvic surgery may have mixed effects on arousal
Female orgasm disorder	Persistent or recurrent distressing compromise of orgasm 1. Frequency – orgasm is decreased frequency or absent 2. Intensity – orgasm occurs with less intensity 3. Timing – orgasm occurs too soon or too late 4. Pleasure – orgasm occurs with decreased or absent pleasure	As above
Genitopelvic pain penetration disorder	Persistent or recurrent difficulties with 1. Vaginal penetration during intercourse 2. Significant vulvovaginal or pelvic pain during genital contact 3. Significant fear or anxiety about vulvovaginal or pelvic pain	As above in genitopelvic pain or penetration disorder

(continued on next page)

Table 1 (continued)	
	in anticipation of, during, or as a result of genital contact 4. Marked hypertonicity or overactivity of pelvic floor muscles with or without genital contact
Persistent genital arousal disorder	Persistent or recurrent, unwanted or intrusive feelings of genital arousal or on the verge or orgasm not associated with sexual interest, thoughts, or fantasies
Female orgasmic illness syndrome	Characterized by peripheral and/or central aversive symptoms that occur before, during, or after orgasm not related to a compromise or orgasm quality

Data from Refs.[1,2,5]

nomenclature for the DSM-V and International Society for the Study of Women's Sexual Health, which can be applied to the geriatric population with special considerations.[1,2,5]

As women age, sexual activity decreases. In women aged 65 to 74 years, 40% report being sexually active compared with 20% of women aged 75 to 85 years.[3] Normal, expected changes occur as women age. The most common symptoms after menopause include decreased libido, sexual pain (dyspareunia), and decreased lubrication.[3,6] Studies suggest the main predictors of sexual satisfaction in elderly women include a partner and good functional and mental status.[7] Despite the decreasing frequency of sexual activity with age, the majority of women report that it is important to them.[3,4]

Health care providers must screen for sexual dysfunction. Concerns may be unaddressed owing to a patient's hesitancy, shame, and/or the provider's lack of training or confidence.[3,4] Providers should create a comfortable setting and develop patient rapport. Normalizing the topic of sexual function in the elderly population is crucial. Using open-ended questions invites the patient to discuss concerns. The PLISSIT approach can be implemented by asking permission to discuss sexual activity, providing limited information about basic anatomy and function, giving specific suggestions and offering intensive therapy with a specialist.[1] **Box 1** outlines the PLISSIT model and offers examples of questions or phrases.[1,8,9]

Various screening tools are available to identify patients with sexual dysfunction. The Female Sexual Function Index is a validated 19-item questionnaire to screen for sexual function in females aged 21 to 69 years.[10] The Female Sexual Function Index specifically addresses symptoms over the last 4 weeks and assesses arousal, desire, orgasm, and pain. The patient can complete the questionnaire privately, which can be easily accessed online here (https://www.fsfiquestionnaire.com/). The Decreased Sexual Desire Screening (DSDS) is a validated, 5-item questionnaire used to identify hypoactive sexual desire disorder.[11] Although the DSDS was validated in women up to age 50 in long-term heterosexual relationships, it can be used for older women (**Box 2**).[11]

Box 1
Permission, Limited Information, Specific Suggestions, Intensive Therapy (PLISST) model for addressing sexual health concerns

PLISST	Notes
P	Permission
	Many of my patients express concerns with their sexual health; would it be Okay to as you some questions about your sexual health?
	Sexual concerns are common; are there sexual concerns you wish to discuss?
LI	Limited Information
	Provide information on basic genital anatomy
	Described age related changes
SS	Specific Suggestions
	How women with (ie, diabetes, cardiovascular disease) handle changes in sexual feelings and function
	Consider changing medication (ie, selective serotonin reuptake inhibitor), if appropriate
IT	Intensive Therapy
	Refer to appropriate specialty
	For example, a neurologist, sexual health specialist, pelvic floor physical floor therapist

Data from Refs.[1,8,9]

Box 2
DSDS

Question

1. In the past, was your level of sexual desire or interest good and satisfying you?   Yes   No
2. Has there been a decrease in your level of sexual desire or interest?   Yes   No
3. Are you bothered by your decreased level of sexual desire or interest?   Yes   No
4. Would you like your level of sexual desire or interest to increase?   Yes   No
5. Please circle all of the factors that you feel may be contributing to your current decrease in sexual desire or interest:
    a. An operation, depression, injuries, or other medical condition
    b. Medications, drugs, or alcohol you are currently taking
    c. Pregnancy, recent childbirth, menopausal symptoms
    d. Other sexual issues you may be having (pain, decreased arousal or orgasm)
    e. Your partner's sexual problems
    f. Dissatisfaction with your relationship or partner
    g. Stress or fatigue

If the patient answers "yes" to questions 1–4, the diagnosis of acquired hypoactive sexual dysfunction disorder may be met.

Adapted from Clayton AH, Goldfischer ER, Goldstein I, Derogatis L, Lewis- D'Agostino DJ, Pyke R. Validation of the Decreased Sexual Desire Screener (DSDS): a brief diagnostic instrument for generalized acquired female hypoactive sexual desire disorder (HSDD). J Sex Med. 2009;6(3):730-738; with permission.

When considering sexual dysfunction, it is critical to obtain a full medical, psychiatric, and medication history. Some information in the history may indicate factors that may be modifiable or reversible. Common medical conditions may affect the sexual response, including cardiovascular disease (CVD), diabetes, and neurologic disorders. Previous gynecologic surgeries (hysterectomy) or radiation therapy may affect the sexual response. **Box 3**[1,3,12] summarizes the relevant components of a patient's history.

There is limited literature to adequately represent the diversity of the patient population. Unfortunately, research regarding sexual health in the elderly is limited to cisgender females in heterosexual relationships with cisgender males. There is a paucity of data for sexual health in lesbian, bisexual, and transgender elderly patients. Regardless of race, gender, sexual orientation, or marital status, health care providers should individualize their evaluation and management to focus on the patient's goals.

VULVOVAGINAL HEALTH AND ANATOMY
Vulvovaginal Health

The personal hygiene industry provides misleading information regarding the maintenance of healthy genitalia. Expensive, scented, and sometimes irritating products are promoted by pharmacies. Magazines and social media suggest the female genitalia must be "managed" to be healthy and satisfy sexual partners. Preservatives, such as parabens, are extremely common in these products and can cause vaginitis or vulvar symptoms. The vulva and vagina do not require scents or chemical products. **Table 2** includes a list of "do's" and "don'ts" of vulvovaginal hygiene that can be provided to patients. Understanding what disrupts the normal flora of the vulva and vagina is helpful in preventing vulvovaginitis syndromes owing to irritants. Cotton materials (underwear, panty liners) and topical products (lotions, soaps, creams) without synthetic plastics or preservatives will decrease the risk of developing reactions. Douching is unnecessary for routine care and is almost never recommended as a treatment because it can make symptoms worse.[13]

Box 3
Medical history associated with sexual dysfunction

Medical and psychiatric conditions
  Cardiovascular disease
  Diabetes
  Emphysema
  Neurologic disorder (ie, stroke, spinal cord injury)
  Urinary incontinence
  Breast, ovarian, uterine, and cervical cancer
  Depression
  Anxiety

Surgeries or procedures
  Pelvic radiation
  Hysterectomy and/or oophorectomy
  Mastectomy

Medications
  Antidepressants (ie, selective serotonin reuptake inhibitors, serotonin norepinephrine reuptake inhibitors)
  Antihypertensives, particularly beta-blockers

Data from Refs.[1,3,12]

Table 2
Vulvovaginal hygiene do's and don'ts

Do...	Don't...
Use unscented, hypoallergenic, and chemical-free products when possible.	Use products with preservatives or other irritants such as: • Parabens • Propylene glycol • Perfumes and fragrances These can be found in: • Soaps • Lotions/creams • Personal lubricants • Vaginal medication preparations • Clothing detergents, fabric softeners, and dryer sheets • Sanitary and incontinence pads
Gently wash the outside of the vulva with warm water with or without a plain, hypoallergenic, unscented soap. A soft wash cloth can be used to carefully clean between the labial folds.	Exfoliate the vulva with harsh scrubs or sponges. Douche, because it is rarely indicated medically, just temporarily masks symptoms, and can make the issue worse.
Wear cotton or other natural, breathable material underwear.	Wear synthetic material underwear or tight fitted clothing, particularly when wet (ie, change out of sweaty gym clothes, wet bathing suit, etc)
Consider leaving pubic hair where it is! It acts as a protective barrier for your vulva and removal methods can do more harm than good. If removal is preferred by the patient, trimming is the least disruptive to the vulva's health.	Shave with a razor, wax, or use chemical hair removal products; these methods are particularly harsh on skin and can cause infected ingrown hairs or chemical burns.
Always wash sex enhancement toys and devices after each use with warm soap and water. Change condoms when switching between oral, vaginal, or anal intercourse.	

Vulvovaginal Anatomy

The vulva is a commonly overlooked and underrepresented region of the female anatomy (**Fig. 1**). It is bordered by the mons pubis anteriorly, the intercrural folds laterally, and the gluteal cleft posteriorly. The labia majora are hair-bearing, fatty structures with sebaceous glands covered by a layer of stratified squamous epithelium. The labia minora are thinner, of varied lengths, and are considered to be a "keratinized mucosa."[14] They extend anteriorly, forming the frenulum and free edge of the clitoral hood, which covers the glans clitoris to varying degrees. The glans clitoris is a highly vascular structure that transmits much of the input for female sexual arousal via the dorsal nerve of the clitoris.[15]

The vestibule is a squamous mucosal epithelium that is bordered by Hart's line, the transition from tissue that arises from ectoderm to that which arises from endoderm.

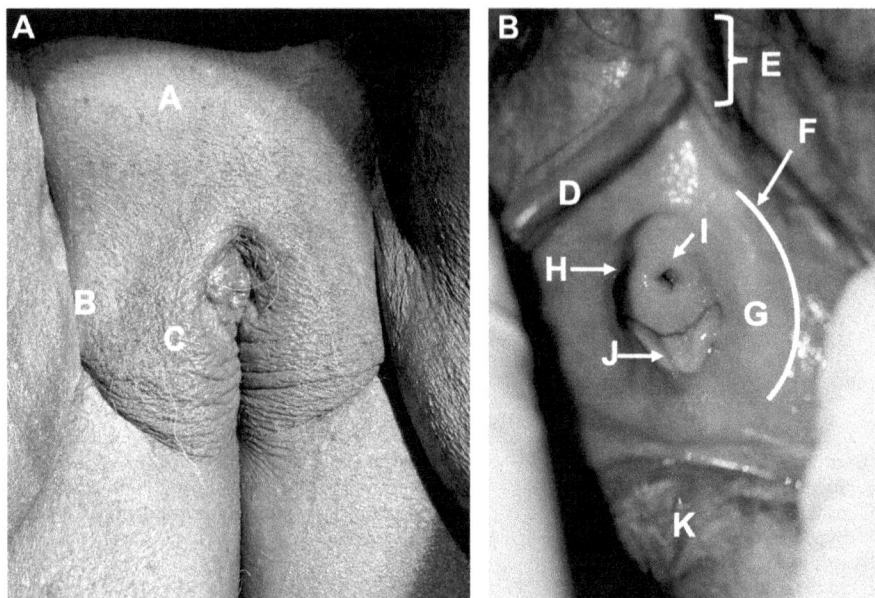

Fig. 1. Vulvar anatomy. (*A*) Labeled structures of vulva including the mons pubis (A), inter-crural folds (B), and labia majora (C). (*B*) Labeled structures of vulva including the labia mi-nora (D), clitoral hood and glans clitoris (E), Hart's line (F), vestibule (G), vestibular glands (H), urethral meatus (I), hymen (J), and perineum (K). ([*A*] Printed with permission of An-drew Goldstein, MD, FACOG.)

The vestibule has multiple gland openings, including the mucus-secreting vestibular glands anteriorly and the Bartholin's glands posteriorly. In a well-estrogenized state, the vestibule is pink, moist, and sensitive to touch. The urethral meatus is anterior to the hymenal ring. The hymenal ring is the medial border of the vestibule and marks the transition from endoderm-derived tissue to the mesoderm-derived tissue of the vaginal mucosa.

The vagina is a tubular structure extending cephalad and posteriorly toward the sacrum, connecting the introitus to the cervix. It has numerous gland openings and is colonized by commensal bacteria that create an acidic environment. Vaginal secre-tions have a pH of 3.5 to 4.5. The walls of the vagina in a well-estrogenized state exhibit rugae and a pink, moist appearance. The vestibule and vagina are both extremely hormonally sensitive and therefore play a large role in sexual dysfunction af-ter menopause.[14]

Normal Changes with Aging

As women age, they may develop some or all of the following changes in the vulva: loss of fullness of the labia majora and minora, narrowed introital opening, and thin-ning and/or graying of pubic hair (**Fig. 2**) These structures can become more sensi-tive and friable owing to a loss of collagen, elasticity, and water-retaining ability.[16] The clitoris may become less sensitive to stimulation owing to a decrease in blood flow, slowing of neurophysiologic response, and decreased sensation. Orgasm, the pleasurable contractions of the uterus and surrounding muscles, can also become less intense or even painful with aging.[17] Although these changes are

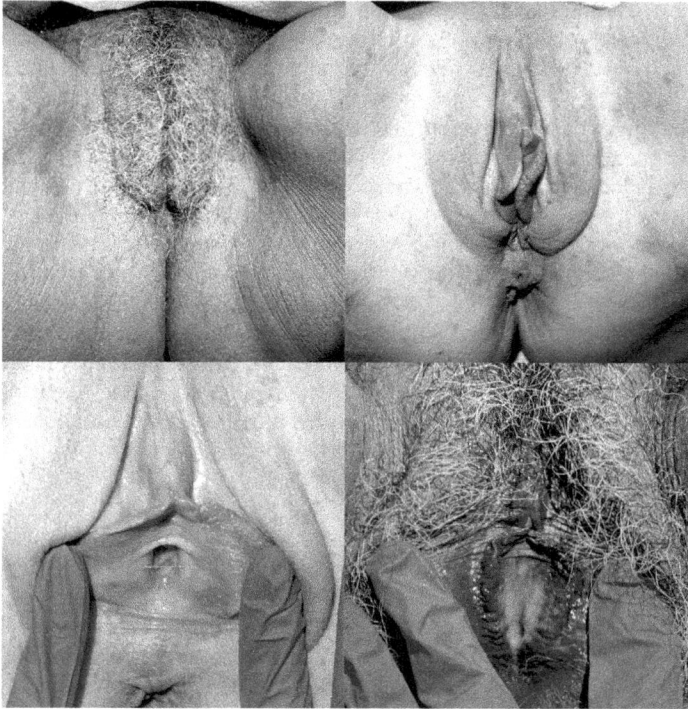

Fig. 2. Examples of menopausal vulvas and vestibules. Note the loss of fullness in labia majora, narrow-appearing introitus, pallor, and erythema of vestibule (evidence of the genitourinary syndrome of menopause), and prominence of urethral meatus. These changes are all a result of low estrogen status and aging.

considered "normal," in many cases they may lead to challenges in sexual function. For example, a narrowing of the introitus causing pain with vaginal intercourse can be reversed using graduated dilators. Thinned, dry vulvar skin can be more sensitive to irritants and friction; applying a barrier ointment can help to moisturize and protect the keratinized vulvar epithelium. The vestibule and vagina, which rely on hormones for their health, also change dramatically in the absence of premenopausal hormone levels.[16]

SYNDROME OF MENOPAUSE
Pathophysiology

Genitourinary syndrome of menopause (GSM, previously called vulvovaginal atrophy) affects 27% to 84% of postmenopausal women. With the onset of menopause comes a decrease in the levels of estrogen, progesterone, and testosterone. These hormones play a role in the health and function of the vulva and vagina, and their decline leads to atrophy and inflammation of the vulvovaginal tissues. The urethra and vestibule can exhibit pallor with overlying erythematous blood vessels owing to thinning of the mucosa. Outgrowth of the urethral meatus, also known as a caruncle, is a commonly seen lesion with GSM. The vaginal mucosa loses rugal folds and becomes pale and increasingly friable and thin. Blood vessels are easily disrupted, making examinations traumatic for patients. Glands produce less secretion to keep the vagina moist. In the setting of low estrogen levels, squamous cells do not mature and deposit glycogen. *Lactobacilli* species rely on glycogen to survive and may no longer create the acidic environment that helps to prevent colonization and infection with fecal and other bacteria and yeast.

These changes can result in pain with vaginal penetration, dysuria, frequent urinary tract infections, and discomfort with activities of daily living owing to decreased lubrication and elasticity. The discomfort associated with these changes can lead to pelvic floor dysfunction and additional provoked or unprovoked pain. Pelvic floor dysfunction is often due to involuntary tightening of the muscles surrounding the introitus and vagina, often in anticipation of sexual activity, such as penetration or touch.[18]

Diagnosis

A diagnosis of GSM can be made with a microscopic examination of discharge from the vaginal fornixes with normal saline. In patients with GSM, the vaginal pH is elevated (>4.5). Microscopic evaluation reveals a decrease in lactobacilli, more than one white blood cell per epithelial cell, and immature (parabasal) vaginal epithelial cells.

Treatment

There are a variety of treatments for GSM, but in a study of 1858 postmenopausal women with GSM, only 50% had used any treatment for their symptoms.[19] This low rate of use is likely linked to discomfort regarding the initiation of conversations about sexuality and intimacy by patients and providers. Apprehension about potential adverse effects of hormones can delay intervention.[18] **Table 3** provides an overview of treatment options.[2,18,20]

Hormone-Free Treatments

Personal lubricants are used to decrease friction during penetration. Lubricants are typically used during sexual encounters, but are not helpful in addressing urinary symptoms or discomfort with daily activities. The osmolarity of lubricants can affect the vaginal environment. Hyperosmolar products have been found to be more damaging to the superficial mucosal cells, whereas iso-osmolar lubricants (<1200 mOsm/kg) are safer for the vagina. When recommending oil-based lubricants, patients must be counseled that they can erode condoms.[18]

Vaginal moisturizers containing bioadhesives such as hyaluronic acid and polycarbophil hold water molecules and provide a long-lasting layer of moisture in the vagina, which can decrease vulvovaginal discomfort. These products can be applied internally or externally to keep the mucosa and skin supple. They are typically used 2 to 3 times per week, and are helpful for patients with cancer who are not candidates for hormone-containing therapies after pelvic surgery, chemotherapy, chemoprophylaxis, or radiation that affects the vulvovaginal tissues.[18]

Newer treatments for GSM, such as laser and radiofrequency devices, are currently under investigation and are used off-label. Energy-based treatments are thought to cause microtrauma, which stimulates collagen formation, angiogenesis, and tissue thickening. This process leads to thicker, moister vulvovaginal tissues. They may be considered for women who have contraindications to hormone-containing medications and have not had success with hormone-free methods.[18]

Hormonal Treatments

Hormone-containing treatment for GSM is considered first line, safe, and effective. Approaches include topical formulations, vaginal suppositories, hormone-releasing

Table 3
Treatments for GSM

	Purpose	Common Dosing	Types	Advantages	Disadvantages
Hormone-free topical treatments					
Personal lubricants	Reduce friction with penetrative acts	Use liberally as needed on both the vulva and object to be inserted (eg, dilator, finger, penis, sex toy)	Water based	Safe to use with latex condoms	Can "dry up" quickly, requiring reapplication, but can "reactivate" by spraying water on genitals
			Oil-based (including coconut or olive oils)	Unlikely to be irritating, natural oils are inexpensive	Erosive to latex condoms, can be messy and stain sheets
			Silicone based	Safe to use with latex condoms	Expensive, cannot use with silicone dilators or toys
Vaginal moisturizers	Bioadhesive-containing solution that holds water to improve moisture in treated skin and mucosa	Use 2–3 times per week vaginally, can also apply to external vulva	Hyaluronic acid Polycarbophil	Longer lasting than lubricants, can be used in addition to lubricants	Can be expensive and messy
Type	Active Ingredient	Common Initial Dosing	Common Maintenance Dosing	Advantages	Disadvantages
Hormone-containing treatments (FDA approved)					
Vaginal creams	17B-estradiol 0.01% Conjugated estrogens (0.625 mg/g)	0.5–1.0 g/d for 2 wk	0.5–1.0 g 1–3 times per week	Can direct application where needed (ie, behind pessary, on vestibule)	Variable absorption
Vaginal inserts	17B-estradiol inserts	4–10 μl/d for 2 wk	1 insert twice per week	Consistently low systemic absorption	Harder to direct the medication to particular tissue
	Estradiol hemihydrate inserts	10 μl/d for 2 wk	1 insert twice per week	Consistently low systemic absorption	
	Prasterone (DHEA) inserts	6.5 mg/d	1 insert per day	Consistently low systemic absorption, converts to both estrogen and testosterone in the tissue	

(continued on next page)

Table 3
(continued)

Vaginal silicone ring	17B-estradiol	2-mm ring (7.5 µ/d released) Replace ring every 90 d	Infrequent need for replacement, helpful for patients with difficulty remembering daily/weekly administration schedules	Ring can be stiff and difficult to remove and replace. May fall out more easily for patients with prolapse or hysterectomy.
Oral tablet	Ospemifene (estrogen agonist/antagonist)	60 mg/d	60 mg/d	Only oral product available for GSM, helpful for patients with difficulty placing vaginal products	Limited data on systemic estrogen levels

Abbreviation: FDA, US Food and Drug Administration.

Data from Crean-tate KK, Faubion SS, Pederson HJ, Vencill JA, Batur P. Management of genitourinary syndrome of menopause in female cancer patients: a focus on vaginal hormonal therapy. Am J Obstet Gynecol. 2020;222(2):103-113. https://doi.org/10.1016/j.ajog.2019.08.043; The 2020 genitourinary syndrome of menopause position statement of The North American Menopause Society. *Menopause J North Am Menopause Soc.* 2020;27(9):976-992. https://doi.org/10.1097/GME.0000000000001609.

devices, and oral pills. **Table 3** organizes these options by route and clinical consideration. For example, an oral formulation may work best for a woman who has difficulty placing anything vaginally owing to physical limitations or vaginal discomfort. A hormone-releasing ring may be preferable for a woman who desires a longer acting option. Topical creams are ideal for those needing targeted treatment of the vestibule and patients using a pessary (can apply to the pessary during placement). Patients should be counseled on the side effects of local hormone therapy. Temporary breast soreness, nausea, and headaches typically resolve after the first 2 weeks of treatment with topical estrogens and are due to the transient increased absorption of the medication. A slight increase in vaginal discharge can be expected from any vaginal formulation.[18] Systemic hormone therapy is typically not sufficient for initial treatment of GSM. For women given systemic hormone therapy, local treatment of GSM can be initiated and discontinued once symptoms have improved. Although nonhormonal agents are preferred for patients with a history of hormone-sensitive malignancy, low-dose topical treatment of GSM can be considered on a case-by-case basis after a discussion of the risks and benefits with the patient and coordination with their oncologist.[20] Patients should be counseled regarding available options, considering safety, convenience, and affordability.

Dilators, Devices, and Toys

An effective option for women who have developed introital and/or vaginal narrowing owing to atrophy is graduated vaginal dilators, which slowly increase the ability of the vagina to accommodate penetration. Treating the underlying atrophic changes and dryness is imperative to tolerate dilator therapy. Dilators can also be helpful for pelvic floor dysfunction in conjunction with treatment by a certified pelvic floor physical therapist. Devices such as vibrating dilators, pelvic trainers, and curved pelvic wands can be helpful, particularly for patients who are receiving pelvic floor physical therapy for hypertonic or hypotonic muscle dysfunction. These devices are typically recommended by physical therapists, and patients should receive detailed instruction before initiation.

Sexual enhancement devices (also known as "sex toys" or "adult lifestyle products") such as vibrators, penetrative devices (dildos), penis rings, anal-specific devices, can be helpful for optimizing arousal and achieving orgasm. More than one-half of all women in the United States have ever used a vibrator. Women who have sex with women use vibrators at a rate of 75%. Normalizing use of devices to aid in sexual function is critical as patients sometimes consider them taboo or promiscuous.[21]

Sexual devices can also assist in treating the effects of aging. For example, vibrators can decrease length of time to achieve orgasm for women with decreased clitoral sensitivity. A collision dyspareunia aid is a soft, donut-shaped ring that fits around a penis or other penetrative device that can help women who experience pain during penetration owing to vaginal shortening or pelvic floor dysfunction.[21] Rubin and colleagues[21] provide an excellent review of these devices, including common uses, proper care, and precautions. A Woman's Touch (https://sexualityresources.com/) is a patient-centered online resource for those interested in sexual enhancement devices.

Sexually transmitted infections

Although sexually transmitted infections (STIs) in the elderly population are less common, they are an important consideration in the differential diagnosis of vaginitis symptoms. The Centers for Disease Control and Prevention recommend screening older women if there is a new sex partner, more than 1 sex partner, a sex partner with multiple partners, or a partner who has a STI.[3] In the last decade, the rates of STIs, including syphilis, gonorrhea, and chlamydia, in adults older than 65 years have more than doubled.[22] Few longitudinal studies have been published for this population. Of the data available, increasing rates of STIs is likely due to decreased screening, ignoring sexual health, and a knowledge gap among patients and providers.[22,23] Patients should not be assumed to be low risk for STIs, especially those living in congregate settings or those who are widowed or divorced.[22,23] Elderly patients are at risk for complications of STIs, including pelvic inflammatory disease, abscess formation, and sepsis. Prompt diagnosis and treatment of STIs is important for maintaining health of this population.[24] The Centers for Disease Control and Prevention has a full guide to diagnosis and treatment of STIs that can be accessed online at https://www.cdc.gov/std/tg2015/default.htm.[25]

Common vulvar dermatoses in the geriatric population

Postmenopausal women may delay reporting vulvar skin concerns to primary care providers or gynecologists owing to embarrassment. Providers who are not as familiar with examining the vulvar skin may not recognize the signs of common and treatable conditions in the early phase. This lack can lead to delayed diagnosis and irreversible harm.[13] The most common dermatoses in this population include vulvar lichen sclerosus, lichen planus, contact dermatitis, and lichen simplex chronicus. Less common but most dangerous are vulvar intraepithelial neoplasia and carcinoma.[13] Biopsy is critical for an accurate diagnosis and is performed with topical or subcutaneous anesthesia. Referral to a provider who is experienced in performing vulvar biopsies is recommended, particularly if the patient does not respond to initial conservative treatments. Reducing incorrect diagnoses can avoid delays in treatment, potential harm from incorrect treatment, irreversible scarring and architectural changes of the vulva, and even life-threatening sequelae such as vulvar carcinoma.

EVALUATION AND MANAGEMENT OF SEXUAL DYSFUNCTION

The diagnostic criteria for sexual dysfunction are outlined in **Table 1**. If more than 1 dysfunction exists, it is important to establish the relationship between the domains.[2]

Box 4
Common medications in the elderly and associated FSD

Drug	Effect on:			
	Desire	Arousal	Orgasm	Pain
Selective serotonin reuptake inhibitor	X	X	X	
Cardiovascular drugs				
Statin	X			
Beta-blocker	X			
Antihistamines		X		
Tamoxifen	X	X		
Chemotherapeutic agents	X	X		

Modified from Clayton AH, Goldstein I, Kim NN, et al. The International Society for the Study of Women's Sexual Health Process of Care for Management of Hypoactive Sexual Desire Disorder in Women. Mayo Clin Proc. 2018;93(4):467-487. https://doi.org/10.1016/j.mayocp.2017.11.002; with permission.

Once a diagnosis is made, the provider must elucidate characteristics such as the onset, duration, and level of distress and avoidance. If the dysfunction can be attributed to GSM, it is imperative to treat those symptoms, because an improvement in desire, arousal, orgasm, and pain may result. Polypharmacy is common in the elderly, and assessing each medication can help to rule out other causes of sexual dysfunction. More adult women aged 40 to 79 years use 1 or more prescription drug when compared with men. Among US adults aged 60 to 79 years, the most commonly used types of prescription drugs are lipid-lowering drugs, antidiabetic agents, beta-blockers, angiotensin-converting enzyme inhibitors, and proton pump inhibitors.[26] **Box 4** provides a reference for common medications in the elderly and their effects on sexual function.[8] In addition to medical management, counseling or psychotherapy may be considered for each domain, as described in greater detail elsewhere in this article.

Desire

Decreased sexual desire occurs with age; however, the associated level of distress varies. Approximately 80% of postmenopausal women do not discuss symptoms of decreased desire with providers, usually owing to embarrassment.[27] The DSDS (see **Box 2**) is a screening tool for low sexual desire.[11] Once a diagnosis is made, shared decision-making can determine the appropriate management. Although medications approved by the US Food and Drug Administration for hypoactive sexual desire disorder are only approved for premenopausal women, their use in postmenopausal women can be considered. The off-label use of hormone therapy with estrogen and testosterone is summarized in **Table 4**.[27–31] Some providers may be hesitant to prescribe estrogen therapy owing to findings from the Women's Health Initiative in which more than 160,000 postmenopausal women aged 50 to 79 years were randomized to treatment with estrogen plus progestin or placebo. In a subgroup of women, quality-of-life indicators, including sexual satisfaction, were analyzed. The results suggested that there was no difference in sexual satisfaction between hormone therapy and placebo.[32] It is reasonable, however, to use systemic hormone therapy to treat vasomotor symptoms that may affect a menopausal woman's desire, or topical estrogen to manage decreased desire related to GSM symptoms.

Arousal

Arousal describes the physiologic response of female genitalia, including lubrication, engorgement, and sensitivity, and is different from desire.[33] Disorders may occur in older women owing to poor vascularization or decreased lubrication associated with decreased hormones. Although there are no medications approved by the US Food and Drug Administration for female genital arousal disorders, there is a medical device approved by the US Food and Drug Administration called the EROS. The EROS uses gentle suction to increase clitoral blood flow and stimulation.[7] It can be prescribed by a provider, but the cost can be prohibitive.[34]

Orgasm

Female orgasm disorder describes decreased intensity, duration, frequency, or pleasure from orgasm. Female orgasm may be achieved through vaginal, clitoral, skin, breast, or nipple stimulation as well as imagery and fantasy.[35] A variety of techniques can be used, such as oral stimulation, a partner's hand, or masturbation.[36] Although female orgasm disorder is the second most common female sexual disorder, it is often found in combination with other complaints.[37] Orgasm may be affected by decreased

Table 4
FSD: desire

Medication	Administration	Mechanism of Action	Advantages	Disadvantages
FDA approved				
Flibanserin	100 mg by mouth at bedtime	Increases sexual desire by increasing dopamine and norepinephrine levels and decreasing serotonin levels	FDA approved treatment for HSDD Improvement in satisfying sexual events	FDA approved for premenopausal women only Adverse effects of dizziness, somnolence, nausea, fatigue, insomnia, dry mouth Cannot be used with alcohol
Bremelanotide	1.75 mg subcutaneous injection at least 45 min before anticipated sexual activity	Melanocortin receptor agonist; exact mechanism unknown	FDA approved treatment for HSDD Improves sexual desire and satisfaction Can decrease side effects because it is administered only before anticipated activity	FDA approved for premenopausal women only Adverse reactions of nausea, emesis, flushing, headache, hyperpigmentation Do not use in women with uncontrolled hypertension or cardiovascular disease
Vaginal dehydroepiandrosterone 1% (DHEA; Prasterone)	6.5 mg per vagina at bedtime	Precursor for androgens and estrogens	FDA approved for dyspareunia in postmenopausal women Improvement in sexual desire Low systemic absorption	Caution in women with breast cancer (recommend consultation with oncologist)
Off-label medications				

Treatment		Mechanism	Benefits	Considerations
Estrogen therapy (supplement with progesterone in women with a uterus; see **Table 3**)	Oral	Undergoes hepatic metabolism ("first-pass effect")	Manage vasomotor symptoms	Increases amount of sex hormone–binding globulin thereby decreasing free testosterone (Santoro et al,[29] 2016)
	Transdermal	Absorbed into systemic circulation via the skin and bypasses the gut and first pass of the liver	Manage vasomotor symptoms Less decrease of testosterone Lower risk of thromboembolism	Prescribe in conjunction with oncologist if applicable
	Local/topical	Improves peripheral blood flow, nerve function and vaginal lubrication (Santoro et al,[29] 2016)	Improve GSM May choose cream, tablet, ring	Prescribe in conjunction with oncologist if applicable
Transdermal testosterone	300 μg/d May be given to supplement estrogen therapy	Improves testosterone availability, which regulates sexual desire	Improves desire and sexual satisfaction Decreases personal distress	Not FDA approved Long-term safety data not available Androgenic adverse effects (hair growth, acne)

Abbreviation: FDA, US Food and Drug Administration.
Data from Refs.[27–31]

desire or arousal, stress, emotional connection to a partner, or partner sexual dysfunction. Cognitive and behavioral therapies are recommended by sexual health experts for orgasm disorder. Multiple studies have found that time to orgasm is shorter with masturbation than intercourse.[36] Directed masturbation has well-established efficacy, and therapy focused on genital stimulation, role play, and sexual fantasy may improve arousal and orgasm. Sex education, anxiety reduction, and cognitive behavioral therapy also help.[37] Supplemental testosterone may be used to improve sexual satisfaction. Limited data exist regarding hormone therapy in women with orgasm disorder as the primary concern.

Pain

Pain during sex has been reported in 25% of postmenopausal women.[29] Sexual pain disorders include vaginal pain during penetration (dyspareunia), involuntary spasms of the pelvic floor muscles, or pelvic pain during intercourse. Pain may lead to fear and anxiety. GSM also contributes to sexual pain, especially in the elderly. Other considerations include pelvic organ prolapse and urinary or bowel incontinence. Pelvic floor disorders are more common in the geriatric population owing to physiologic changes in muscle tone and vascularization.[7] When pain is the main concern, referral to a sexual pain specialists and pelvic floor physical therapists should be offered.[2] It is important to treat the pain before treating complaints of desire, arousal, and orgasm.

SEXUAL HEALTH AND COMORBID MEDICAL CONDITIONS

Many medical problems are associated with FSD, the majority of which increase with age.[12] The most important are summarized in **Box 5**; however, sexual dysfunction is not limited to these conditions.

Diabetes

FSD occurs more frequently in women with diabetes; however, the pathophysiology is not well-understood. This condition is often comorbid with obesity and depression,

---

Box 5
Tips for improving sexual health in those with chronic comorbid conditions

Chronic Comorbid Condition	Practical Tips for Improving Sexual Health
Diabetes	Weight loss
	Glycemic control
Cardiovascular disease	Blood pressure control
	Do not need to limit sexual activity for hypertension alone
Osteoarthritis	Warm up the joints before sexual activity (exercise, warm shower)
	Take medication before sex
	Use sex toys, especially if osteoarthritis stiffens fingers
	Consider positional pillows, foam wedges, and other support structures to help individuals relax in comfortable positions for sexual activities
Depression and dementia	Screen for depression and trauma
	Openly support the caregiver
Breast and gynecologic cancers	Multidisciplinary approach for treatment
	Try nonhormonal treatments first

which have known associations with FSD.[38] Intact nervous, vascular, and sensory systems are necessary for sexual response. Hyperglycemia can dehydrate mucus membranes, resulting in vaginal dryness and dyspareunia. Diabetes can also induce vascular and nerve damage of the female genitalia, impairing the response to stimuli.[39] A meta-analysis suggests that premenopausal women with diabetes experience FSD more frequently than menopausal women.[38] The effect of diabetes on males is better established, with erectile dysfunction occurring more frequently in diabetic compared with nondiabetic men.[3,39]

Cardiovascular Disease

The correlation between CVD and male sexual dysfunction is well-understood, and erectile dysfunction is an early marker of CVD. In females with CVD, sexual dysfunction is thought to have the same vascular pathophysiology, but does not necessarily predict the development of CVD. Clitoral erectile function requires the same nitric oxide pathway as male penile erectile function.[40,41] Decreased blood flow and atherosclerosis can lead to vaginal and clitoral vascular insufficiency syndrome.[7,41] Poor circulation can cause fibrosis, vaginal dryness, and dyspareunia.[7] Antihypertensives and statins used to can also contribute to sexual dysfunction. Thomas and colleagues[40] investigated antihypertensive use in women more than 50 years of age and the impact on sexual function. Sexual dysfunction was not linked to a single class of medication. Previous data have suggested that FSD could be associated with beta-blockers.[2,12] It is important to understand how medications can negatively impact sexual function and to counsel patients on the potential sexual side effects to decrease nonadherence to medication.[40]

Osteoarthritis

Osteoarthritis (OA) is commonly diagnosed in the primary care setting. The strongest risk factor for its development is age, and OA is more prevalent and severe in females.[42] The pain and inflammation of OA can greatly impact sexual health. Research on OA and sexual health is limited. A recent qualitative study found that, despite a desire to engage in sexual activity, patients felt constrained by hip and knee pain. Decreased hip mobility negatively impacted sexual activity more than decreased knee mobility.[43] OA in the hands is prevalent, and hand stiffness can impact touch and the administration of vulvovaginal medications.[42]

Depression and Dementia

Depression is common in the elderly, and occurs more frequently in those with other health conditions.[44] Depression is a risk factor for sexual dysfunction[2] and its relationship should be viewed as bidirectional. A review by Atlantis and colleagues[45] evaluated this relationship and found that individuals with depression had up to a 70% increased risk of developing sexual dysfunction and those with sexual dysfunction had a 130% to 210% increased risk of developing depression. Practitioners should screen for depression in patients who report sexual dysfunction and vice versa.[45] Patients should be screened for a history of trauma, which may contribute to low desire or pain.[8,27] Survivors of violence, especially sexual trauma, are at an increased risk of sexual dysfunction.[12] Trauma-informed care and referral to a mental health specialist are critical.

Dementia can affect both the patient and their partner. Dementia may decrease sexual desire, but uninhibited sexual behavior may also be observed.[8,9] Approximately two-thirds of caregivers of those with dementia are the spouse or partner. When the caregiver is also the partner, it can be particularly straining on intimacy. Autonomy and consent in patients with dementia can impact the sexual experience. As dementia progresses, intimacy may cease. Loss of communication and reciprocity may be especially challenging.[46] Normalizing sex in the elderly can help the patient and caregiver find the support they deserve.

Breast and Gynecologic Cancers

Cancer and its relationship with sexual function is multifaceted and often overlooked. Cancer and treatment may directly influence sexual function, and may also affect

Table 5
Addressing sexual health

Products and education		
A Woman's Touch	A sexuality resource center for information and products	https://sexualityresources.com/
National Vulvodynia Association	Not-for-profit organization that offers education, supports research, and has patient stories and additional referral resources	https://www.nva.org/
Memorial Sloan Kettering	A helpful webpage with instructions on how to use a vaginal dilator for patients	https://www.mskcc.org/pdf/cancer-care/patient-education/how-use-vaginal-dilator?mode=large
Finding a specialist		
North American Menopause Society	Menopausal information for both patients and professionals Also helps locate a menopause practitioner	www.menopause.org
American Physical Therapy Association-Section on Women's Health	Locate a pelvic floor physical therapist	https://ptl.womenshealthapta.org/
American Association of Sexuality Educators, Counselors, and Therapists	Locate sex therapists, counselors and educators	https://sstarnet.org/find-a-therapist/
Pelvic Guru	Online directory for sexual medicine specialists in variety of fields.	https://pelvicguru.com/
Professional organizations		
International Society for the Study of Women's Sexual Health	A multidisciplinary, academic, and scientific organization for women's sexual health	www.isswsh.org
International Society for Sexual Medicine		www.issm.info
Sexual Medicine Society of North America		www.smsna.org

mood, interpersonal relationships, and body image. Up to 80% of women with breast cancer report decreased sexual desire.[8]

Real or perceived changes in body image after cancer treatment can impact sexual function. Chemotherapy can induce alopecia and weight changes, which may affect desire.[20] Chemotherapy and radiation can impact ovarian function and exacerbate GSM.[20] Surgery on the breasts or other organs can impact body image and lead to decreased sensitivity.[20] Mastectomy leads to greater sexual dysfunction than breast-conserving surgery.[3] Nonhormonal treatments for GSM are the first-line therapy for those with hormone-dependent cancer, including lubricants, dilators, and physical floor therapy (see **Table 3**). If nonhormonal therapies do not improve symptoms, hormonal options may be considered.[20]

SEXUAL HEALTH AND ISSUES WITH PARTNER

Aging has adverse effects on sexual function in men and women. The term "couplepause" refers to situations in which both partners are experiencing changes related to menopause and/or andropause. The concept is an evolution of the couple-oriented approaches of Masters and Johnson and others.[47] Simultaneous biological changes in the aging couple can amplify the sexual dysfunction of individuals. The presence of GSM may be compounded by a partner's sexual dysfunction, especially erectile dysfunction. Restoring an individual's sexual function while ignoring partners' issues can lead to increased frustration. Couplepause is a paradigm for addressing the sexual health needs of a couple as a whole and should be the standard used by clinicians in an aging population.[47]

Treatment plans should reflect the interdependence of intimate relationships. In addition to the personal changes impacting female sexual function, women are negatively impacted by diminished sexual function in their male partners.[48] Visits to male sexual function clinics are often initiated by female partners. Despite this circumstance, female partners are rarely screened for sexual dysfunction while their partners are treated. Erectile dysfunction of males in heterosexual relationships causes difficulty with orgasms for older women.[49] Treating clinicians should encourage acts of intimacy that not only focus on penetration, but also promote ways to achieve female orgasm without penetration. Vibrators and clitoral stimulation can improve sexual satisfaction when penetration is not possible. It is helpful to counsel patients to encourage other forms intimacy to decrease frustration, disappointment, or shame for both parties. Sexual relationships do not always involve heterosexual partners seeking penile penetration. It is also important to treat GSM in women who have sex with women.

ADDRESSING SEXUAL HEALTH AS A HEALTH CARE PROVIDER

Women's sexual health is a challenging area of medicine owing to its multifactorial nature and its complexity is intensified in the elderly population owing to lack of research and education. Simple steps to address sexual health may be taken by clinicians caring for older adults. Inviting the patient to openly disclose sexual concerns helps patients receive the care they need to improve their quality of life. Screening tools, such as the Female Sexual Function Index and the DSDS, can be administered to assist in identifying the areas of sexual function that are impaired. There are safe and effective treatments available for many sexual concerns and multidisciplinary specialists nationwide to address issues that may be out of the scope of the primary provider's expertise (**Table 5**).

CLINICS CARE POINTS

- The geriatric patient population is less sexually active overall, but assumptions should not be made about an individual's current sexual practices based on that generalization.
- There are specific, clear criteria to aid in diagnosis of sexual dysfunction as outlined by International Society for the Study of Women's Sexual Health and the DSM-V.
- There are a variety of effective and evidence-based treatments for women with sexual concerns in the geriatric population.
- The selection of treatments should include a consideration of the patient's physical and mental abilities and limitations.
- Comorbid conditions and their treatments can be key players in sexual dysfunction.
- The partner's sexual function is an important factor in a patient's function and must be considered as part of the evaluation.
- There are numerous resources available to aid in diagnosis, management, and referral for geriatric patients with sexual dysfunction.

DISCLOSURE

The author certify that all my affiliations with or financial involvement in, within the past 5 years and foreseeable future, any organization or entity with a financial interest in or financial conflict with the subject matter or materials discussed in this article are completely disclosed (eg, employment, consultancies, honoraria, stock ownership or options, expert testimony, grants or patents received or pending, royalties).

REFERENCES

1. Hoffman BL, Schorge JO, Halvorson LM, et al. Psychosocial issues and female sexuality. In: Williams gynecology. 4th edition. McGraw-Hill Education; 2020. Available at: http://accessmedicine.mhmedical.com/content.aspx?aid=1171529751.
2. Parish SJ, Hahn SR, Goldstein SW, et al. The International society for the study of women's sexual health process of care for the identification of sexual concerns and problems in women. Mayo Clin Proc 2019;94(5):842–56.
3. Granville L, Pregler J. Women's sexual health and aging. J Am Geriatr Soc 2018; 66(3):595–601.
4. Sinković M, Towler L. Sexual aging: a systematic review of qualitative research on the sexuality and sexual health of older adults. Qual Health Res 2019;29(9): 1239–54.
5. Sexual Dysfunctions. In: The Diagnostic and Statistical Manual of Mental Disorders (5th Ed, DSM-5).
6. Hoffman BL, Schorge JO, Halvorson LM, et al. Menopause and the mature woman. In: Williams gynecology. 4th edition. McGraw-Hill Education; 2020. Available at: http://accessmedicine.mhmedical.com/content.aspx?aid=1171531513.
7. Walsh KE, Berman JR. Sexual dysfunction in the older woman an overview of the current understanding and management. Drugs Aging 2004;21(10):655–75.
8. Clayton AH, Goldstein I, Kim NN, et al. The international society for the study of women's sexual health process of care for management of hypoactive sexual

desire disorder in women. 2018;93(4):467–87. https://doi.org/10.1016/j.mayocp.2017.11.002.

9. Wallace MA. Assessment of sexual health in older adults: using the PLISSIT model to talk about sex. Am J Nurs 2008;108(7):52–60.

10. Rosen R, Brown C, Heiman J, et al. The Female Sexual Function Index (FSFI): a multidimensional self-report instrument for the assessment of female sexual function. J Sex Marital Ther 2000;26(2):191–208.

11. Clayton AH, Goldfischer ER, Goldstein I, et al. Validation of the decreased sexual desire screener (DSDS): a brief diagnostic instrument for generalized acquired female hypoactive sexual desire disorder (HSDD). J Sex Med 2009;6:730–8.

12. Thomas HN, Neal-Perry GS, Hess R. Female sexual function at midlife and beyond. Obstet Gynecol Clin North Am 2018;45(4):709–22.

13. Spadt SK, Kusturiss E. Vulvar dermatoses: a primer for the sexual medicine clinician. Sex Med Rev 2015;3(3):126–36.

14. Edwards L. Genital anatomy. In: Genital dermatology atlas and manual. 3rd edition. Wolters Kluwer; 2018. p. 1–9.

15. Kelling JA, Erickson CR, Pin J, et al. Anatomical dissection of the dorsal nerve of the clitoris. Aesthet Surg J 2020;40(5):541–7.

16. Calleja-Agius J, Brincat MP. The urogenital system and the menopause. Climacteric 2015;18(Suppl 1):18–22.

17. Kingsberg SA. The impact of aging on sexual function in women and their partners. Arch Sex Behav 2002;31(5):431–7.

18. The 2020 genitourinary syndrome of menopause position statement of the North American Menopause Society. Menopause 2020;27(9):976–92.

19. Kingsberg SA, Krychman M, Graham S, et al. The women's EMPOWER survey: identifying women's perceptions on vulvar and vaginal atrophy and its treatment. J Sex Med 2017;14(3):413–24.

20. Crean-tate KK, Faubion SS, Pederson HJ, et al. Management of genitourinary syndrome of menopause in female cancer patients: a focus on vaginal hormonal therapy. Am J Obstet Gynecol 2020;222(2):103–13.

21. Rubin ES, Deshpande NA, Vasquez PJ, et al. A clinical reference guide on sexual devices for obstetrician – gynecologists. Obstet Gynecol 2019;133(6):1259–68.

22. Smith ML, Bergeron CD, Goltz HH, et al. Sexually transmitted infection knowledge among older adults: psychometrics and test–retest reliability. Int J Environ Res Public Health 2020;17(7). https://doi.org/10.3390/ijerph17072462.

23. Bodley-Tickell A, Olowokure B, Bhaduri S, et al. Trends in sexually transmitted infections (other than HIV) in older people: analysis of data from an enhanced surveillance system. Sex Transm Infect 2008;84(4):312–7.

24. Workowski KA. Centers for disease control and prevention sexually transmitted diseases treatment guidelines. Clin Infect Dis 2015;61(Suppl 8):759–62.

25. Prevention C for DC and. 2015 Sexually transmitted diseases treatment guidelines. Available at: https://www.cdc.gov/std/tg2015/default.htm. Accessed January 22, 2021.

26. Hales CM, Servais J, Martin CB, et al. Prescription drug use among adults aged 40-79 in the United States and Canada. NCHS Data Brief 2019;(347):1–8.

27. Clayton AH, Kingsberg SA, Goldstein I. Evaluation and management of hypoactive sexual desire disorder. Sex Med 2018;6(2):59–74.

28. Dhillon S, Keam SJ. Bremelanotide: first approval. Drugs 2019;79(14):1599–606.

29. Santoro N, Worsley R, Miller KK, et al. Role of estrogens and estrogen-like compounds in female sexual function and dysfunction. J Sex Med 2016;13(3): 305–16.

30. Shifren JL, Davis SR, Moreau M, et al. Testosterone patch for the treatment of hypoactive sexual desire disorder in naturally menopausal women: results from the INTIMATE NM1 Study. Menopause 2006;13(5):770–9.

31. Labrie F, Archer D, Fortier M, et al. Effect of intravaginal dehydroepiandrosterone (Prasterone) on libido and sexual dysfunction in postmenopausal women. Menopause 2009;16(5):923–31.

32. Hays J, Ockene JK, Brunner RL, et al. Effects of estrogen plus progestin on health-related quality of life. N Engl J Med 2003;348(19):1839–54.

33. Althof SE, Meston CM, Perelman MA, et al. Opinion paper: on the diagnosis/classification of sexual arousal concerns in women. J Sex Med 2017;14(11): 1365–71.

34. Josefson D. FDA approves device for female sexual dysfunction. BMJ 2000; 320(7247):1427.

35. Levin RJ. The pharmacology of the human female orgasm — its biological and physiological backgrounds. Pharmacol Biochem Behav 2014;121:62–70.

36. Shaeer O, Skakke D, Giraldi A, et al. Female orgasm and overall sexual function and habits: a descriptive study of a cohort of U. S. Women. J Sex Med 2020; 17(6):1133–43.

37. Laan E, Rellini AH, Barnes T. Standard operating procedures for female orgasmic disorder. J Sex Med 2013;10(1):74–82.

38. Pontiroli AE, Cortelazzi D, Morabito A. Female sexual dysfunction and diabetes: a systematic review and meta-analysis. J Sex Med 2013;10(4): 1044–51.

39. Maiorino MI, Bellastella G, Esposito K. Diabetes and sexual dysfunction: current perspectives. Diabetes Metab Syndr Obe 2014;7:95–105.

40. Thomas HN, Evans GW, Berlowitz DR, et al. Antihypertensive medications and sexual function in women: baseline data from the SBP intervention trial (SPRINT). J Hypertens 2016;34(6):1224–31.

41. McCall-Hosenfeld JS, Freund KM, Legault C, et al. Sexual satisfaction and cardiovascular disease: the women's health initiative. Am J Med 2008;121(4): 295–301.

42. Neogi T, Zhang Y. Epidemiology of osteoarthritis. Rheum Dis Clin North Am 2013; 39(1):1–19.

43. Strid EN, Ekelius-hamping M. Experiences of sexual health in persons with hip and knee osteoarthritis: a qualitative study. BMC Musculoskelet Disord 2020; 5:1–9.

44. CDC. Depression is not a normal part of growing older. 2017. Available at: https:// www.cdc.gov/aging/mentalhealth/depression.htm.

45. Atlantis E, Sullivan T. Bidirectional association between depression and sexual dysfunction: a systematic review and meta-analysis. J Sex Med 2012;9(6): 1497–507.

46. Youell J, Callaghan JEM, Buchanan K. "I don't know if you want to know this": carers' understandings of intimacy in long-term relationships when one partner has dementia. Ageing Soc 2016;36(5):946–67.

47. Jannini EA, Nappi RE. Couplepause: a new paradigm in treating sexual dysfunction during menopause and andropause. Sex Med Rev 2018;6(3): 384–95.

48. Goldstein I, Fisher WA, Sand M, et al. Women's sexual function improves when partners are administered vardenafil for erectile dysfunction: a prospective, randomized, double-blind, placebo-controlled trial. J Sex Med 2005;2(6): 819–32.
49. Fisher WA, Rosen RC, Eardley I, et al. Sexual experience of female partners of men with erectile dysfunction: the female experience of men's attitudes to life events and sexuality (FEMALES) study. J Sex Med 2005;2(5):675–84.

Issues in the Lives of Older Lesbian, Gay, Bisexual, Transgender, and/or Queer Women

Joy A. Laramie, MSN, NP, ACHPN

KEYWORDS

- LGBTQ • Lesbian • Transgender • Barriers to health care

KEY POINTS

- The increasing diversity of the older population is reflected not only in race and ethnicity but also in sexual and gender identities.
- Lesbian, gay, bisexual, transgender, and/or queer (LGBTQ) individuals face health disparities linked to social stigma, discrimination, and denial of their civil and human rights.
- The availability of a supportive social network provides protective factors and increases resilience, decreasing the odds of psychological and physical health challenges.
- Physical health and function in later years are influenced by social aspects and variants throughout our lives, including family structure, socioeconomic status, and housing stability. Each of these factors may look different in the lives of older LGBTQ women because of isolation, inability to marry, not having children, job insecurity and pay inequality, and housing discrimination.
- To promote health equity, practitioners need to assess their own biases regarding LGBTQ persons, and understand how these, as well as the lives of LGBTQ persons, have been and continue to be shaped by contested, shifting sociocultural and historical discourses.

INTRODUCTION

The changing demographics and increasing diversity of the older population will be a defining feature of the twenty-first century. This diversity is reflected not only in race and ethnicity but also in sexual and gender identities. Individuals who openly self-identify as lesbian, gay, bisexual, transgender, and/or queer (LGBTQ) are estimated to compromise 2.4% of the US older adult population, or 2.7 million individuals.[1–3]

When also considering same-sex behavior and diverse, nonbinary genders, the number of LGBTQ adults ages 50 years and older doubles to more than 6% of the

The author has nothing to disclose.
4812 20th Place North, Arlington, VA 22207, USA
E-mail address: joylaramie@aol.com

Clin Geriatr Med 37 (2021) 579–591
https://doi.org/10.1016/j.cger.2021.05.005
0749-0690/21/Published by Elsevier Inc.

population. Given the fast growth of older adults, LGBTQ adults will account for more than 20 million older adults in the United States by 2060.[4]

Sexuality is complex and core to being human. Sexual orientation and gender identity can be fluid in individuals and change over time. Persons have the right to decide and explore their sexual orientation and gender identity.

LGBTQ older adults are of increasing interest to gerontologists, researchers, and policy makers as a vulnerable and underserved population. Although the acronym LGBTQ unintentionally may signal a single population, these individuals not only are unique unto themselves but also comprise a variety of subpopulations defined by sexual orientation, gender identity, and other factors.[5]

GLOSSARY

Bisexual

A person emotionally, romantically, or sexually attracted to more than 1 sex, gender, or gender identity although not necessarily simultaneously, in the same way or to the same degree.

Cisgender

A person whose sex assigned at birth and gender identity correspond in the expected way.

Closeted

Describes an LGBTQ person who has not disclosed their sexual orientation or gender identity.

Coming Out

The process in which a person first acknowledges, accepts, and appreciates their sexual orientation or gender identity and begins to share that with others.

Gay

A person who is emotionally, romantically, or sexually attracted to members of the same gender.

Gender Dysphoria

Clinically significant distress caused when a person's assigned birth gender is not the same as the one with which they identify.

Gender Expression

External appearance of one's gender identity, usually expressed through behavior, clothing, haircut, or voice and which may or may not conform to socially defined behaviors and characteristics typically associated with being either masculine or feminine.

Gender-Fluid

Describes an identity that may change or shift over time; relating to a person having or expressing a fluid or unfixed gender identity.

Gender Identity

The internal perception of one's gender and how they label themselves. Not to be conflated with biological sex or sex assigned at birth.

Gender Nonconforming

A broad term referring to people who do not behave in a way that conforms to the traditional expectations of their gender or whose gender expression does not fit neatly into a category.

Genderqueer

A gender identity label often used by people who do not identify with the binary of man/woman. People who identify as "genderqueer" may see themselves as being both male and female, being neither male nor female, or falling completely outside these categories.

Intersex

Term for a combination of chromosomes, gonads, hormones, internal sex organs, and genitals that differs from the 2 expected patterns of male or female. In some cases, these traits are visible at birth, and, in others, they are not apparent until puberty. Some chromosomal variations may not be physically apparent at all. Formerly known as hermaphrodite (or hermaphroditic), but these terms now are outdated and derogatory.

Lesbian

A woman who is emotionally, romantically, or sexually attracted to other women.

Living Openly

A state in which LGBTQ people are comfortably out about their sexual orientation or gender identity—where and when it feels appropriate to them.

Nonbinary

An adjective describing a person who does not identify exclusively as a man or a woman. Nonbinary people may identify as being both a man and a woman, somewhere in between, or falling completely outside these categories.

Outing

Exposing someone's lesbian, gay, bisexual, or transgender identity to others without their permission. Outing someone can have serious repercussions on employment, economic stability, personal safety, religious, or family situations.

Queer

An umbrella term to describe individuals who do not identify as straight and/or cisgender and often can be used interchangeably with LGBTQ. Due to its historical/ongoing use as a derogatory term, it is not embraced or used by all LGBTQ people.

Transgender

A term for people whose gender identity and/or expression is different from cultural expectations based on the sex they were assigned at birth or for someone who has transitioned (or is transitioning) from living as one gender to another. Transgender people may identify as straight, gay, lesbian, or bisexual.[6–14]

Sexual orientation and gender identity questions rarely are asked on most health surveys, making it difficult to estimate the true number of LGBTQ individuals within a population and to understand their health needs and challenges. The medical community is lacking the data needed to understand how and why this community is impacted by various social issues and medical illnesses and how best to approach solutions. These data are critical to help guide the data-driven response of states and the nation in their response to health crises—most recently noted with the COVID-19 pandemic.

The assumption of heterosexuality by medical providers serves to reinforce hetero-normative thinking and practice. Older LGBTQ adults thus are rendered invisible. LGBTQ persons often are viewed by medical professional only in relation to their sexuality. This leads to health conditions being diagnosed in relation to the medical professionals' assumptions about sexuality rather than the whole person.[15,16]

Groups and government representatives have proposed legislation to require such data collection and reporting. Assessment must include level of education, lifestyle, work history, level of physical activity, and responsibilities that have an impact on their demands on their time and resources. The AARP report *Caregiving in the United States 2020*[17] found that 8% of caregivers self-identify as lesbian, gay, bisexual, and/or transgender.

LGBTQ individuals face health disparities linked to social stigma, discrimination, and denial of their civil and human rights. Civil and human rights, which has been associated with higher rates of psychiatric disorders, substance abuse, and suicide.[18] This community also faces higher rates of respiratory issues, HIV and AIDS, cancer, and homelessness, putting its members at high risk of greater health impacts from all types of illness.

Research illustrates that older adults from socially and economically disadvantaged populations are at high risk of poor health and premature death. It was only in Healthy People 2020 that LGBTQ people were for the first time identified in the United States as an at-risk population.

A commitment of the National Institutes of Health (NIH) is to reduce and eliminate health disparities for communities that have encountered systemic obstacles to health as a result of social, economic, and environmental disadvantages.[18] Based on the mounting evidence of health disparities across all ages of LGBTQ populations, the NIH launched the Sexual & Gender Minority Research Office in 2015.[2]

The landmark study, *Aging with Pride: National Health, Aging, and Sexuality/Gender Study,* is the first federally funded longitudinal national project designed to better understand the aging, health, and well-being of LGBTQ midlife and older adults and their families. It is funded through a federal grant from the NIH and the National Institute on Aging. With more than 2400 LGBTQ adults ranging in age from 50 to over 100, this project hopes to deepen the understanding of how various life experiences are related to changes in aging, health, and well-being over time. The findings paint a vivid portrait of the lives of LGBTQ midlife and older adults, documenting the interplay of risk and resilience to further understand those reaching their full aging and health potential and those most at risk of health, social, and economic disparities. This project is a collaboration with 17 community agencies serving LGBTQ older adults in every census division throughout the United States.[1,2]

Although most Americans face challenges as they age, LGBTQ elders have the added burden of a lifetime of stigma; familial relationships that lack legal recognition; and unequal treatment under laws, programs, and services designed to support and protect older Americans. Furthermore, the lack of financial security, health care, and social and community support is a fearful reality for a disproportionate number of LGBTQ older adults.[19–22] Older lesbians came of age during a time when same-sex relationships were severely stigmatized and even criminalized, and same-sex identities were socially invisible.[23,24] That said, a positive experience of "coming out" and developing an affirmative lesbian, gay, bisexual (LGB) identity enables individual to develop strengths and strategies that can be used in later life.[15] It is important to understand how a lifetime of experience has an impact on the health and well-being of these individuals as they age.

CLINICAL CARE
Psychological Aspects

The prevalence of depression and anxiety may be higher in sexual minority older adults who have experienced a lifetime of chronic stress and challenges, including concealment of one's true identity; internalized stigma; gender dysphoria; social isolation; abandonment by family, friends, and religious communities; discrimination in the workplace, in housing opportunities, and by local and national government; and psychological, emotional, and physical victimization.

Even bereavement over the loss of a partner is different for sexual minority older adults and can have an impact on their psychological well-being and adjustment to loss. A study by Ingham and colleagues[25] demonstrated 3 themes:

1. Being alone encapsulated feelings of isolation and exclusion.
2. Navigating visibility centred on how homophobia led to a lack of recognition of the women's grief.
3. Finding new places to be authentic related women's need to develop new relationships in which they could comfortably be themselves.

The availability of a supportive social network provides protective factors and increases resilience, decreasing the odds of psychological and physical health challenges.

It is critical that future efforts include recognition of the unique challenges and needs for survivors of same-sex partner loss and creating competencies and strategies for culturally competent bereavement care.

Social Aspects

Physical health and function in later years are influenced by social aspects and variants throughout individuals' lives, including family structure, socioeconomic status, and housing stability. Each of these factors may look different in the lives of older LGBTQ women because of isolation, inability to marry, not having children, job insecurity and pay inequality, and housing discrimination.

Social determinants affecting the health of LGBTQ individuals largely relate to oppression and discrimination. Examples identified by Healthy People 2020 include the following:

- Legal discrimination in access to health insurance, employment, housing, marriage, adoption, and retirement benefits
- Lack of law protecting against bullying in schools
- Lack of social programs targeted to and/or appropriate for LGBTQ youth, adults, and elders
- Shortage of health care providers who are knowledgeable and culturally competent in LGBTQ health

Although older LGBTQ adults are more likely to be partnered, they are less likely to be married, which may have implications for health care advocacy, caregiving, and the availability of financial resources as they age.[23,24]

Thus, the social support system of older lesbians differs from other older women, because they are more likely to depend on friends and partners, their "Family of Choice," than relatives for support. It is important to explore and respect this nontraditional network in determining available supports and caregivers and in development of a successful plan of care for aging lesbian women.

Although studies have shown differing accounts of financial status and stability among older LGBTQ persons, these factors may contribute to financial challenges in later years and in retirement. The *Caring and Aging with Pride* study[40] revealed that most LGBTQ older adults in the United States reported experiencing disadvantages and discrimination in work environments, which have fostered long-term economic inequities and may have resulted in an elevated need for full-time employment among the oldest LGBTQ adults.[1,2] They found significant differences between age cohorts of LGBTQ older adults, with approximately 40% of those older than age 80 living at or below the federal poverty level.[5]

An emerging concern for many LGBTQ older adults is competent and compassionate long-term care. As older LGBTQ adults age, fear and anxiety of being outed, disrespected, mistreated, and harmed are compounded by their vulnerability in requiring assistance for daily needs. A study by Stein and colleagues[26] found that older LGBTQ adults living in both the community and in long-term care facilities feared being mistreated or ostracized by peers as well as the staff in those facilities. Older LGBTQ adults who move into skilled nursing homes often choose to stay closeted. This loss of a safe space, a true home, where one can fully be oneself, is detrimental to quality of life and overall well-being.[27]

The SAGE National LGBT Elder Housing Initiative provides advocacy and services for LGBTQ elders. They report that 48% of older same-sex couples have experienced housing discrimination. Initiated in New York City, the program expanded nationwide in 2015 to identify LGBTQ-friendly housing that provides affordable, sensitive, respectful, and compassionate care.

In the past 2 decades, there has been significant strides in support and recognition of the rights of same-sex couples, including the legalization of marriage resulting from the 2015 Supreme Court decision mandating the constitutional right to marry. A notable event was the endorsement of same-sex civil unions (but not marriage) by Catholic Pontiff, Pope Francis, in October 2020. These advances are under relentless fire from various groups, however, and are in constant peril because the right to marry could be overturned by a Supreme Court who majority members do not deem this case to be settled law, leaving LGBTQ persons feeling vulnerable and even fearful for their rights and safety.

Medical Aspects

It has been postulated that lifetime experiences of victimization among sexual minority older adults affects their mental health later in life and that the physiologic impact of these chronic stressors may partially account for higher rates of disability among older LGBTQ adults.[23,24] Many LGBTQ older adults have historically avoided and delayed receiving health care out of fear of being mistreated, disrespected, and even harmed by health care providers.[27]

Communication skills are critical so that mixed messages are not unintentionally sent that may be perceived as negative judgments. Part of becoming more competent, welcoming, and inclusive providers of care to LGBTQ individuals is cultivating an awareness of personal beliefs and biases toward LGBTQ persons and their families.[27] To improve the health and care of LGBTQ persons, Healthy People 2020 encourages the training of medical, nursing, and other health students in the provision of culturally competent care.

It is important to ask in an appropriate and supportive way about a patient's sexual orientation and gender identity to enhance the patient-provider interaction and care relationship. Individuals, however, should never be forced to disclose this information. This critical communication may be complicated further by issues, such as language and hearing or visual impairments, and the appropriate accommodations must be made thoughtfully.

Several studies have shown that older LGBTQ persons have higher rates of risk behaviors, including excessive drinking, smoking, and obesity, which may, at least in part, result from a lifetime of isolation and victimization. In addition, older lesbian and bisexual women are less likely to have health insurance than their heterosexual female peers.[5] These factors contribute to higher rates of medical illness, including cardiovascular disease, diabetes, and cancer.

Although there have been mixed findings, lesbian and bisexual women may be at risk of not utilizing preventive health care and screenings (eg, routine checkups, mammograms, and Pap tests). Lesbians are less likely to get preventive services for cancer, as reported by Healthy People 2020.

A higher incidence of malignancies of the breast is thought to be attributable to elevated prevalence of obesity, substance use, and nulliparity. And malignancies of the lung are likely associated with higher rates of smoking.

Clinical Care Points

- LGBTQ older adults face many of the same health challenges as other older adults and also may have additional medical, psychological, and social needs.
- LGBTQ older adults often are underserved by the health care system. LGBTQ adults may have difficulty in disclosing sexual orientation because of prior negative experiences in the health care system and/or as a result of experiencing and fearing societal discrimination. Lack of disclosure can lead to poor access to care and sometimes inappropriate care.
- As transgender adults age, they may be more likely to encounter health issues that correspond to their biological sex; these patients may need help in coping with a disease or condition associated with their prior gender. In addition, providers must be aware of potential effects and screening guidelines based on prior surgical or hormonal treatments.
- LGBTQ older adults are more likely to live alone, be single, and not have children. They may rely more on extensive networks of friends rather than family. As they age, they may be at greater risk of isolation. As they become more reliant on others, their sense of vulnerability may enhance their fears of discrimination, especially in nursing home, assisted living and home health settings.[28,29]

WOMEN VETERANS

A 2020 study in the *Journal of Traumatic Stress* has found that military veterans who identify as LGBTQ are twice as likely to experience incidents of sexual assault while on active-duty compared with non-LGBTQ service members. The significantly higher rate of sexual assault experienced by these demographics increases the likelihood of enduring symptoms of posttraumatic stress disorder or depression later in life. Of the lesbian and bisexual female veterans who participated in the study, 57.5% reported experiencing sexual assault, compared with 37.4% of non-LGBTQ female veterans.

TRANSGENDER ISSUES

The term, transgender, generally refers to people whose gender identity is at odds with the gender they were assigned at birth according to the physiologic characteristics of their bodies. For example, a transgender woman is a person who was born physiologically male but whose deepest sense of self is as female. The critical point for transgender individuals is that there is incongruence between their gender identity and their birth sex. The intensity of this incongruence can vary, and transgender individuals may choose varying degrees of transition.[30–32]

It is important not to conflate sexual and gender identity because they are separate constructs (eg, transgender individuals may have a heterosexual, bisexual, lesbian, or gay sexual identity).[33]

Transgender individuals have unique health needs, and the approach to their care generally is lacking in medical school curricula. Because of estrangements from their families, lack of affordable housing, mental health and addiction problems, and emotional and physical abuse, as many as 1 in 5 transgender youth becomes homeless. They have fewer legal protections from job and housing discrimination, and some turn to sex work, increasing their risk for exposure to sexually transmitted disease and physical violence.[30]

In a 2019 review by Fredriksen and colleagues,[33] transgender older adults compared with nontransgender counterparts had the highest rates of victimization and discrimination, with reports ranging from 57% to 69% of participants. Rate of lifetime discrimination and victimization were associated with poorer physical health, disability, chronic illness, depression, and lower mental health–related quality of life.

There are multiple antitrans bills being reviewed in the US government. These measures target transgender and nonbinary people for discrimination, such as by barring access to or even criminalizing the use of appropriate facilities, including restrooms, restricting transgender students' ability to fully participate in school and sports, barring health care for transgender youth, allowing religiously motivated discrimination against trans people, or making it more difficult for trans people to get identification documents with their name and gender.[34–38]

According to the Human Rights Campaign, at least 22 transgender and nonconforming people—almost all were black transgender women—were killed in 2019 in the United States.[6] Twenty-six percent of transgender and gender nonconfirming individuals have been physically assaulted and 10% have been sexually assaulted. In 1 study, 78% experienced gender-related psychological abuse and 50% experienced gender-related physical abuse. The Transgender Day of Remembrance is held in November of each year to memorialize those who were killed due to antitransgender hatred or prejudice.[30]

The American Society of Plastic Surgeons 2016 annual report included 1759 male-to-female (MTF) patients undergoing gender-confirmation surgery (GCS). In addition, many surgeries are performed by other surgical subspecialties (eg, urologist, obstetricians/gynecologist, and maxillofacial surgeons). In 1 large study, among MTF individuals, 10% had vaginoplasty or labiaplasty, 9% orchiectomy, 8% augmentation mammoplasty, and 6% facial surgery.[30]

Because GCS can cost in the range of $30,000 in the United States and generally is not covered by health insurance, many transgender individuals have gone abroad for surgery, Thailand being a common destination.[30]

Social and medical history must be approached in a supportive, nonjudgmental manner that communicates sensitivity and empathy and will facilitate trust. Improving access can be facilitated by providing a welcoming environment for transgender patients: adding a "transgender" option to checklists on patient visit records; referring to body parts with gender-neutral language whenever possible, such as "chest" and "genitals"; and avoiding using gender-based pronouns. Ask how the patient would like to be addressed, by what pronoun, and what name. Guidelines for creating a welcoming office environment for transgender patients have been developed by the Gay and Lesbian Medical Association and can be found online at http://www.glma.org.[30]

Important information to obtain when caring for transgender persons includes all medications, including hormone use (past or present) and silicone injections (often done by nonmedical persons using nonmedical grade or contaminated materials with a shared needle); a full review of systems (transgender persons may be hesitant to report chest pain or dyspnea as they fear that the provider will stop estrogen therapy); lifestyle and health care practices (smoking, alcohol use, diet, exercise, safe sex, and so forth); surgical procedures (past or planned); mental health issues; and history of sexually transmitted illness.

IMPORTANT ASPECTS OF THE PHYSICAL EXAMINATION FOR TRANSGENDER WOMEN

- Evaluation for signs of blood clots
- Scarring from surgeries or silicone injections
- Malignancy of sex organs
- Annual prostate examination (it is not removed in GCS surgery)
- Pap test to screen for squamous cell carcinoma (the glans penis is used to create a clitoris)
- Screening for heart disease, cancer, and adverse effects of hormone therapy (blood clots, diabetes, blood pressure changes, and cancer) is critical.
- Laboratory work should include screening for transmissible diseases, such as hepatitis and human immunodeficiency virus, and an annual prolactin level.

With regard to breast cancer screening, transgender women differ from nontransgender women in the length of exposure to estrogens as well as variable exposure to progestogens. It is recommended that screening not commence in transgender women until after a minimum of 5 years of feminizing hormone use, regardless of age. Some providers may choose to discuss the risks and unknowns with patients and delay screening until after up to 10 years of feminizing hormone use. It is recommended that screening mammography be performed every 2 years, once the age of 50 and 5 years to 10 years of feminizing hormone use criteria have been met. Providers and patients should engage in discussions that include the risks of overscreening and an assessment of individual risk factors.[39]

Aging postoperative MTF patients may have increased risk for genitourinary complications caused by the compounded effects of aging and postsurgical complications. Complaints of frequent, hesitancy, urgency, and dysuria should be assessed, keeping in mind that the complaints could be prostate related.[30]

It also is important to have a working knowledge of a person's insurance coverage to avoid unexpected expenses that may create obstacles to care.

Providing medical care for transgender persons may feel uncomfortable or intimidating due to a lack of familiarity with their particular care needs. It is important to understand limitations and biases and to be able to respectfully refer patients to providers who are more experienced and can provide the competent and culturally sensitive care they deserve, if needed.

FUTURE RESEARCH

Many health-related organizations and publications, including the Centers for Disease Control and Prevention, Healthy People 2020, and the Institutes of Medicine, have identified health disparities related to sexual orientation as one of the main gaps in current health research.

Although there has been more research on the health issues of LGBTQ persons in recent years, there remains a dearth of research regarding the oldest in this community as well as bisexuals, nonbinary older adults, persons of color, and those living in poverty.[1,2]

AREAS FOR FUTURE RESEARCH

- Cardiovascular risk/diagnosis/interventions (including minorities)
- Benefits/opportunities/protective factors of "family of choice"
- Risk factors contributing to obesity
- Relationship between internalized stigma, disability, and poor general health
- Heterogeneity within LGBTQ communities
- LGBTQ wellness model

SUMMARY

It is crucial for gerontological practitioners to be aware of and sensitive to the specific histories and needs of LGBTQ older adults, including issues of lifetime and current victimization, and the effect those experiences have on access to care, safety, and quality of life.[5]

To shift practice to promote health equity, practitioners need to assess their own overt and covert biases regarding LGBTQ persons and understand how these, as well as the lives of LGBTQ persons, have been and continue to be shaped by contested, shifting sociocultural and historical discourses. Practitioners must use their practice knowledge and commitment to social justice to advocate for policy change and equitable access to services.[33]

RESOURCES/COMMUNITY ADVOCATES

Fenway Health (LGBT Aging Project)
    https://fenwayhealth.org
GLMA: Health Professionals Advancing LGBTQ Equality (previously known as the Gay & Lesbian Medical Association): 1133 19th Street NW, Suite 302, Washington, DC 20036; (202) 600-8037
    http://glma.org/
Healthy People 2020
    https://www.healthypeople.gov/
Human Rights Campaign
    https://www.hrc.org/
Lambda Legal
    https://www.lambdalegal.org/
Movement Advancement Project
    https://www.lgbtmap.org/
National Coalition for LGBT Health
    https://healthlgbt.org/
National Gay and Lesbian Taskforce
    https://www.thetaskforce.org/
NIH Sexual & Gender Minority Research Office
    https://dpcpsi.nih.gov/sgmro
National Resource Center on LGBT Aging (a project of www.sageusa.org)

https://www.lgbtagingcenter.org/
Safe Zone Project
https://thesafezoneproject.com
SAGE national headquarters: 305 7th Avenue, 15th Floor, New York, NY 10001; (212) 741-2247
https://sageusa.org
Transgender Law Center
https://transgenderlawcenter.org/
World Professional Association of Transgender Health
https://www.wpath.org/

REFERENCES

1. Fredriksen Goldsen KI, Jen S, Muraco A. Iridescent life course: LGBTQ aging research and blueprint for the future - a systematic review. Gerontology 2019; 65(3):253–74.
2. Fredriksen Goldsen K, Kim HJ, Jung H, et al. The evolution of aging with pride-national health, aging, and sexuality/gender study: illuminating the iridescent life course of LGBTQ adults aged 80 Years and older in the United States. Int J Aging Hum Dev 2019b;88(4):380–404.
3. Gay and Lesbian Medical Association. Available at: http://www.glma.org. Accessed November 3, 2020.
4. Fredriksen Goldsen & Kim, 2017.
5. Emlet CA. Social, economic, and health disparities among LGBT older adults. Generations 2016;40(2):16–22.
6. Human Rights Campaign. Available at: https://www.hrc.org/. Accessed November 3, 2020.
7. Ingham division of health research, faculty of health and medicine, Lancaster University, Lancaster, England. Available at: UKCorrespondencecharlotteingham@me.com.
8. Eccles CF, Armitage JR, Murray CD. Same-sex partner bereavement in older women: an interpretative phenomenological analysis. Aging Ment Health 2016; 21(9):917–25.
9. Kushalnagar P, Miller CA. Health disparities among mid-to-older deaf LGBTQ adults compared with mid-to-older deaf non-LGBTQ adults in the United States. Health Equity 2019;3(1):541–7.
10. Legislation affecting LGBT rights across the country. 2020. Available at: ACLU.org. Accessed August 1, 2020.
11. LGBTQ Rights. Milestones fast facts. Atlanta (GA): CNN Editorial Research; 2020.
12. Safe Zone project. Available at: https://thesafezoneproject.com. Accessed November 12, 2020.
13. Schuyler AC, Klemmer C, Marney MR, et al. Experiences of sexual Harassment, stalking, and sexual assault during military service among LGBT and non-LGBT service members. J Trauma Stress 2020;33(3):257–66.
14. Services and Advocacy for GLBT Elders. Understanding and meeting the needs of LGBT elders. New York: SAGE News; 2010.
15. Cronin A, King A. Power, inequality and identification: exploring diversity and intersectionality amongst older LGB adults source. Sociology 2010;44(5):876–92.
16. Caceres BA, Brody A, Luscombe RE, et al. A systematic review of cardiovascular disease in sexual minorities. Am J Public Health 2017;107(4):e13–21.

17. AARP and National Alliance for Caregiving. Caregiving in the United States 2020. Washington, DC: AARP; 2020. https://doi.org/10.26419/ppi.00103.003. Available at:.

18. Healthy People 2020 [Internet]. Washington, DC: U.S. Department of Health and Human Services, Office of Disease Prevention and Health Promotion. Available at: https://www.healthypeople.gov/2020. Accessed September 14, 2020.

19. Orel NA. Investigating the needs and concerns of lesbian, gay, bisexual, and transgender older adults: the use of qualitative and quantitative methodology. J Homosex 2014;61(1):53–78.

20. Peel E, Taylor H, Harding R. Sociolegal and practice implications of caring for LGBT people with dementia. Nurs Old People 2016;28(10):26–30.

21. Poteat T. Top 10 Things lesbians should discuss with their healthcare provider. GLMA; 2012. Available at: http://www.glma.org. Accessed July 14, 2020.

22. Services and Advocacy for GLBT Elders. Understanding and meeting the needs of LGBT elders. SAGE News 2010; Available at: https://www.sageusa.org/.

23. Fredriksen Goldsen KI, Emlet CA, Kim HJ, et al. The physical and mental health of lesbian, gay male, and bisexual (LGB) older adults: the role of key health indicators and risk and protective factors. Gerontologist 2013;53(4):664–75.

24. Fredriksen Goldsen KI, Kim HJ, Barkan SE, et al. Health disparities among lesbian, gay, and bisexual older adults: results from a population-based study. Am J Public Health 2013;103(10):1802–9.

25. Ingham CF, Eccles F, Armitage JR, et al. Same-sex partner bereavement in older women: an interpretative phenomenological analysis; Aging & Mental Health 2016; p. 917–25.

26. Stein GL, Beckerman NL, Sherman PA. Lesbian and gay elders and long-term care: identifying the unique psychosocial perspectives and challenges. J Gerontol Soc Work 2010;53(5):421–35.

27. Steelman E. Person-centered care for LGBT older adults. J Gerontol Nurs 2018; 44(2):3–5.

28. Harper GM, Lyons WL, Potter FJ. Geriatrics review syllabus (10th edition): Lesbian, gay, bisexual, transgender health. New York: American Geriatrics Society; 2019.

29. Hughes TL, Veldhuis CB, Drabble LA, et al. Research on alcohol and other drug (AOD) use among sexual minority women: a global scoping review. PLoS One 2020;15(3):e0229869.

30. Mesics S. Clinical care of the transgender patient. Sacramento (CA): NetCE; 2018.

31. Molnar F, Frank CC. Optimizing geriatric care with the GERIATRIC 5Ms. Can Fam Physician 2019;65(1):39.

32. National Institutes of Health. Sexual & gender minority research office. Available at: https://dpcpsi.nih.gov/sgmro. Accessed November 2, 2020.

33. Fredriksen Goldsen KI, Simoni JM, Kim H-J, et al. The health equity promotion Model: reconceptualization of lesbian, gay, bisexual, and transgender (LGBT) health disparities. Am J Orthopsychiatry 2014;84(6):653–63.

34. American Civil Liberties Union. 2020. Available at: https://www.aclu.org/legislation-affecting-lgbt-rights-across-country. Accessed November 3, 2020.

35. Blosnich JR, Silenzio VM. Physical health indicators among lesbian, gay, and bisexual U.S. veterans. Ann Epidemiol 2013;23(7):448–51.

36. Brennan-Ing M, Seidel L, Larson B, et al. Social care networks and older LGBT adults: challenges for the future. J Homosex 2014;61(1):21–52.

37. Brodeur N. Are LGBTQ seniors dying of loneliness? It's possible, Research says. Washington, DC: The Seattle Times; 2019. Local News.
38. Cancer facts for lesbian and bisexual women. American Cancer Society; 2020. Available at: https://www.cancer.org. Accessed July 2020.
39. Deutsch MB. Screening for breast cancer in transgender women. UCSF transgender care. Available at: https://transcare.ucsf.edu/guidelines/breast-cancer-women. Accessed November 3, 2020.
40. Fredriksen-Goldsen KI, Kim H-J, Emlet CA, et al. The Aging and Health Report: Disparities and Resilience among Lesbian, Gay, Bisexual, and Transgender Older Adults - Key Findings Fact Sheet. Seattle (WA): Institute for Multigenerational Health; 2011.

Brain Health

Tania Alchalabi, MD, Christina Prather, MD*

KEYWORDS

- Brain health • Aging • Women • Healthy brain • Dementia • Cognitive impairment

KEY POINTS

- Brain health is the preservation of mental and cognitive function with the goal of optimal cognitive, emotional, psychological, and behavioral functioning.
- Developing and maintaining a healthy brain requires healthy development, the ability to adapt and respond to stress and adversity, promotion of healthy behaviors, and building resilience to contend with the variable demands of everyday life.
- The healthy aging brain continues to function to meet a variety of needs, including cognition, motor function, emotional regulation, and tactile function.
- Although aging itself is not associated with loss of brain health, age is a risk factor for many conditions associated with memory loss and other disorders of cognition.
- Many chronic conditions that are more common among older adults, such as diabetes mellitus, advanced renal disease, and heart failure, are associated with cognitive loss.

INTRODUCTION
Overview

According to the World Health Organization (WHO), between 2015 and 2050 the proportion of the world's population older than 60 years will nearly double, from 12% to 22%.[1] In 2015, the number of persons aged 60 years and older was 900 million and is expected to increase to 2 billion by 2050.[1] The overall pace of population aging is much faster than in the past.[1] Although aging itself is not associated with increased disease, many conditions associated with memory loss and other disorders of cognition have age as a risk factor. Older persons are at increased risk of memory loss and other disorders of cognition, including Alzheimer disease (AD) and related dementias (ADRD). Related dementias include other neurodegenerative conditions, such as dementia with Lewy body (DLB), frontotemporal dementia (FTD), and vascular dementia. Cognitive loss is increasingly associated with other chronic conditions that are more common among older adults, such as diabetes mellitus, advanced renal disease, and heart failure.[2,3] Other late life conditions, such as Parkinson disease, also can be associated with impaired cognitive functioning. As the number of older individuals

Division of Geriatrics and Palliative Medicine, The George Washington University School of Medicine and Health Sciences, 2300 M Street Northwest, Suite 3-335, Washington, DC 20037, USA
* Corresponding author.
E-mail address: cprather@mfa.gwu.edu

Clin Geriatr Med 37 (2021) 593–604
https://doi.org/10.1016/j.cger.2021.05.006
0749-0690/21/© 2021 Elsevier Inc. All rights reserved.

increases, the prevalence of conditions associated with increased risk of cognitive loss will increase and efforts to improve and maintain brain health will be critical.

What Is Brain Health

A healthy brain is important for individuals to maintain independence, to engage in what matters most to them, and to be able to participate in life. Currently, there is no consensus definition for the term brain health. The Centers for Disease Control and Prevention (CDC) defines brain health as the ability to perform all the mental processes of cognition, including the ability to learn and judge, use language, and remember.[4] The American Heart Association uses a functional definition of brain health grounded in performance, defining brain health as "average performance levels among all people at that age who are free of known brain or other organ system diseases in terms of decline from function levels, or as adequacy to perform all activities that the individual wishes to undertake."[5] The WHO provides a more fluid definition of brain health, describing it as "an emerging and growing concept that encompasses neural development, plasticity, functioning, and recovery across the life course."[1]

We propose a definition of brain health in line with Wang and colleagues,[6] who describe it as "the preservation of optimal brain integrity and mental and cognitive function and the absence of overt neurologic disorders." The term brain health, as used in this article, emphasizes the preservation of optimal brain integrity and mental and cognitive function with the goal of enabling every individual to optimize their cognitive, emotional, psychological, and behavioral functioning. Developing and maintaining a healthy brain requires healthy development, the ability to adapt and respond to stress and adversity, promotion of healthy behaviors, and building resilience to contend with the variable demands of everyday life.[1]

In this article, we present the normal aging brain and factors that contribute to maintaining brain health in later life. We highlight the differences between a normal aging brain and abnormal aging. This article is limited to an overview of factors that can contribute to brain health and should serve as an introduction that fuels additional reading and deeper learning on topics of interest.

AGING AND COGNITION
Neurogenesis

The aging brain continues to evolve, adapt, and develop new connections. A key mechanism through which this occurs is neurogenesis, the process of forming new neurons from neural stem cells. In the healthy aging brain, neurogenesis continues throughout life. Neurogenesis occurring in the dentate gyrus of the hippocampus is associated with important cognitive processes that remain essential for aging adults, such as memory encoding, mood regulation, pattern separation, and cognitive flexibility.[7] Increasing evidence suggests that when neurogenesis in the hippocampus is dysregulated, these processes become dysfunctional, presenting as cognitive decline in neurologic conditions, and increased psychological symptoms in psychiatric conditions.[7] This process is shown in **Fig. 1**.

Neurogenesis occurs through a process of regulatory feedback informed by the microenvironment surrounding neural stem cells. The main components of this microenvironment are mature neurons, neuronal progenitors, endothelial cells, ependymal cells, astrocytes, and microglia. This microenvironment is essential to the normal functioning of stem cells, including coordinating their behavior and interactions with their surroundings. The microenvironment is also essential to establishing control of cell proliferation, differentiation, and apoptosis.[3] Through this regulation, intermediate

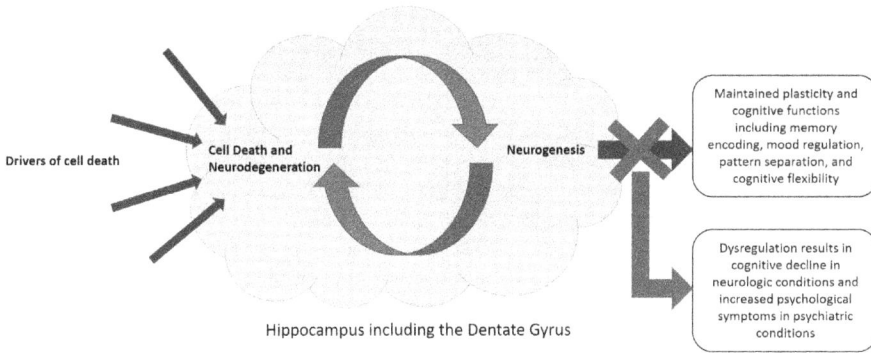

Fig. 1. Neurogenesis and cognition hypothesis.

progenitors and neuroblasts are amplified, growing into neurons that are subsequently integrated into existing neural circuits.[7]

The specific role newly formed neurons play in learning and memory remains controversial, with variable acceptance regarding their role in direct learning and memory. Some hypotheses propose that neurogenesis is more crucial for complex tasks, such as pattern recognition and cognitive flexibility.[8] Regardless of the specific role newly formed neurons play, it is well recognized that impaired neurogenesis is abnormal, and plays an important role in loss of normally functioning cognitive processes. Research that explores the influencing factors on neurogenesis will be important in the understanding of brain health in the years to come.

Normal Aging Brain

Normal aging of any organ or organism is impacted by numerous factors. Some factors that influence aging include the environment, genetics and epigenetics, education, nutrition, trauma, stress and inflammation, socioeconomic status, social factors, sex, ethnicity, and disease. **Fig. 2** shows a limited selection of factors that influence aging.

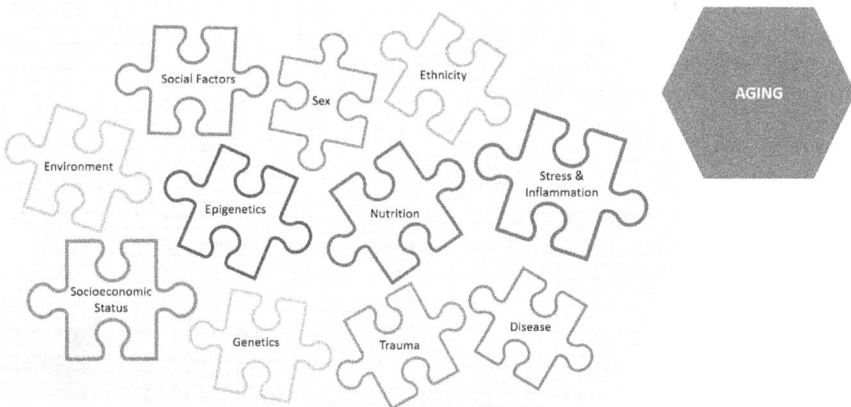

Fig. 2. Factors that influence brain health through their influence on aging.

Each contribute collectively to how we age and their impact on the brain is no exception. Research increasingly shows each of these factors inform cognition, one of the many functions of the extraordinarily complex human brain. Less well understood is how each of these factors interact and to what degree they affect the brain's function, but what is widely agreed on, is that each contributes to brain health.

The aging brain undergoes predictable changes. At the cellular level, cell death occurs leading to loss of synaptic contacts, the points at which neurons connect, which can provoke decline in cognitive functioning. In the healthy aging brain, neurogenesis overcomes predictable cell death, enabling the ongoing ability for remodeling and retraining neural connections. This enables healthy older adults to maintain brain health with fully affective and intellectual capabilities despite advanced age.

Aging in the brain is also influenced by the cardiovascular system and the complex highways of vascular networks that are essential for brain health. Changes in cardiac output related to heart disease, as well as atherosclerosis and loss of elasticity in aging blood vessels, impact the delivery of nutrients, as well as waste and potential toxins, to the brain. Changes resulting from luminal occlusions and atherosclerosis in blood vessels involved in cerebrovascular flow can cause microischemic changes. In some studies, these changes have been seen in up to 28% of cognitively healthy older adults.[2] Aging brains in adults without cognitive complaints also may show signs of white matter changes and dilated perivascular spaces with microbleeds on MRI.[2]

Inflammation, chronic illnesses such as obesity and diabetes, and poor nutrition also influence the aging brain. Each of these is a risk factor for stroke and cardiovascular disease, which are well-established risk factors for poor brain health that may manifest through cognitive impairment and, in advanced functional loss, dementia.[5] Independently each of these factors also influences the health of neurons through impacts on the microenvironment at the cellular level. Each should be recognized for their role in contributing to brain health and the potential to disrupt healthy brain aging.

Last, volume loss or atrophy of the overall brain is also normal within limits during the aging process. In general, atrophy occurs relatively symmetrically across the brain and without localization to regions of critical function. Localized atrophy, such as in the hippocampus or frontal lobe, is a sign of neurologic disease and is not consistent with healthy brain aging. Generalized atrophy is expected and should not preclude older adults from having ongoing integrity of essential brain functioning.

The healthy aging brain permits the brain to continue to function to meet a variety of essential needs, including cognition, motor function, emotional regulation, and tactile function. New signs of dysregulation, dysfunction, or functional dependence are abnormal and should prompt clinical evaluation.

Cognition: What Is It?

Cognition is the mental action or process of acquiring knowledge and understanding through thought, experience, and the senses. It describes the process by which we receive signals from the environment, through touch, sound, sight, hearing, and smells. The brain receives this information while simultaneously applying filters and patterns, or algorithms, to enhance understanding and recognition. These algorithms are generated through a lifetime of learning and continue to evolve across the lifespan. These signals are encoded and stored in the brain as discrete types of information. Data can be stored in the brain in a variety of ways, and retrieval of stored information is informed by how it is stored. Words, for example, can be stored in the brain structurally (how they look), phonemically (how they sound), or semantically (based on meaning). Disorders of cognition can impair data recall, for example, primarily impairing recall of semantic data over phonemic data, such as in AD.

The breadth of cognitive tasks attributed to the brain are routinely described as cognitive domains. Memory is only one domain of cognition, albeit one of the most complex cognitive domains. It includes short-term memory, also called working memory, and describes information held in the brain not yet stored. This can be verbal, spatial, emotional, auditory, tactile, or other types of information. Episodic memory, prospective memory, procedural memory, and semantic memory are types of memory more often associated with the term "long-term memory." Encoding, storage, and retrieval of information all occur within the domain of memory. In addition to memory, the brain performs several other critical cognitive tasks. These fall into the domains of sensation, perception, motor skills and construction, attention and concentration, executive functioning, processing speed, and language.[9] Each of these informs who we are, how we function, and how we interact with the world around us.

Cognitive Changes in Normal Aging

Although the healthy aging brain maintains integrity of many cognitive processes, aging has been shown to result in decline of certain types of cognitive functions across adulthood. Cognitive abilities that are impacted by aging can be described as fluid abilities or crystallized abilities. Fluid abilities primarily rely on processing aspects of cognition, and include things like psychomotor speed, memory, and abstract reasoning. Crystallized abilities describe processes that rely on declarative and procedural knowledge acquired through one's lifetime and include knowledge of vocabulary, social norms, literacy, and acquired skills or facts.[10] Fluid cognitive abilities decline with advancing age, whereas crystallized abilities increase through middle adulthood and are less impacted by advanced age.[10] These changes often manifest as increased wisdom, knowledge, and experience in older adults, while simultaneously presenting with slowed processing, impaired multitasking, and challenges with short-term recall.

Presented another way, the brain processes information differently as we age. For example, if a task is given to both a 20-year-old and an 80-year-old, both may succeed in performing the task, but their brains complete the task differently. The 80-year-old's brain is more likely to exhibit bilateral recruitment of prefrontal regions while completing the task, whereas the 20-year-old's brain exhibits lateral recruitment of the same regions. This demonstrates the hypothesis that older adults may compensate for emerging cognitive challenges by additionally recruiting contralateral regions to contribute to the ongoing task.

The important part to take from this section is that a healthy aging brain evolves and compensates to enable ongoing integrity of essential cognitive functions. Although older brains may perform a task or process information differently from younger brains, healthy older brains are still able to perform the task. This should be emphasized when discussing healthy aging and brain health with older adults, as memory loss in general, and dementia in particular, are not consistent with normal aging.

Optimizing and Maintaining Brain Health

Brain health in later life is positively influenced by minimizing risks to the aging brain and optimizing conditions in which the aging brain thrives. Maintaining a healthy brain is inseparable from maintaining a healthy body and mind overall. Habits that optimize cognition function include quality sleep and good sleep hygiene, mindfulness, exercise, nutrition, and purposeful living. Each of these factors both independently and collectively can lead to better brain health. Conversely, avoiding factors that negatively impact brain health, such as excess alcohol and other potential toxins, smoking, polypharmacy, high-risk medications, purposeless living, and poor nutrition, can minimize risk to brain health. A third component of brain health is attentive management of disease-specific risk factors that confer risk of cognitive loss, notably conditions associated with vascular disease, including obesity, diabetes, hypertension, hypercholesterolemia, heart disease, and stroke. Managing chronic health conditions like hypertension and diabetes mellitus can promote a healthier brain and prevent further cell damage. These factors are presented collectively in **Fig. 3**.

To emphasize the importance of controlling and managing vascular risk factors to optimize brain health, one need look no further than the popular trial, the Systolic Blood Pressure Intervention Trial (SPRINT) Memory and Cognition in Decreased Hypertension (SPRINT MIND). In this 9000-person study of community-dwelling older adults, intensive blood pressure lowering measurably decreased the incidence of mild cognitive impairment (MCI). Lack of observed change in incident dementia is attributed to the short duration of follow-up. Secondary outcomes importantly included increased risk of falls, a potentially devastating outcome in older adults.[11] This study highlights the importance of thoughtfully considering application of novel literature to older adults who often have multicomplexity that necessitates person-centered, priority-driven care plans that align with what matters most to individual patients.

Developing a plan to optimize brain health is personal and must align with individual patient priorities as well as possibilities. It is important to emphasize that there is no single pill or medication that eliminates memory changes or improves brain health. When we discuss strategies to minimize or slow memory loss and other cognitive changes with patients, we emphasize there is no magic pill. Instead, for each individual we discuss collective efforts involving different aspects of life that might lead to better overall well-being and consequently, improved brain health. These efforts are grounded in the essential components critical to maintaining a healthy brain: exercise, nutrition, purpose, mindfulness, quality sleep, toxin avoidance, and management of medical risk factors.

Nutrition and Brain Health

Nutrition plays a critical role in brain health. Nutrition directly informs the micronutrients neurons receive through blood flow and influences neurogenesis through manipulation of the microenvironment essential to the birth and integration of new

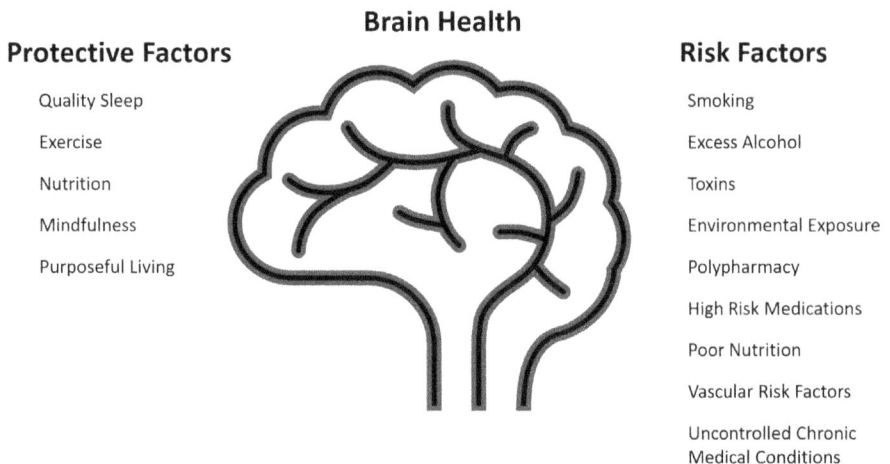

Brain Health

Protective Factors

Quality Sleep

Exercise

Nutrition

Mindfulness

Purposeful Living

Risk Factors

Smoking

Excess Alcohol

Toxins

Environmental Exposure

Polypharmacy

High Risk Medications

Poor Nutrition

Vascular Risk Factors

Uncontrolled Chronic
Medical Conditions

Fig. 3. Influential clinical factors on brain health.

neurons throughout the lifespan. In addition, inflammation, micronutrient deficiencies or excess, and macronutrient metabolism are some of the mechanisms by which brain health is affected by nutrition.

Nutrition also plays an important role in the development of chronic conditions, such as diabetes mellitus and obesity, which are precursors to vascular disease, which is itself an independent risk factor for cognitive loss. Unfortunately, disparate food access and health deserts in predominantly underserved communities highlight health disparities through lack of access to nutritious food and resultant increased incidence of conditions associated with vascular disease and other conditions that increase risk to brain health.

The modern Western diet, which is high in saturated fats and low in whole and plant-based foods, is shown in some studies to be potentially detrimental to cognitive health. In one rodent study, a traditional Western diet impaired hippocampal-dependent cognitive function.[12] In another study, it resulted in dysfunction of the blood–brain barrier (BBB) and dysfunctional glucose regulation in the central nervous system. Conversely, intermittent ketosis, atypical in the Western diet, may have protective effects on the hippocampus and BBB.[13] This finding has fueled interest in intermittent fasting as a protective mechanism for cognitive loss and to delay ongoing cognitive impairment.

Diets that are high in omegas and whole and plant-based foods have claimed neuroprotective benefits. Some studies suggest that diets such as the Mediterranean Diet and MIND Diet may positively impact brain function, promote better brain health, and prevent memory loss.[12] In populations studied outside their native diet, dementia rates mimic those of western or European ancestry, as was shown in a study on incidence of dementia in Japanese Americans compared with native Japanese.[14] Increasingly, whole food and plant-based diets are shown to improve cardiovascular risk factors, which are inferred to decrease risk to brain health through improvement of underlying risk factors, such as hypertension, obesity, hypercholesterolemia, and chronic inflammation, and directly through increased consumption of anti-inflammatory and other foods important in brain health.

ALZHEIMER DISEASE AND RELATED DEMENTIAS
The Dementia Syndrome

The dementia syndrome represents failing brain health and atypical aging of the adult brain. Dementia, clinically classified as Major Neurodegenerative Disorder, is defined as significant cognitive decline from a previous level of performance in one or more cognitive domains (including complex attention, executive function, learning and memory, language, perceptual-motor, or social cognition). Individuals must demonstrate substantial impairment in cognitive performance on validated testing methods and either the individual or a knowledgeable informant must endorse concern for a significant decline in cognitive function. Cognitive deficits must be sufficient to interfere with independence in daily activities and not occur in the presence of an acute or fluctuating change in mentation, such as delirium, nor can they be better explained by a different psychiatric condition.

AD is a well-recognized cause of the dementia syndrome. AD is one of several neurologic conditions associated with degeneration of cells of the nervous system that causes the dementia syndrome, which classically includes memory loss, personality change, impaired executive function, and ultimately, functional dependence. Other neurodegenerative processes that result in the dementia syndrome include DLB, FTD or frontotemporal lobar degeneration, and vascular dementia. Although each has its own unique pathologies and clinical trajectories, their clinical syndromes are devastatingly similar in that the result is an insult to brain health that ultimately strips individuals of autonomy and independence without present options for meaningful pharmacologic treatment or disease-modifying therapies.

In addition to the neurodegenerative disorders mentioned, a dementia-like syndrome can result from a broad variety of conditions that result in injury to the brain. Through traumatic brain injury, intracranial bleeding, or diffuse axonal injury, cognitive changes can occur. In other conditions of neurodegeneration, such as Parkinson's disease, amyotrophic lateral sclerosis, and multisystem atrophy, the dementia syndrome also can occur. This list represents a small number of conditions that pose a risk to brain health, which also tend to occur in later life.

Preventing Alzheimer Disease and Related Dementias and Loss of Brain Health

Given the limited options presently available to slow or abort disease progression for many of the underlying causes of the dementia syndrome, increasingly efforts are focused on disease prevention. As currently understood, for each type of dementia, there is associated a putative protein or set of proteins, or underlying pathology such as vascular disease, which has been implicated in the cause and progression of the neurodegenerative process. Whether it is the amyloid plaques and tau neurofibrillary tangles associated with AD, the tau or ubiquitin proteins of frontotemporal dementia, or the cytoplasmic α-synuclein inclusion bodies of DLB and Parkinson's disease dementia, it is the accumulation of these proteins or protein aggregates within the brain that set off a cascade of events that directly impact neuronal function and ultimately cause cell death in a disease-specific pattern.

Ongoing efforts to better understand the genetics and environmental influences driving these mechanisms represent the best opportunity to understand the evolution of these neurodegenerative disorders that undermine brain health. Many of these destructive mechanisms appear to be well under way in the brain decades before any pathology is clinically identifiable. Current research efforts are focused on understanding these pathologic processes in their earliest and most insidious stages, hopefully providing us with knowledge and tools to prevent dementia altogether.

Prevention of dementia, especially AD, is an active area of research. The general premise driving innovative research is understanding risk and protective factors thought to have an impact on cognitive function. Potential factors that have been identified can be classified according to lifestyle and physical environmental factors (smoking, alcohol, diet, physical activity, education, cognitive and social activity) and vascular risk factors (hypertension, hyperlipidemia, diabetes, obesity, vascular insults, and neuronal damage). An additional area of increased interest includes head trauma, which is thought to disrupt neuronal synapses and predispose to β-amyloid formation. Last, depression and mental health may be important risk factors for dementia. The role of depressive symptoms in cognition was highlighted in the Women's Health Initiative Memory Study, which followed 6376 women ages 65 to 79 for approximately 5 years. This study revealed that depressive symptoms at baseline were associated with significant increased risk for MCI and probable dementia. Research continues to explore how to mitigate the risks of and exploit protective factors to prevent cognitive decline.

Research in healthy older adults has found encouraging although at times inconclusive evidence to support interventions that can slow cognitive aging or slow clinical dementia. Blood pressure management for persons with hypertension is thought to be able to prevent, delay onset, or slow dementia. Similarly, treatment of poorly controlled diabetes mellitus can improve vascular risk factors that are associated with end organ damage, such as stroke and dementia. Treatment of obstructive sleep apnea and other sleep disorders can also improve cognition. Individuals should be educated about the importance of managing chronic conditions to avoid vascular damage to the brain that might lead to vascular memory loss, as well as the potential to improve brain health through management of other medical conditions.

Some models of aging suggest that brain structure and function adapt and reorganize in response to cognitive and physical training, suggesting that cognitive training may also provide benefit in improving brain health and memory by delaying or slowing cognitive decline. One meta-analysis demonstrated benefits of either cognitive or physical training on cognition in older adults.[15] It is hypothesized that these interventions drive plasticity in the aging brain to support or improve cognitive function and to delay neurodegenerative process through benefits inherent to each specific intervention.

Physical activity is also highly encouraged, whether the benefits stem from increasing numbers of blood vessels and synapses, increasing brain volume, or decreasing age-related brain atrophy, have all been reported. In addition, positive localized effects in brain areas related to thinking and problem solving have also been reported, including increases in the number of new nerve cells and increases in proteins that help these neurons survive and thrive. In recent years, cognitive improvements also have been demonstrated with low-intensity mind-body exercises such as in some forms of yoga and tai chi, as well as with resistance (ie, weight) training.

It is important when discussing healthy aging and brain health to consider the body as a whole and not focus singularly on the brain. In addition to neurodegenerative conditions that can cause dementia, brain health can be affected by other age-related changes in the brain, including through injuries such as stroke or traumatic brain injury, as well as through mood disorders such as depression, or substance use disorder or addiction. Although some factors affecting brain health cannot be changed, there are many lifestyle changes that might make a difference to improve brain health.

The same applies when discussing prevention of ADRD or delaying disease progression for individuals already diagnosed with dementia. When discussing brain health, we emphasize the importance of improving circumstances that can lead to a healthier brain through a healthier body. This includes increased physical activity, improved nutrition, quality sleep, avoiding smoking and excessive alcohol, treating comorbid anxiety or depression, and following a healthy lifestyle. We also focus on factors that may negatively impact brain health and try to eliminate or control these factors.

Several randomized controlled trials are beginning to test multicomponent interventions that target several of these risk factors simultaneously. Reviews suggest that interventions including diet, exercise, cognitive training, and vascular risk monitoring could improve or maintain cognitive functioning in at-risk individuals. Although we do not have a magic pill to prevent dementia, we increasingly understand that damage to the brain builds up over a lifetime, and the earlier we can intervene to improve brain health, the better positioned we will be to prevent ADRD and other conditions detrimental to brain health.

Women and Risk of Alzheimer Disease and Related Dementias

Two-thirds of clinically diagnosed cases of ADRD occur in women. There have been multiple theories to explain this, including increased longevity of women compared with men and increased numbers of women relative to men; however, these hypotheses only begin to explain this disparate statistic.

Worldwide, women live longer than men. Given that the rate of dementia doubles every 5 years after the age of 65 and is increasingly prevalent after age 80, this is especially significant as women age. Women also outnumber men worldwide, with 55% of adults older than 60 years in 2007 being women.[16] As women outlive men, the disproportionate number of women as compared with men continues to increase with age, especially in those older than 80, which is the age in which women are more likely to be affected by dementia.[16,17] In many parts of the world, including Europe, Latin America, Australia, and areas outside of the Pacific region of Asia, female gender independently predicted a higher prevalence of dementia by approximately 20%. Last, women outnumber men in both developed and undeveloped countries, so increased prevalence of dementia in women is not a problem isolated to the developed world.[16,17]

AD disproportionately affects women in both prevalence and severity. Some studies have shown that at a similar stage of AD, women have more pronounced cognitive deficits than men[18]; however, the underlying mechanisms for these differences are unknown. In one metanalysis it was found that men with AD outperform women across multiple cognitive domains, with cognitive deficits in women being more pronounced in both severity and number of domains affected.[16] There is also evidence that women may experience more rapid cognitive deterioration in the early stages of AD. Age-related estrogen loss in women is one of many theories for this difference.

Risk factors for progression of disease may also be more present in women, including more severe periventricular white matter abnormalities on neuroimaging and poorer global cognitive functioning.[16] Older age, worse depressive symptoms, and being positive for APOE4 were risk factors for more rapid progression in women. Recent research has found that hippocampal volume decreased more rapidly in women with AD as compared with men. Last, lack of caregivers may further negatively impact the clinical course of AD in women. It has been reported that women often lack access to caregivers compared with men, as their spouse may already be deceased or unwilling or unable to serve as a caregiver.[16]

The current published literature describes several different hypotheses regarding sex-specific biological and gender-specific sociocultural factors that might increase women's vulnerability for dementia compared with men's.[16–20] Ultimately, understanding gender-specific trends in ADRD may help identify preclinical factors that can be intervened on to lower risk of onset differentially in men and women,[18] as well as guide options for treatment and disease management.

SUMMARY

Brain health describes the preservation of optimal brain integrity and mental and cognitive function with the goal of enabling optimal cognitive, emotional, psychological, and behavioral functioning. Developing and maintaining a healthy brain requires healthy development, the ability to adapt and respond to stress and adversity, promotion of healthy behaviors, and building resilience to contend with the variable demands of everyday life. Maintaining brain health in later life is contingent on factors that influence aging, including the environment, genetics and epigenetics, education, nutrition, trauma, stress and inflammation, socioeconomic status, social factors, sex, ethnicity, and disease. A healthy aging brain evolves and compensates to enable ongoing integrity of essential cognitive functions. Although older brains may complete tasks or process information differently from younger brains, task integrity is maintained through late life across most cognitive domains. Memory loss and cognitive impairment are not consistent with normal aging.

Loss of brain health can manifest as cognitive impairment or the syndrome of dementia. Women are disproportionately affected by dementia, both as persons with disease and as caregivers for those with dementia. Cognitive impairment and dementia are influenced by potential factors that can be classified according to lifestyle and physical environmental factors (smoking, alcohol, diet, physical activity, education, cognitive and social activity) and vascular risk factors (hypertension, hyperlipidemia, diabetes, obesity, vascular insults, and neuronal damage). In other scenarios, dementia seemingly rises unpredictably in otherwise healthy individuals in the later decades of life. Multidimensional interventions that focus on eliminating or managing factors that may negatively impact brain health as well as factors that improve brain health, such as increased physical activity, improved nutrition, quality sleep, avoiding smoking and excessive alcohol, treating comorbid anxiety or depression, and following a healthy lifestyle, are important in the care of individuals with cognitive impairment and dementia as well as for those seeking to optimize brain health.

CLINICS CARE POINTS

- Brain health describes the preservation of optimal brain integrity and mental and cognitive function with the goal of enabling optimal cognitive, emotional, psychological, and behavioral functioning.
- A healthy aging brain evolves and compensates to preserve cognitive functions. Memory loss and cognitive impairment are not consistent with normal aging.
- The dementia syndrome affects complex attention, executive function, learning and memory, language, perceptual-motor, or social cognition, and ultimately results in loss of autonomy and progressive functional dependence.
- Women are disproportionately affected by dementia with increasing prevalence by the eighth decade of life.
- Although some factors affecting brain health cannot be changed, there are many lifestyle changes that may make a difference to improve brain health.

DISCLOSURE

The authors have nothing to disclose.

REFERENCES

1. World Health Organization. Ageing and health. 2018. Available at: https://www.who.int/news-room/fact-sheets/detail/ageing-and-health. Accessed December 30, 2020.
2. Grajauskas LA, Siu W, Medvedev G, et al. MRI-based evaluation of structural degeneration in the ageing brain: pathophysiology and assessment. Ageing Res Rev 2019;49:67–82.
3. Isaev NK, Stelmashook EV, Genrikhs EE. Neurogenesis and brain aging. Rev Neurosci 2019;30(6):573–80.
4. CDC: Centers for Disease Control and Prevention. Healthy aging. What is a healthy brain? New research explores perceptions of cognitive health among diverse older adults. Available at: https://www.cdc.gov/aging/pdf/perceptions_of_cog_hlth_factsheet.pdf. Accessed December 30, 2020.
5. Gorelick PB, Furie KL, Iadecola C, et al, American Heart Association/American Stroke Association. Defining optimal brain health in adults: a presidential advisory

from the American Heart Association/American Stroke Association. Stroke 2017; 48(10):e284–303.

6. Wang Y, Pan Y, Li H. What is brain health and why is it important? BMJ 2020;371: m3683.

7. Toda T, Parylak SL, Linker SB, et al. The role of adult hippocampal neurogenesis in brain health and disease. Mol Psychiatry 2019;24(1):67–87.

8. Cameron HA, Glover LR. Adult neurogenesis: beyond learning and memory. Annu Rev Psychol 2015;66:53–81.

9. Harvey PD. Domains of cognition and their assessment. Dialogues Clin Neurosci 2019;21(3):227–37.

10. Lövdén M, Fratiglioni L, Glymour MM, et al. Education and cognitive functioning across the life span. Psychol Sci Public Interest 2020;21(1):6–41.

11. SPRINT MIND Investigators for the SPRINT Research Group, Williamson JD, Pajewski NM, Auchus AP, et al. Effect of intensive vs standard blood pressure control on probable dementia: a randomized clinical trial. JAMA 2019;321(6): 553–61.

12. Davidson H. Inter-relationships among diet, obesity and hippocampal-dependent cognitive function. Neuroscience 2013;253:110–22.

13. Grammatikopoulou G. To keto or not to keto? A systematic review of randomized controlled trials assessing the effects of ketogenic therapy on Alzheimer disease. Adv Nutr 2020;11(6):1583–602.

14. White L, Petrovitch H, Ross GW, et al. Prevalence of dementia in older Japanese-American men in Hawaii: the Honolulu-Asia aging study. JAMA 1996;276(12): 955–60.

15. Karssemeijer E, Aaronson JA, Bossers WJ, et al. Positive effects of combined cognitive and physical exercise training on cognitive function in older adults with mild cognitive impairment or dementia: a meta-analysis. Ageing Res Rev 2017;40:75–83.

16. Derreberry TM, Holroyd S. Dementia in women. Med Clin North Am 2019;103(4): 713–21.

17. Beam CR, Kaneshiro C, Jang JY, et al. Differences between women and men in incidence rates of dementia and Alzheimer's disease. J Alzheimers Dis 2018; 64(4):1077–83.

18. Dumas JA, Filippi CG, Newhouse PA, et al. Dopaminergic contributions to working memory-related brain activation in postmenopausal women. Menopause 2017;24(2):163–70.

19. Rettberg JR, Yao J, Brinton RD. Estrogen: a master regulator of bioenergetic systems in the brain and body. Front Neuroendocrinol 2014;35(1):8–30.

20. Roberts R, Knopman DS. Classification and epidemiology of MCI. Clin Geriatr Med 2013;29(4):753–72.

Advance Care Planning

Anca Dinescu, MD[a,b]

KEYWORDS

- Advance care planning • End of life • Life-sustaining treatments
- State-authorized portable documents • Women's health

KEY POINTS

- Advance care planning (ACP) is becoming an increasingly important aspect of women's health care and has recently been approved for reimbursement.
- Women, with their longer life expectancy, and high potential for end-of-life poverty and institutionalization, are especially vulnerable to the risks of absent ACP.
- ACP is a continual, dynamic process that needs to be refined over time, as one's life is a journey, and priorities shift.
- Identifying the appropriate timing for ACP conversations is complicated, with the surprise question representing a good trigger.
- The ACP conversation is better suited for outpatient visits and for the practitioner who has the most trusted relationship with the person.

Advance care planning (ACP) is the process by which individuals anticipate and discuss how their personal medical condition(s) or changes to their health may affect them in the future and, if they wish, negotiate and document their preferences for the future care plans.[1,2] Comprehensive, person-centered ACP includes attention to clinical, emotional, cultural, spiritual, and legal dimensions.

ACP is becoming an increasingly important aspect of health care, for patients and providers alike. ACP aims to ensure receipt of medical care aligned with patients' values and satisfaction. ACP has recently been approved for insurance reimbursement and is often recommended as a quality indicator in clinical practice guidelines. In the last several years, increasing numbers of people, especially older adults, are documenting their wishes for the care they would like to receive, or specifically not receive, near the end of their lives through various available forms and templates. In 1 recent study,[3] people aged 65 and older more frequently completed any advance directive (45.6%) compared with younger adults (31.6%). Additionally, the Nurses' Health Study reported that women are more likely than male counterparts to complete

[a] Geriatrics and Palliative Care Department, Washington DC Veteran Administration Medical Center, 50 Irving Street NW, Washington, DC, 20422, USA; [b] Internal Medicine, George Washington University, Washington, DC, USA
E-mail address: anca.dinescu@va.gov

Clin Geriatr Med 37 (2021) 605–610
https://doi.org/10.1016/j.cger.2021.06.001
0749-0690/21/© 2021 Elsevier Inc. All rights reserved.

an advance directive; 84% of women in this study reported ACP documentation, surpassing the rate of completion by men.[4] Despite increasing availability and acceptance of ACP, the overall rate of ACP in the general population remains low, hovering around 35%, and engagement remains especially low among minorities and patients with limited health literacy and English proficiency.[5] As well, the ability to universally support ACP is hindered by a myriad of health care system deficiencies, including inadequate standardization of such documents, provider comfort with the ACP process, communication skills, and time.

DEMOGRAPHICS

Women, with their longer life expectancy, and high potential for end-of-life poverty, disability, and nursing home dependency/institutionalization, are especially vulnerable to the risks of absent ACP.

As a group, women account for 56% of adults aged 65 and older and 67% of adults older than the age of 85 in the United States.[6] Nowadays, women have an increased life expectancy (+5 years) compared with men, and those who reach age 65 can expect to live an average of 20 more years, while those who reach age 75 can expect to live an additional 13 years.[7] Along with an increased life expectancy, older women are living with higher rates of disability and chronic health problems and lower incomes than men on average. When unable to live independently or provide for their care at home, many older, disabled and seriously ill women are cared for in nursing homes. Currently more than 70% of nursing home residents are women; their average age at admission is 80 years. For those who live in a nursing home, ACP documentation takes on an even more important role, in order to assure that health care preferences will be honored in the institutional setting.[7]

The female survival advantage also creates challenges in identifying a surrogate decision maker when necessary. It is not uncommon for seriously ill older women to have outlived a husband and siblings. Older women may need to rely on their adult children for support and surrogacy, often complicated by responsibilities and challenges of families, professional careers, and geography.

Women tend to be caregivers to their spouses, an activity documented well as a main cause of poor health among the caregiver spouses. Many times the overly burdened spouse, who is in more cases the woman in the couple, neglects personal health, including planning for end of life[7,8]

ADVANCE CARE PLANNING, A CONTINUAL PROCESS

The general approach of eliciting and documenting wishes for medical care at the end of life remains largely un-unified and under continual refinement. The most current approach, supported by various professional associations involved in end-of-life care, supports the idea that ACP it is not a static snapshot of someone's wishes for end-of-life care, but a continual, dynamic process that needs to be refined over time. This new understanding of ACP is rooted in the understanding that one's life is a journey, and priorities change as life unfolds.

The process should start early in someone's adult life, with a broad scope of defining what matters most for that person and focus on establishing a trusting relationship between the practitioner and the patient. At this initial stage, the ACP is usually recorded in an advance directive document or a living will and might include as little as naming a health care proxy (HCP).

Over time, the initial broad framework defining someone's life priorities could be refined to include more specific limitations of specific medical procedures and interventions, as chronic conditions approach more advanced stages or new serious illness is diagnosed. The specific decisions resulting from the refinement of initial goals are more recently documented in State authorized portable orders (SAPO) documents and can be readily actionable as needed. These medical orders for limiting certain life-supporting treatments, as opposed to the initial framework represented by the advance directives, represent a more concrete way for the individual person to assert self-determination. Decisions made in the context of advance illness would also have a higher chance to accurately represent the person's views about what gives quality to life. Ultimately, a previously recorded SAPO or advance directive document may and should be reviewed at all points of care in serious illness to help design a plan for personalized care consistent with one's values and preferences.

ADVANCE CARE PLANNING COMPONENTS

In the last several years, there has been more consensus about what the content of ACP documentation should be, beyond the simplistic and outdated equation of ACP with code status. This recent standardization was brought by the many states' efforts to create SAPOs. Generally, all ACP documentation today includes the naming of an HCP or agent and preferences regarding life-sustaining treatment interventions (previously known under the name life-support) such as cardiopulmonary resuscitation (CPR), invasive ventilatory support, intensive care unit admission, intravenous hydration and nutrition, and includes other, more disease specific, interventions, such as chemotherapy, hemodialysis, and surgeries.

Clear communication with providers and understanding of one's expected disease trajectory are integral parts of ACP, as decisions to accept or limit certain interventions should be discussed in the setting of person-centered medical facts and science. Low patient health literacy is often cited as a key barrier to ACP conversations and is associated with lower rates of advance directives completion, higher rates of aggressive treatment in the last month of life, and death in hospitals. Women have been reported to have higher health literacy compared to men, with two-fifths of women demonstrating poor health literacy, compared with half of men in one study.[9] Even in a cohort of well-educated people, the risk of low health literacy was high (43.4%).

Procedurally, all ACP discussions, documented on an advance directive form or an SAPO, should be approached with the same level of informed consent as any other medical intervention. Before opening an ACP discussion, providers must determine a person's capacity and document ability to make decisions about naming an HCP and health care intervention preferences. Conversations about ACP may be accomplished over several visits and may be coded for reimbursement by Medicare.

ADVANCE CARE PLANNING, THE PROCESS
Designing Advance Care Directives – Initial Approach

The initial process should focus mainly on eliciting a history of what matters for the individual, what are one's wishes for health, and what gives one's life meaning and quality. One useful way to accomplish this task is by using the Magic Questions (Appendix 1).[10] These questions are designed to elicit important information about the person's life-long values, beliefs, attitudes, and hopes in the context of advancing age and serious illness.

Studies show that the practitioner who has the most trusted relationship with the person should be the one initiating ACP. The primary care provider is traditionally the practitioner with the closest relationship with the patient, but certain specialists such as oncologists or nephrologists develop continuity relationships with their patients by the nature of the chronicity of the specific disease or diagnosis, and may initiate the discussion.

The initiation of the ACP discussion is better suited for outpatient visits. The outpatient setting offers the advantage of a less stressful environment, as opposed to an emergency department, acute care hospital ward, or intensive care unit. Another advantage of starting ACP in the outpatient setting is the possibility of inviting the patient's surrogate to be present for the discussion, which may in turn be a key factor in the later process of honoring patient stated wishes, as the surrogate may be called on to work collaboratively with the hospital team to make decisions on the patient's behalf.

The role of an outpatient palliative care team in initial ACP remains controversial, as the palliative care team does not have usually a long-standing relationship with the patient. One advantage of an outpatient palliative care team would be an expert knowledge of resources, such as hospice, for the seriously ill person. Another advantage of early involvement of a palliative care specialist would be development of a new trusted relationship with the patient, that over time could be beneficial to discuss, document, and ensure provision of care consistent with patient preferences[11,12].

State Authorized Portable Orders Documents– Final Stage of Advance Care Planning

Over time, the initial broad framework defining someone's life priorities (as recorded in the Advance Directive) could be later refined to include more specific limitations of life-sustaining treatment interventions and document them as orders in an SAPO, as chronic conditions advance and/or a new serious illness is diagnosed and a person's risk of dying increases.

For example, an initial preference "to spend more time with family" documented in an advance directive for a person with advanced serious illness, might transfer to SAPO orders "do not attempt cardiopulmonary resuscitation," and "limit use of prolonged ventilatory support" as the disease progresses.

The ideal setting for SAPO order review and documentation remains the outpatient office, for the same reasons cited before: trusted provider, nonurgent medical necessity, no overwhelming symptoms, less stressful environment, increased chance of attendance by the surrogate decision maker, and longer time to plan after. Nonetheless, initial ACP conversations often occur in emergency departments, acute hospital wards, or intensive care units. In a similar manner with the initial phase of ACP, these difficult discussions leading to an SAPO, are best when conducted by the primary practitioner known to and trusted by the patient, with another specialist, palliative care provider, or geriatrician also appropriate choices.

Identifying the appropriate timing for ACP conversations and exploration of wishes about life-sustaining treatment interventions is complicated by prognostication challenges. Although various mortality/risk of death calculators exist, individual prognostication cannot always fit cleanly into an algorithm. Progression to an advanced stage of cancer, entering the end stage of one of the main chronic disorders that account for the top causes of death in United States, heart failure, chronic obstructive pulmonary disease, cardiovascular disease and extreme age, are typical triggers for ACP conversations and SAPO completion. One of the most wildly used approaches to define if a person is at high risk of dying in the next 6 month to a year is the surprise question: 'Would you be surprised if this person would die in the next 6 months to a year?' A negative response to the surprise question is associated with sensitivity 67%, a specificity 80.2% and has a positive predictive value 83% for cancer patients. As issues persist with the with lower positive predictive values in noncancer population (around 30%), generally the surprise question represents a good trigger for ACP and SAPO documentation if indicated.[13]

TYPES OF ADVANCE CARE PLANNING DOCUMENTS

ACP documents have achieved more standardization in the last several years. Documentation of the person's capacity to make decisions about proxy and preferences, and identification of a health care agent or proxy are embedded in all types of ACP. Specific preferences for or against many life-sustaining interventions, such as CPR, ventilatory support, intravenous hydration, and artificial nutrition are present with variations in terminology and detail.

In various states, SAPOs carry different names (eg, POLST, physician order for life-sustaining treatments and MOLST, medical order for life-sustaining treatments). The largest comprehensive US health care system, Veteran Administration, recently adopted the LSTDI (life-sustaining treatment decisions initiative) as a uniform way to elicit, document and honor veterans' preferences for care near the end of life with great success. Advance directives and SAPO differ in that that the latter is an explicit and actionable set of orders that can be used directly by the practitioner to honor patient preferences at the point of care. SAPO orders are designed to be more specific than the more general framework of an advance directive. Providers must use caution interpreting the SAPO, as the specificity carries danger of misunderstanding. A recent study auditing the accuracy of POLST documents demonstrated 25% of patients and/or their surrogates were unaware of the "do not attempt resuscitation" orders recorded in their own SAPO; 50% were unsure of their prognosis, and another 40% felt their condition was not terminal. Overall, 44% of the time, the existing POLST orders were discordant with patient wishes, and 38% were rescinded.[14]

ACP is an important, comprehensive, person-centered, continual process that can help elicit, document ,and honor peoples' preferences for future medical care, such as when illness is serious and life-expectancy is limited. Universal access to quality ACP is critical for women in order to ensure they understand their possible future health care trajectory, have opportunity to name a surrogate decision maker, and share their preferences for care based on personal values and what gives meaning to their lives.

CLINICS CARE POINTS

- ACP is becoming an increasingly important aspect of women's health care and has recently been approved for reimbursement.

- Women, with their longer life expectancy, and high potential for end-of-life poverty and institutionalization, are especially vulnerable to the risks of absent ACP.

- ACP is a continual, dynamic process that needs to be refined over time, as one's life is a journey, and priorities shift.

- Identifying the appropriate timing for ACP conversations is complicated, with the surprise question representing a good trigger.

- The ACP conversation is better suited for outpatient visits and for the practitioner who has the most trusted relationship with the patient.

- Generally, ACP documentation includes the naming of an HCP, preferences regarding life-sustaining treatment interventions, and other, more disease specific, interventions, such as chemotherapy, hemodialysis, and surgeries.

DISCLOSURE

The authors have nothing to disclose.

REFERENCES

1. McMahan RD, Tellez I, Sudore RL. Deconstructing the complexities of advance care planning outcomes: what do we know and where do we go? a scoping review. J Am Geriatr Soc 2021;69(1):234–44.
2. Sudore RL, Lum HD, You JJ, et al. Defining Advance Care Planning for Adults: A Consensus Definition From a Multidisciplinary Delphi Panel. J Pain Symptom Manage. 2017 May;53(5):821–32.e1. https://doi.org/10.1016/j.jpainsymman.2016.12.331. Epub 2017 Jan 3. PMID: 28062339; PMCID: PMC5728651.
3. Yadav KN, Gabler NB, Cooney E, et al. Approximately one in three US adults completes any type of advance directive for end-of-life care. Health Aff (Millwood) 2017;36(7):1244–51.
4. Kang JH, Bynum JPW, Zhang L, et al. Predictors of advance care planning in older women: the nurses' health study. J Am Geriatr Soc 2019;67(2):292–301.
5. Sudore RL, Schillinger D, Katen MT, et al. Engaging diverse English- and Spanish-speaking older adults in advance care planning: the PREPARE randomized clinical trial. JAMA Intern Med 2018;178(12):1616–25.
6. Thompson K, Shi S, Kiraly C. Primary care for the older adult patient: common geriatric issues and syndromes. Obstet Gynecol Clin North Am 2016;43(2):367–79.
7. Blackstone K. AARP, Accessed January 24, 2021.
8. Williams LA, Giddings LS, Bellamy G, et al. 'Because it's the wife who has to look after the man': a descriptive qualitative study of older women and the intersection of gender and the provision of family caregiving at the end of life. Palliat Med 2017;31(3):223–30.
9. Nouri SS, Barnes DE, Volow AM, et al. Health literacy matters more than experience for advance care planning knowledge among older adults. J Am Geriatr Soc 2019;67(10):2151–6.
10. Magic questions. Available at: http://www.cherp.research.va.gov/promise/PROMISESummer2013Newsletter.pdf.
11. Clayton JM, Hancock K, Parker S, et al. Sustaining hope when communicating with terminally ill patients and their families: a systematic review. Psychooncology 2008;17(7):641–59.
12. Back AL, Young JP, McCown E, et al. Abandonment at the end of life from patient, caregiver, nurse, and physician perspectives: loss of continuity and lack of closure. Arch Intern Med 2009;169(5):474–9.
13. Downar J, Goldman R, Pinto R, et al. The "surprise question" for predicting death in seriously ill patients: a systematic review and meta-analysis. CMAJ 2017;189(13):E484–93.
14. Mirarchi FL, Juhasz K, Cooney TE, et al. TRIAD XII: are patients aware of and agree with DNR or POLST orders in their medical records. J Patient Saf 2019;15(3):230–7.

APPENDIX 1

Magic Questions script for eliciting life-long values during ACP
   "It helps me to be a better doctor for you when I know about you as a person.

1. Tell me about yourself (your loved one).
2. What makes you (or your loved one) happy these days?
3. What worries you (or your loved one) for the future?"

Breast Cancer in Women Over 65 years- a Review of Screening and Treatment Options

Parth Desai, MD, Anita Aggarwal, DO, PhD*

KEYWORDS

- Breast cancer • Elderly • Screening • Treatment

KEY POINTS

- Incidence of breast cancer in older women is rising. Comprehensive geriatric assessment, life expectancy and comorbidities should be considered for appropriate management in these patients.
- Breast conservation with adjuvant endocrine therapy should be offered to HR+ early breast cancer. Those with limited life expectancy, primary endocrine therapy may be offered.
- Adjuvant radiation can be avoided for some early stage tumors.
- Sentinel node biopsy and axillary staging can be avoided in clinically node-negative otherwise early stage tumors during surgery.
- Less cytotoxic chemotherapy, HER-2 targeted therapy, immunotherapy, and newer molecularly targeted therapy should be considered for advanced/recurrent disease whenever possible.
- Primary endocrine therapy may be offered to those with early hormone receptor-positive breast cancer with limited life expectancy.
- Less cytotoxic chemotherapy, HER-2 targeted therapy, immunotherapy, and newer molecularly targeted therapy should be considered for advanced/recurrent disease whenever possible.

INTRODUCTION

Breast cancer remains a major epidemiologic challenge. Approximately 1 in 8 women will be diagnosed with invasive breast cancer in their lifetime, and 1 in 39 women will die from breast cancer.[1] Breast cancer incidence and death rates increase with age until about the seventh decade, after which they tend to decrease, primarily thought to reflect lower screening rates.[2] The median age of diagnosis of breast cancer is 62 years, and hence a significant proportion of women are diagnosed with invasive breast cancer after 65 years.

Hematology/Oncology Division, Veterans Affairs Medical Center, 50 Irving Street Northwest, Washington, DC 20422, USA
* Corresponding author.
E-mail address: Anita.aggarwal@va.gov

Clin Geriatr Med 37 (2021) 611–623
https://doi.org/10.1016/j.cger.2021.05.007
0749-0690/21/Published by Elsevier Inc.

National Comprehensive Cancer Network (NCCN) is a not-for-profit alliance of leading cancer centers that provides evidence-based cancer guidelines. NCCN defines older adults based on their functional status rather than chronologic age; however, those aged 65 years and older are generally considered older adults. The number of Americans age 65 years and older in the United States is projected to be 88.5 million by 2050. Age 80 years and older, a rapidly expanding group, now comprises 9 million members of the US population.[3] The aging population and projected increased cancer incidence indicate that there will be about a 67% increase in cancer incidence for patients age 65 years and older between 2010 and 2030.[4] Evidence-based treatment guidelines for older adults are lacking because of the paucity of clinical data from persistent under-representation of older adults in clinical trials.[5] Clinicians face challenges in treating the elderly because of a lack of the information needed to estimate the likelihood of toxicities and effectiveness that can be life-changing in older adults. Few guidelines, now relatively outdated, exist, which are derived mainly from expert consensus and observational data available to guide oncologists in delivering optimal care to these vulnerable patient populations.[6]

BREAST CANCER CHARACTERISTICS IN OLDER WOMEN

Infiltrating ductal carcinoma is the most common pathologic subtype in older women, who are more likely to have estrogen (ER)- and progesterone receptor (PR)-positive luminal breast cancer with or without the human epidermal growth factor 2 (HER-2) overexpression compared with younger women.[7] Almost 85% of tumors in women greater than 80 years express ER/PR receptor, and less than 10% have HER-2 positive overexpression at diagnosis.[8] Clinically, older women at presentation have larger tumors and nodal involvement, likely because of the delay in diagnosis. The incidence of breast cancer in women greater than 80 years is slightly lower (400 cases/100,000 population) than in women younger than 80 years, but the mortality rates are comparatively higher, likely because of lack of screening mammography, higher stage of cancer at presentation, undertreatment, and multiple comorbidities.[9]

BREAST CANCER SCREENING IN OLDER WOMEN

Screening mammography reduces breast cancer mortality by 19% among women 40 to 69 years of age, but its usefulness is unknown for women older than 70 years. As per some statistical models, screening may prevent 1 to 2 breast cancer deaths per 1000 women aged greater than 70 years.[10]

Current breast cancer screening recommendations vary in terms of starting age and frequency. As per the American Cancer Society (ACS), women aged 40 to 49 years should have the choice for annual screening mammogram with the option to transition to biennial screening until age 75 years. ACS also recommends to continue screening mammography biennially if women are in good health and their life expectancy is more than 10 years.[11] The American College of Obstetricians and Gynecologists (ACOG) recommends screening mammography starting at 40 years with the decision to stop screening be based on a shared decision-making process that includes a discussion of the woman's health status and longevity as per ACOG. US Preventive Services Task Force (USPSTF) recommends biennial screening mammograms starting at age 50 and none for women older than 75 years.[12] In summary, screening recommendations must be tailored based on patient's age, goals, and expected life expectancy.

PRETREATMENT CONSIDERATIONS IN OLDER WOMEN

Management of any cancer presents unique challenges in older adults, and in many cases, treatment is denied because of age, although many can benefit if the right decision-making tools are used. As with any cancer management approach in the senior population, a comprehensive geriatric assessment (CGA) is of paramount importance.[13] This ideally should include a geriatrician; however, if not available, it can be performed by an oncologist using widely available guidance and online assessment plans.[14] CGA uses functional status revolving around the patient's current activities of daily living (ADLs & IADLS), gait assessment, visual/hearing status, performance status, socioeconomic status, psychological status, comorbidity scores, nutritional status, polypharmacy, and cognitive status.[15] CGA or any available screening tools must be used as a minimum.[16,17] Vulnerable Elders Survey VES-13 score particularly was found to be predictive of functional decline and death in early breast cancer patients,[18] which allows oncologists to tailor management approaches and chemotherapy decisions depending on baseline deficits. Medication reconciliation with attention to the indication for each medication should be critically reviewed periodically to prevent medication interaction-related adverse effects.

An honest discussion with the patient and close family members should take place for cancer workup and treatment approaches. Well-validated life expectancy calculators are available online, which could be a good starting point to present different management approaches.[19,20] Advance care planning incorporates information about the patient's preferences for care and health care proxies. Decision-making capacity should be assessed at the outset and periodically. Health care proxies should be formally identified. Goals of care are likely to evolve over time in the event of disease progression. Family meetings are helpful to ensure communication between the patient and health care proxies about preferences for care. In essence, care planning at the primary visit should ideally be a patient-centered, collaborative effort including a breast oncologist, oncology pharmacists, nutritionists, social workers, the psychology department, and a palliative care team to help guide patients on the best treatment options/routes.

TREATMENT CONSIDERATIONS IN OLDER WOMEN WITH BREAST CANCER

From epidemiologic data, it appears that following a new diagnosis of breast cancer, older women often receive less aggressive treatment or less often receive therapies as per guidelines compared with younger women worldwide.[21–23] These disparities persist despite adjusting for differences in tumor characteristics.[21] In the most extensive study including over 120,000 women, increasing age was associated with decreased rates of breast-conserving surgery, axillary dissection, and radiotherapy, and there was increased use of upfront mastectomy and primary endocrine therapy.[24] Interestingly, according to another study done in the United Kingdom (UK), the low rates of surgery were not explained by patients actively opting out of surgery.[22] The treatment of individuals who are age 65 years and older is complex and involves clearly defining the goals and value of treatment while also weighing risks, such as the potential effects of treatment on functional loss and quality of life.[25] The knowledge gap in caring for these older patients and the need for increased research efforts have been well defined by the Institute of Medicine, the American Society of Clinical Oncology, and the Cancer and Aging Research Group (CRAG).[26]

EARLY STAGE CANCER (STAGE I-III)

Breast cancer treatment is multimodal and multidisciplinary. In general, patients with early stage breast cancer are curable, and definitive local treatment should include primary surgery lumpectomy/mastectomy and regional nodes assessment with or without radiation therapy (RT). Adjuvant systemic therapy may be offered based on primary tumor characteristics, such as tumor size, grade, number of involved lymph nodes, the status of ER/PR, and HER-2 receptors.

Surgery

Advanced chronologic age was considered a poor prognostic and predictive factor in surgical oncology.[27,28] In the mid-1990s, based on functional age, comorbidities, the difference in physiology, response to anesthesia, and stress, older patients were denied appropriate surgical treatment more often than younger patients.[29] In subsequent years, Preoperative Risk Estimation in Onco-geriatric Surgical Patients (PREOP) developed a risk score tool to provide a decision measure based on 3 common geriatric screening tools: The Timed Up and Go Test, Nutritional Risk Screening, and the ASA classification.[30] The preoperative Assessment of Cancer in the Elderly (PACE) score can also be used to determine the surgical suitability of older patients.[31] The contribution of geriatricians has resulted in a significant reduction in surgical complications in older patients such as acute delirium and long-term disability.[32]

Traditionally most older women choose mastectomy because of recurrence fear and no local RT.[33] One of the more debatable points is knowing the axillary lymph node status and removal in older patients, given associated morbidity around it. Sentinel lymph node biopsy in clinically node-negative women greater than 70 years of age with early stage hormone receptor (HR)-positive, HER-2 negative breast cancer is not recommended by Choosing Wisely Campaign and Society of Surgical Oncology given the fact that it is unlikely to change management.[34,35] There is evidence that women age 80 years or older overall tolerate breast cancer-related surgery well with low complication rates depending on their comorbidities. Delayed wound healing was the only complication noted in 6% in 1 study of 129 women aged 80 years and older. Thirty-two percent had a simple mastectomy; 27% had breast conservation, and 6% had axillary dissection.[36] According to a study presented at the 12th European Breast Cancer Conference-12, women over 70 who are fit can benefit from surgery, whereas their less fit, frailer counterparts may be treated with oral hormone therapy alone.[37,38] Older women with estrogen receptor-positive breast cancer have poorer survival than younger women, but this gap might be closed by offering surgery to women over 70 who are fit and have resectable tumors.

Radiation

The role of radiation to achieve loco-regional control and recurrence of disease continues to evolve. Partial mastectomy followed by radiation has been the standard of treatment and is well tolerated.[39,40]

Adjuvant breast-conserving therapy and endocrine therapy without breast radiation are viable options in some older women who have small (≤3 cm, margins >1 mm) node-negative, ER/PR positive and HER-2 negative tumors but at a higher risk of in-breast recurrence. In a randomized trial (CALGB 9343) of women age 70 years and older with T1N0M0 tumors, there was a 10% local-regional recurrence rate after breast conservation in those who received tamoxifen alone versus 2% for those who received tamoxifen and radiation.[41] Ten-year overall survival was almost identical, with most patients dying of nonbreast cancer causes. Similarly, the PRIME II trial, which looked at slightly higher risk early breast cancer patients (65 years or older with HR-positive, axillary node-negative, <3 cm tumors), showed similar results of increased local-regional recurrence at 5 and 10 years but no difference in overall survival and distance recurrence.[42,43] Both studies did not include many patients with very high-risk features like tumors larger than 3 cm, high-grade tumors with lymph vascular invasion, and node-positive tumors. For these patients, loco-regional radiation, whenever feasible, should be offered. However, survival benefits usually are not noted until 5 to 10 years after diagnosis, which makes such treatment of marginal or no benefit in those with life expectancies less than 5 years.[44,45] Hypofractionated radiation offers similar loco-regional control and adverse effects as standard radiation to the whole breast with possibly better breast cosmesis.[46] Primary RT without any surgery or chemotherapy in unfit older patients may be an option, with some retrospective evidence suggesting durable local control in doses higher than 60 Gy.[47]

Endocrine Therapy

Most early stage cancers in older women are HR-positive.

Adjuvant endocrine therapy should be offered to all women with ER/PR-positive breast tumors, regardless of age, provided they are candidates for medical therapy. Aromatase inhibitor (AI) is preferred choice of endocrine therapy in older women because of better progression-free survival and fewer thromboembolic risks, and less endometrial thickening and bleeding when compared with tamoxifen.[48,49] However, tamoxifen is preferable for women at risk for cardiovascular complications or bone loss and those unable to tolerate an AI because of toxicity.

When compared to observation alone, the benefit of tamoxifen appears to be maintained in older women including reduction in the 10-year risk of recurrence (23 vs 44%) and breast cancer-specific mortality (20 vs 37%).[50] In the 2010 Early Breast Cancer Trialists' Group (EBCTCG) meta-analysis, adjuvant treatment with tamoxifen versus an AI reported AI given for 5 years resulted in trends toward reduced recurrences compared with tamoxifen in women aged 60 to 69 years (12 vs 14%; relative risk [RR] 0.80) and in women aged 70 years or older (14 vs 17%; RR 0.78). Contrary to in younger women, the optimal duration of endocrine therapy use is not clear. Minimum duration of 5 years of endocrine therapy should be prescribed for most older women. However, longer durations up to 10 years might be appropriate in selected patients, especially those with higher-risk tumor features (eg, nodal involvement, higher tumor grade). Primary endocrine therapy is also considered an option for frail older women with limited life expectancy (<2–3 years) for ER/PR-positive early breast cancer, with a study revealing 40% complete clinical response and overall good duration of clinical response,[51,52] although there is sufficient evidence that surgery with adjuvant endocrine therapy is still the ideal treatment for elderly fit patients with breast cancer with better loco-regional control albeit not much difference in overall survival.[52,53] Endocrine therapy can also be considered in the neoadjuvant setting for elderly breast cancer patients for downstaging large or locally advanced tumors and when patients are not ready for surgery, wherein AIs are better than tamoxifen.[54]

Chemotherapy

Older women with breast cancer are under-represented in clinical trials, and data on the effects of adjuvant chemotherapy in such patients are scant. There is often a general concern among oncologists that older women may not be able to tolerate more intensive chemotherapy regimens, and, therefore, not always offered care consistent with treatment guidelines; such lapses can adversely affect survival.[55] Although adjuvant chemotherapy has improved survival among women with early stage breast cancer,[56] the Oxford Overview analysis of 15-year results included too few patients older than 70 years of age to assess the effect of chemotherapy in that age group accurately. Older women with breast cancer who are in good health may tolerate chemotherapy equally well as younger patients,[57] and the more severe toxicities of chemotherapy in older patients have not meaningfully affected the benefits of adjuvant chemotherapy.[58] Various chemotherapy toxicity assessment tools are available to get an estimate of expected toxicity with chemotherapy regimens in older patients, including chemotherapy risk assessment scale for high-age patients (CRASH)[59] and CARG chemotherapy toxicity calculators.[60] Cardiac function (anthracyclines, trastuzumab), neuropathy (taxanes), renal function, and myelodysplasia (anthracyclines) are important comorbidities to consider before choosing chemotherapy options.

For older women who are fit and candidates for adjuvant chemotherapy, CMF (Cytoxan, methotrexate, 5-fluorouracil [5FU]) combination is still the most used regimen but generally not well tolerated. Replacing 5FU with an oral agent, capecitabine, has not been effective to prevent relapse.[51] The first-line standard doxorubicin and cyclophosphamide (AC) combination regimen is usually not an option for the older patients because of anthracycline-related cardiotoxicity. Taxanes like nab-paclitaxel or docetaxel plus cytophosphamide (TC), are usually well-tolerated, and 4 cycles of adjuvant TC regimen have superior PFS and are better tolerated when compared against AC in older and younger patients with more febrile neutropenia but less anemia.[61] Hematological toxicities leading to dose delays, interruptions, and hospitalizations remain an issue in older patients receiving cytotoxic chemotherapy.

The use of 21 gene recurrence score (Oncotype dx score) to guide chemotherapy decisions is well established in node-negative early stage HR-positive breast cancer patients. However, this score is not well validated in an older patients. Chemotherapy use was not associated with improved survival in the older as opposed to younger patients with high-risk Oncotype dx in a SEER (Surveillance, Epidemiology, and End Results) database study,[62] which had a small proportion of older patients. Some experts recommend the addition of chemotherapy for some with high-risk features and expected life expectancy longer than 5 years.[25]

HER-2 targeted agents have resulted in improved survival in HER-2 amplified breast cancers; however, all the major trials were under-represented by patients older than 65 years. NSABP-31, which compared AC→T ± trastuzumab, had about 16% of patients older than 60 years with significantly improved disease-free survival for all age groups.[63] A systematic review reported a 47% relative risk reduction with the use of trastuzumab in patients older than 60 years but had a 5% rate of clinically significant cardiotoxicity in trastuzumab-receiving patients.[64] Higher cardiotoxicity rates up to 20% have been reported in patients older than 70 years who received trastuzumab but were linked to concomitant use of anthracyclines.[65]

Overall, there are good data to support that adjuvant or neoadjuvant chemotherapy prolongs survival in older patients with breast cancer. The United Kingdom-based PREDICT model and Adjuvant! Online provide 5- and 10-year survival estimates of the benefits of adding chemotherapy, endocrine therapy, or HER-2 targeted therapy based on various demographic and clinical factors.[66–68]

METASTATIC/RECURRENT BREAST CANCER

Metastatic breast cancer in women older than 65 years is managed with the goal of palliation rather than cure. Because of the higher frequency of HR expression, the tendency is toward more indolent tumor growth and without the life-threatening or rapidly progressive disease. These patients can be treated with endocrine therapy successfully. With the availability of several different endocrine agents, treatment should be tried in succession to maximize the quality of life for the longest period. Patients who relapsed after a long time on tamoxifen can be switched to AIs or fulvestrant. The main adverse effects of AIs, including arthralgias, carpal tunnel syndrome, bone loss, and cardiovascular disease risk increase, need to be weighed against the benefits. Hot flashes and venous thromboembolism (VTE) as seen with tamoxifen are less often issues with AI. Bone density assessment and the use of bisphosphonates should be strongly recommended wherever appropriate, especially in patients with lytic bone lesions. Fulvestrant, a monthly intramuscular injection, has a relatively low adverse effect profile and should be an option.

Cyclin-dependent kinase (CDK)4/6 inhibitors in combination with AI or fulvestrant with tolerable adverse effects are available to younger patients as the first line for the treatment of metastatic disease and have proven to prolong PFS and overall survival (OS), but many clinicians are reluctant to give CDK4/6 inhibitors to older patients with breast cancer. To better understand the safety and efficacy of these drugs in geriatric populations, a pooled analysis of clinical trials by the US Food and Drug Administration (FDA) showed that estimated pooled median PFS was 31.1 months in ages 75 years or above (95% confidence interval [CI], 20.2 months to not reached) for those on combination therapy versus 13.7 months (95% CI, 10.9 months to 24.9 months) AI alone but at the cost of grade 3 to 4 adverse events in almost 90% in patients 75 years of age and older.[69] These values should carry over into evolving risk-benefit conversations with older patients.

For HER-2 positive stage IV breast cancer, based on the CLEOPATRA trial, pertuzumab should be combined with trastuzumab in the frontline setting. Of the 808 patients enrolled in this trial, 129 were older than 65 years, and the subgroup analysis of this population showed significant PFS of 21.5 months in the pertuzumab group versus 10.4 months in the placebo group.[70] Diarrhea, fatigue, loss of appetite, and emesis are of concern, but usually manageable toxicities, and there was no additional cardiotoxicity risk to that already incurred by trastuzumab. Ado-trastuzumab emtansine is an antibody drug conjugate approved in HER-2 positive metastatic breast cancer; however, the clinical trials included much younger populations. Fewer cardiotoxicity features of ado-trastuzumab emtansine make it an encouraging option for elderly patients.[71] Lapatinib, an oral dual HER-1/HER-2 blocking agent is approved in combination with capecitabine with HER-2 positive metastatic breast cancer as a second-line agent. The patient group studied in this trial was a median of 69 years, with significant toxicities being diarrhea and fatigue but overall low cardiotoxicities.[72,73]

Depending on comorbidities, performance status, and patient preferences for care, chemotherapy may be considered for breast cancer refractory to endocrine therapy or as first-line therapy if life-threatening or rapidly progressive disease is present, and no other safer targeted options are available. Sequential single-agent treatment is often chosen in older women with metastatic breast cancer. Eribulin as a single agent is also considered as a "less-toxic" chemotherapy patients for elderly patients with metastatic breast cancer with safer side effect profile.[74] Oral chemotherapy like capecitabine has manageable toxicity profiles and reasonable disease control rates.[73,75]

Older patients presenting with de novo advanced/metastatic or recurrent triple-negative (TN) breast cancer should always be tested for PD-L1 and germline, BRCA mutations Targeted chemo-immunotherapy (nab-paclitaxel plus atezolizumab) for PD-L1 high (>1% expression) and PARP inhibitors for BRCA mutated tumors should be offered, which are relatively well tolerated in older patients.[76,77] Additionally, NTRK fusion, PIK3CA mutation, and MSI status should also be checked for nonchemotherapeutic treatment options for these patients.

SUPPORTIVE CARE CONSIDERATIONS

Bone health is of paramount importance in the older patient population and assumes even more importance given the risks associated with breast cancer metastases to bones and treatment-associated bone loss. Osteoclast inhibition significantly reduces the risk of skeletal-related events in women with bone metastases; the choice of agent (ie, a bisphosphonate or denosumab) depends on many factors but should be considered in patients taking AI or having bone metastases. Balancing the risk of osteoporosis-related fracture prevention with bisphosphonate use and the added risk of atypical fractures requires careful consideration.[78] Creatinine in older persons may not be a good indicator of renal function. Avoiding frequent redundant iodine contrast studies and using creatinine clearance by Cockcroft-Gault or MDRD equations is recommended.[79] There are also many other areas of support that an onco-geriatric cancer patient may require to maintain the best quality of life. These are best identified using the CGA discussed earlier and should be addressed from the onset of treatment planning and management. Fall prevention with durable medical equipment and in-home safety evaluations, nausea/vomiting management, frequently addressing polypharmacy, and reducing pill burden are only some of the more important helpful measures. Early involvement of palliative care may be essential for older patients with advanced/metastatic breast cancer with a dismal traditional record of hospice utilization.

In summary, older breast cancer patients represent a unique challenge and opportunity to provide the best possible care in alignment with their goals. As Mahatma Gandhi and Arti Hurria, who was a champion for onco-geriatric patients quoted, "The true measure of any society can be found in how it treats its most vulnerable members." Senior patients with breast cancer require utmost care, empathy, love, and skilled guidance through this miserable disease during the autumn years of their life.

CLINICS CARE POINTS

- Treatment decisions for elderly patients with breast cancer should be based on a comprehensive geriatric assessment, comorbidities, frailty, and expected life expectancy rather merely age.

- For clinically node-negative early stage breast cancer, sentinel lymph node biopsy can be avoided during surgery given there is evidence suggesting that results from this procedure likely do not change the outcome.

- For early stage HR breast cancer patients who undergo conservative surgery, adjuvant RT can be avoided given increased comorbidities and only modest decrease in local recurrence rate.

- For frail elderly women with HR-positive breast cancer (most common type seen in this age group), primary endocrine therapy may be a suitable alternative, and aromatase inhibitors should be considered as a first choice.

- For elderly patients needing chemotherapy for breast cancer, taxane and cyclophosphamide-based regimens are effective and safe, given a favorable cardiac and myelosuppressive profile. Oral capecitabine has proven to be ineffective in the adjuvant setting compared with multiregimen chemotherapy when patients can tolerate it.

- HER-2 targeted immunotherapy and molecularly targetable newer therapies that have favorable toxicity profile should always be considered for eligible elderly patients whenever possible.

- Fit elderly patients should be encouraged to participate in clinical trials to eventually increase the amount and quality of data generated from these that will help inform decision making for these patients in future.

DISCLOSURE

C.O.I.

REFERENCES

 1. Cancer facts & figures 2020. Atlanta (GA): American Cancer Society; 2020.
 2. Howlader N, Noone AM, Krapcho M et al. SEER Cancer Statistics Review, 1975-2012, National Cancer Institute. Bethesda (MD): Available at: , based on November 2014 SEER data submission, posted to the SEER web site, Accessed April1, 2015.
 3. Ortman, Jennifer M, Victoria A. et al. An Aging Nation: The Older Population in the United States, Current Population Reports, P25-1140. U.S. Census Bureau, Washington, DC: 2014.
 4. Smith BD, Smith GL, Hurria A, et al. Future of cancer incidence in the United States: burdens upon an aging, changing nation. J Clin Oncol 2009;27(17):2758–65.
 5. Murthy VH, Krumholz HM, Gross CP. Participation in cancer clinical trials: race-, sex-, and age-based disparities. JAMA 2004;291(22):2720–6.
 6. Biganzoli L, Wildiers H, Oakman C, et al. Management of elderly patients with breast cancer: updated recommendations of the international society of geriatric oncology (S.I.O.G.) and European society of breast cancer specialists (E.U.S.O.M.A.). Lancet Oncol 2012;13(4):e148–60.
 7. Schonberg MA, MArcantomo ER, Li D, et al. Breast cancer among the oldest old: tumor characteristics, treatment choices, and survival. J Clin Oncol 2010;28(12):2038–45.
 8. Eppenberger-Castori S, Moore DH, Thor AD, et al. Age-associated biomarker profiles of human breast cancer. Int J Biochem Cell Biol 2002;34(11):1318–30.
 9. Anderson WF, Katki HA, Rosenberg PS. Incidence of breast cancer in the United States: current and future trends. J Natl Cancer Inst 2011;103(18):1397–402.
10. Walter LC, Schonberg MA. Screening mammography in older women: a review. JAMA 2014;311(13):1336–47.
11. Oeffinger KC, Fontham ETH, Etzioni R, et al. Breast cancer screening for women at average risk: 2015 guideline update from the American Cancer Society. JAMA 2015;314(15):1599–614.
12. Siu AL, USPST Force. Screening for breast cancer: U.S. Preventive Services Task Force recommendation statement. Ann Intern Med 2016;164(4):279–96.
13. Kirkhus L, Benth JS, Rostoft S, et al. Geriatric assessment is superior to oncologists' clinical judgment in identifying frailty. Br J Cancer 2017;117(4):470–7.
14. Mohile SG, Dale W, Somerfield MR, et al. Practical assessment and management of vulnerabilities in older patients receiving chemotherapy: A.S.C.O. guideline for geriatric oncology. J Clin Oncol 2018;36(22):2326–47.
15. Russo C, Giannotti C, Signori A, et al. Predictive values of two frailty screening tools in older patients with solid cancer: a comparison of SAOP2 and G8. Oncotarget 2018;9(80):35056–68.
16. Overcash JA, Beckstead J, Extermann M, et al. The abbreviated comprehensive geriatric assessment (aCGA): a retrospective analysis. Crit Rev Oncol Hematol 2005;54(2):129–36.
17. Extermann M, Aapro M, Bernabei R, et al. Use of comprehensive geriatric assessment in older cancer patients: recommendations from the task force on C.G.A. of the International Society of Geriatric Oncology (S.I.O.G.). Crit Rev Oncol Hematol 2005;55(3):241–52.

18. Owusu C, Marggvucius S, Schluchter M, et al. Vulnerable elders survey and socioeconomic status predict functional decline and death among older women with newly diagnosed nonmetastatic breast cancer. Cancer 2016;122(16): 2579–86.

19. Walter LC, Brand RJ, Counsell SR, et al. Development and validation of a prognostic index for 1-year mortality in older adults after hospitalization. JAMA 2001;285(23):2987–94.

20. Anderson F, Downing GM, Hill J, et al. Palliative performance scale (P.P.S.): a new tool. J Palliat Care 1996;12(1):5–11.

21. Lavelle K, Todd C, Moran A, et al. Non-standard Management of breast cancer increases with age in the U.K.: a population-based cohort of women > or =65 years. Br J Cancer 2007;96(8):1197–203.

22. Lavelle K, Sowerbutts AM, Todd C, et al. Is lack of surgery for older breast cancer patients in the U.K. explained by patient choice or poor health? A prospective cohort study. Br J Cancer 2014;110(3):573–83.

23. Wyld L, Garg DK, Kumar D, et al. Stage and treatment variation with age in postmenopausal women with breast cancer: compliance with guidelines. Br J Cancer 2004;90(8):1486–91.

24. Bastiaannet E, Liefers GJ, de Caren AJ, et al. Breast cancer in elderly compared to younger patients in The Netherlands: stage at diagnosis, treatment and survival in 127,805 unselected patients. Breast Cancer Res Treat 2010;124(3):801–7.

25. Shachar SS, Hurria A, Muss HB. Breast cancer in women older than 80 Years. J Oncol Pract 2016;12(2):123–32.

26. Hurria A, Levit LA, Dale W, et al. Improving the evidence base for treating older adults with cancer: American Society of Clinical Oncology statement. J Clin Oncol 2015;33(32):3826–33.

27. Mueller CB, Ames F, Anderson GD. Breast cancer in 3,558 women: age as a significant determinant in the rate of dying and causes of death. Surgery 1978;83(2): 123–32.

28. Waldron RP, Donovan A, Drumm J, et al. Emergency presentation and mortality from colorectal cancer in the elderly. Br J Surg 1986;73(3):214–6.

29. Fentiman IS. Are the elderly receiving appropriate cancer treatment? Ann Oncol 1996;7(7):657–8.

30. Huisman MG, Audisio RA, Ugolini G, et al. Screening for predictors of adverse outcome in onco-geriatric surgical patients: a multicenter prospective cohort study. Eur J Surg Oncol 2015;41(7):844–51.

31. Audisio RA, Ramesh H, Longo WE, et al. Preoperative assessment of surgical risk in oncogeriatric patients. Oncologist 2005;10(4):262–8.

32. Korc-Grodzicki B, Downey RJ, Shahrokni A, et al. Surgical considerations in older adults with cancer. J Clin Oncol 2014;32(24):2647–53.

33. Sandison AJ, Gold DM, Wright P, et al. Breast conservation or mastectomy: treatment choice of women aged 70 years and older. Br J Surg 1996;83(7):994–6.

34. Martelli G, Miceli R, Daidone MG, et al. Axillary dissection versus no axillary dissection in elderly patients with breast cancer and no palpable axillary nodes: results after 15 years of follow-up. Ann Surg Oncol 2011;18(1):125–33.

35. Giuliano AE, Hunt KK, Ballman KV, et al. Axillary dissection vs no axillary dissection in women with invasive breast cancer and sentinel node metastasis: a randomized clinical trial. JAMA 2011;305(6):569–75.

36. Chatzidaki P, et al. Perioperative complications of breast cancer surgery in older women (>/=80 years). Ann Surg Oncol 2011;18(4):923–31.

37. Wyld L, Reed M, Collins K, et al. Impacts of omission of breast cancer surgery in older women with ER1 early breast cancer. In: 12th European Breast Cancer Conference. 2020.
38. Wyld L, Reed M, Collins K, et al. Cluster randomized trial to evaluate the clinical benefits of decision support interventions for older women with operable breast cancer. In: 12th European Breast Cancer Conference. October 2-3, 2020; Virtual conference.
39. Wyckoff J, Greenberg H, Sanderson R, et al. Breast irradiation in the older woman: a toxicity study. J Am Geriatr Soc 1994;42(2):150–2.
40. Kunkler IH, Audisio R, Belkacemi Y, et al. Review of current best practice and priorities for research in radiation oncology for elderly patients with cancer: the International Society of Geriatric Oncology (SIOG) task force. Ann Oncol 2014; 25(11):2134–46.
41. Hughes KS, Schnaper LA, Bellon JR, et al. Lumpectomy plus tamoxifen with or without irradiation in women age 70 years or older with early breast cancer: long-term follow-up of CALGB 9343. J Clin Oncol 2013;31(19):2382–7.
42. Kunkler IH, et al. Breast-conserving surgery with or without irradiation in women aged 65 years or older with early breast cancer (PRIME II): a randomised controlled trial. Lancet Oncol 2015;16(3):266–73.
43. Kunkler IH, Williams LJ, Jack W, et al. Prime 2 randomized trial (postoperative radiotherapy in minimum-risk elderly): wide local excision and adjuvant hormonal therapy +/- whole breast irradiation in women =/> 65 years with early invasive breast cancer: 10-year results, In: 2020 San Antonio Breast Cancer Symposium. 2020: San Antonio.
44. Clarke M, Collins R, Darby S, et al. Effects of radiotherapy and differences in the extent of surgery for early breast cancer on local recurrence and 15-year survival: an overview of the randomized trials. Lancet 2005;366(9503):2087–106.
45. VanderWalde N, et al. The role of adjuvant radiation treatment in older women with early breast cancer. J Geriatr Oncol 2013;4(4):402–12.
46. Group ST, et al. The U.K. Standardisation of Breast Radiotherapy (START) Trial B of radiotherapy hypofractionation for treatment of early breast cancer: a randomized trial. Lancet 2008;371(9618):1098–107.
47. Arriagada R, Mouriesse H, Sarrazin D, et al. Radiotherapy alone in breast cancer. I. Analysis of tumor parameters, tumor dose and local control: the experience of the Gustave-Roussy Institute and the Princess Margaret Hospital. Int J Radiat Oncol Biol Phys 1985;11(10):1751–7.
48. Mouridsen H,, Chaudri-Ross HA. Efficacy of first-line letrozole versus tamoxifen as a function of age in postmenopausal women with advanced breast cancer. Oncologist 2004;9(5):497–506.
49. Breast International Group 1-98 Collaborative Group, Thürlimann B, Keshaviah A, Coates A, et al. A comparison of letrozole and tamoxifen in postmenopausal women with early breast cancer. N Engl J Med 2005;353(26):2747–57.
50. Wildiers H, Kunkler I, Biganzoli L, et al. Management of breast cancer in elderly individuals: recommendations of the International Society of Geriatric Oncology. Lancet Oncol 2007;8(12):1101–15.
51. Akhtar SS, Allan SG, Rodger A, et al. A 10-year experience of tamoxifen as primary treatment of breast cancer in 100 elderly and frail patients. Eur J Surg Oncol 1991;17(1):30–5.
52. Hind D, Wyld L, Beverley CB, et al. Surgery versus primary endocrine therapy for operable primary breast cancer in elderly women (70 years plus). Cochrane Database Syst Rev 2006;(1):CD004272.

53. Mustacchi G, Ceccherini R, Milani S, et al. Tamoxifen alone versus adjuvant tamoxifen for operable breast cancer of the elderly: long-term results of the phase III randomized controlled multicenter GRETA trial. Ann Oncol 2003;14(3):414–20.

54. Macaskill EJ, Renshaw L, Dixon JM. Neoadjuvant use of hormonal therapy in elderly patients with early or locally advanced hormone receptor-positive breast cancer. Oncologist 2006;11(10):1081–8.

55. Hébert-Croteau N, Brisson J, Latreille J, et al. Compliance with consensus recommendations for systemic therapy is associated with improved survival of women with node-negative breast cancer. J Clin Oncol 2004;22(18):3685–93.

56. Early Breast Cancer Trialists' Collaborative, G. Effects of chemotherapy and hormonal therapy for early breast cancer on recurrence and 15-year survival: an overview of the randomised trials. Lancet 2005;365(9472):1687–717.

57. Christman K, Muss HB, Case LD, et al. Chemotherapy of metastatic breast cancer in the elderly. The Piedmont Oncology Association experience [see comment]. JAMA 1992;268(1):57–62.

58. Muss HB, Berry DA, Cirrincione C, et al. Toxicity of older and younger patients treated with adjuvant chemotherapy for node-positive breast cancer: the Cancer and Leukemia Group B Experience. J Clin Oncol 2007;25(24):3699–704.

59. Extermann M, Boler I, Reich RR, et al. Predicting the risk of chemotherapy toxicity in older patients: the chemotherapy risk assessment Scale for High-age patients (CRASH) score. Cancer 2012;118(13):3377–86.

60. Hurria A, Togawa K, Mohile SG, et al. Predicting chemotherapy toxicity in older adults with cancer: a prospective multicenter study. J Clin Oncol 2011;29(25):3457–65.

61. Jones S, Holmes FA, O'Shaughnessy J, et al. Docetaxel with Cyclophosphamide is associated with an overall survival Benefit Compared with Doxorubicin and Cyclophosphamide: 7-year follow-up of US oncology research trial 9735. J Clin Oncol 2009;27(8):1177–83.

62. Kizy S, Altman AM, Marmor S, et al. 21-gene recurrence score testing in the older population with estrogen receptor-positive breast cancer. J Geriatr Oncol 2019;10(2):322–9.

63. Perez EA, Romond EH, Suman VJ, et al. Trastuzumab plus adjuvant chemotherapy for human epidermal growth factor receptor 2-positive breast cancer: planned joint analysis of overall survival from NSABP B-31 and NCCTG N9831. J Clin Oncol 2014;32(33):3744–52.

64. Brunello A, Monfardini S, Crivellari D, et al. Multicenter analysis of activity and safety of trastuzumab plus chemotherapy in advanced breast cancer in elderly women (70 years). J Clin Oncol 2008;26(Suppl 15):1096.

65. Denegri A, Moccetti T, Moccetti M, et al. Cardiac toxicity of trastuzumab in elderly patients with breast cancer. J Geriatr Cardiol 2016;13(4):355–63.

66. Wishart GC, Bajdik CD, Dicks E, et al. PREDICT Plus: development and validation of a prognostic model for early breast cancer that includes HER2. Br J Cancer 2012;107(5):800–7.

67. Engelhardt EG, Garvelink MM, de Haes JH, et al. Predicting and communicating the risk of recurrence and death in women with early-stage breast cancer: a systematic review of risk prediction models. J Clin Oncol 2014;32(3):238–50.

68. Paridaens RJ, Gelber S, Cole BF, et al. Adjuvant! Online estimation of chemotherapy effectiveness when added to ovarian function suppression plus tamoxifen for premenopausal women with estrogen-receptor-positive breast cancer. Breast Cancer Res Treat 2010;123(1):303–10.

69. Howie LJ, Singh H, Bloomquist E, et al. Outcomes of older women with hormone receptor-positive, human epidermal growth factor receptor-negative metastatic breast cancer treated with a CDK4/6 Inhibitor and an Aromatase Inhibitor: an FDA Pooled analysis. J Clin Oncol 2019;37(36):3475–83.
70. Swain SM, Kim SB, Cortés J, et al. Pertuzumab, trastuzumab, and docetaxel for HER2-positive metastatic breast cancer (CLEOPATRA study): overall survival results from a randomised, double-blind, placebo-controlled, phase 3 study. Lancet Oncol 2013;14(6):461–71.
71. Krop IE, Kim SB, González-Martín A, et al. Trastuzumab emtansine versus treatment of physician's choice for pretreated HER2-positive advanced breast cancer (TH3RESA): a randomised, open-label, phase 3 trial. Lancet Oncol 2014;15(7):689–99.
72. Geyer CE, Forster J, Lindquist D, et al. Lapatinib plus capecitabine for HER2-positive advanced breast cancer [published correction appears in N Engl J Med. 2007 Apr 5;356(14):1487]. N Engl J Med 2006;355(26):2733–43.
73. Bajetta E, Procopio G, Celio L, et al. Safety and efficacy of two different doses of capecitabine in the treatment of advanced breast cancer in older women. J Clin Oncol 2005;23(10):2155–61.
74. Crivellari D, Aapro M, Leonard R, et al. Breast cancer in the elderly. J Clin Oncol 2007;25(14):1882–90.
75. Rousseau F, Retornaz F, Joly F, et al. Impact of an all-oral capecitabine and vinorelbine combination regimen on functional status of elderly patients with advanced solid tumours: a multicentre pilot study of the French geriatric oncology group (GERICO). Crit Rev Oncol Hematol 2010;76(1):71–8.
76. Schmid P, Rugo HS, Adams S, et al. Atezolizumab plus nab-paclitaxel as first-line treatment for unresectable, locally advanced or metastatic triple-negative breast cancer (IMpassion130): updated efficacy results from a randomised, double-blind, placebo-controlled, phase 3 trial. Lancet Oncol 2020;21(1):44–59.
77. Robson M, Im SA, Senkus E, et al. Olaparib for metastatic breast cancer in patients with a Germline BRCA Mutation. N Engl J Med 2017;377(6):523–33 [published correction appears in N Engl J Med. 2017 Oct 26;377(17):1700].
78. Saita Y, Ishijima M, Kaneko K. Atypical femoral fractures and bisphosphonate use: current evidence and clinical implications. Ther Adv Chronic Dis 2015;6(4):185–93.
79. Lichtman SM, Wildiers H, Launay-Vacher V et al.

The Science of Frailty
Sex Differences

Caroline Park, MD, PhD[a], Fred C. Ko, MD[b,c,*]

KEYWORDS

- Frailty • Sex differences • Sex-frailty paradox • 5 Ms

KEY POINTS

- Frailty is an important clinical syndrome of age-related decline in physiologic reserve and increased vulnerability and is associated with numerous adverse clinical outcomes.
- Frailty is driven by dysregulation of neuroendocrine, inflammatory, and metabolic pathways.
- Frailty is more prevalent in older women.
- Sex-specific differences in frailty is an emerging area of investigation.
- The 5 Ms (multicomplexity, mind, mobility, medications, and matters most) of geriatric medicine can be integrated in the clinical management of frail older adults to improve care.

DEFINITIONS, INCIDENCE, AND RISK FACTORS OF FRAILTY

The aging process in an older adult is driven by multidimensional inputs that contribute to an individual's overall progressive decline and ultimately death. These inputs span biological, environmental, and gene-environment interactions factors as well as changes in an individual's social and behavioral characteristics (**Fig. 1**). Importantly, this age-associated decline has an impact on multiple physiologic systems, leading to a state of decreased reserve and compromised resistance to stressors, which in turn contributes to increased vulnerability and adverse outcomes. Frailty is a clinical syndrome that captures this state of vulnerability and decline frequently seen in older adults.

Although frailty has many operational definitions, a majority of these definitions are embedded within 2 conceptual frameworks. The first framework conceptualizes frailty as a syndrome with a distinct physical phenotype with measurable clinical features. This physical frailty is best exemplified by the Fried phenotype, which characterizes

[a] Section of Geriatrics, Division of Primary Care & Population Health, Stanford School of Medicine, Stanford Senior Care, 211 Quarry Road. Suite 4C, Palo Alto, CA 94304, USA; [b] Brookdale Department of Geriatrics and Palliative Medicine, Icahn School of Medicine at Mount Sinai, One Gustave L. Levy Place, Box 1070, New York, NY 10029, USA; [c] Geriatric Research Education and Clinical Center, James J. Peters VA Medical Center, Bronx, NY, USA
* Corresponding author. Brookdale Department of Geriatrics and Palliative Medicine, Icahn School of Medicine at Mount Sinai, One Gustave L. Levy Place, Box 1070, New York, NY 10029.
E-mail address: Fred.ko@mssm.edu

Clin Geriatr Med 37 (2021) 625–638
https://doi.org/10.1016/j.cger.2021.05.008
0749-0690/21/Published by Elsevier Inc.

geriatric.theclinics.com

THE AGING OLDER ADULT

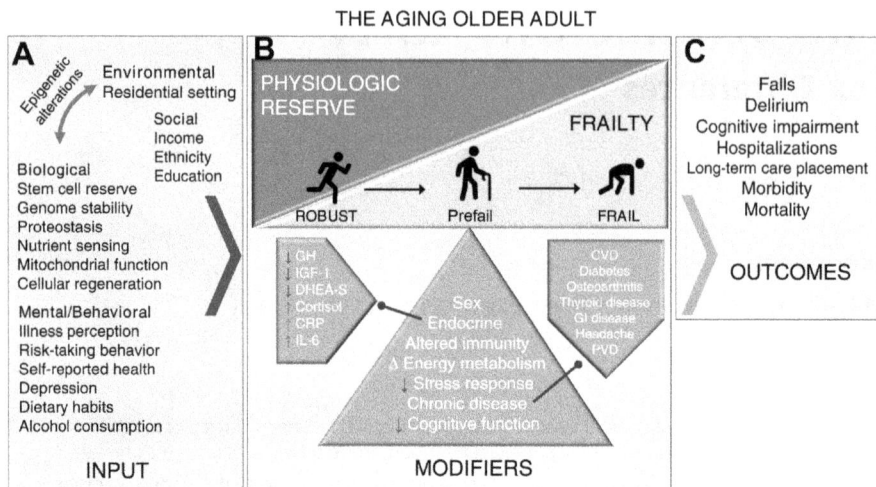

Fig. 1. Model pathway for frailty and contributing factors: (A) input, (B) modifiers, and (C) outcomes. Also shown (B) is the progression of frailty (yellow shaded area) from robust to prefrail to frail, as physiologic reserve (blue shading) declines. CVD, cardiovascular disease; GI, gastrointestinal; PVD, peripheral vascular disease.

frailty by unintentional weight loss ($\geq$5% of body weight in the past year), self-reported exhaustion, weakness (as measured by decreased grip strength), slow walking speed, and low physical activity.[1] Specifically, those who meet greater than or equal to 3 of these criteria are considered frail, whereas those meeting 1 to 2 criteria are prefrail, and those without any of these characteristics are robust (see Fig. 1B). The second framework conceptualizes frailty as a state of vulnerability due to deficit accumulation that can be ascertained through cumulative comorbidities, disease states, functional and cognitive deficits, and psychosocial factors.[2,3] These deficits can be tallied to determine a frailty index (FI), with a higher number of deficits yielding a higher FI score.

Despite the lack of a gold standard definition, frailty, as operationally defined previously, has been demonstrated to increase risks for adverse clinical outcomes, including falls, surgical complications, institutionalization, disability, and death.[4] For instance, in a prospective observational study in older adults agee 85 and older, baseline frailty is found associated with a more than 2-fold risk of mortality after 7 years compared with those who are nonfrail.[5] Moreover, frailty leads to increased health care utilization and associated total health care costs, of 54% to 101%.[6] Thus, frailty in late life is a serious medical condition that needs to be managed carefully.

This association between older age and frailty is important, particularly given that society is rapidly aging. According to the 2019 United Nations World Population Ageing Highlights, there are an estimated 703 million persons ages 65 years and older, which is projected to double by 2050.[7] It is anticipated that this large increase in the geriatric population will correspond to a proportional increase in older adults who are frail. To this end, the epidemiology, prevalence, and incidence of frailty have been determined in many population-based studies worldwide. The mean prevalence of frailty among the community-dwelling population ages 65 years and older is approximately 10% but can range widely from 4.0% to 59.1%, depending on the frailty criteria used.[8] A recent meta-analysis of 120,805 adults 60 years or older across 28 countries reported that the estimated global incidence of frailty, as determined by the Fried phenotype, in community-dwelling older adults is 40 cases per 1000 person-years over a median follow-up of 3 years (95% CI, 34.5–48.5; I^2 = 98.2%).[9] Factors that are associated with an increased prevalence of frailty include African American or Hispanic ethnicity, lower income and education level, poorer health, and higher rates of comorbid chronic diseases and disability.[1]

Given that frailty in older adults is common and leads to a multitude of adverse outcomes, a deeper understanding of the science of frailty is a critical first step to help design effective interventions that prevent or attenuate frailty-induced sequelae. Part of such in-depth understanding of frailty also involves recognizing that sex differences in frailty do exist. In community-dwelling older adults more than 65 years of age, frailty was found more common in women and in greater severity (as determined by FI, which is a known predictor of all-cause mortality[3]) compared with men for any age group.[10] Despite the greater likelihood of being frail, however, risk of mortality was lower in women. Therefore, because such sex discrepancies in frailty exist, it is important to understand the causes of these differences so that sex-specific frailty interventions can be developed further as part of providing the best possible patient-centered care for frail older adults. This article reviews the proposed pathophysiology of frailty in general as well as hypothesized contributing factors of sex-specific differences in frailty. Similar reviews have been published previously.[10–12]

PATHOPHYSIOLOGY OF FRAILTY

The pathophysiology of frailty is an active area of research. Although the precise pathogenesis of frailty remains unknown, available evidence suggests that physical frailty is in part driven by dysregulation of neuroendocrine, inflammatory, and metabolic pathways (see **Fig. 1**A, B). For example, age-related hormonal changes that are associated with frailty include decreased levels of growth hormone (GH), insulinlike growth factor 1 (IGF-1), and dehydroepiandrosterone sulfate (DHEA-S)[13] as well as increased cortisol levels.[14] Additionally, due to the anabolic and immunity-modulating effects of these hormones, alterations in these hormones likely have direct or indirect impacts on skeletal muscles, therefore causing dysregulated glucose metabolism and insulin signaling, and sarcopenia (ie, age-related loss of muscle mass and strength).[15,16] Furthermore, chronic low-grade inflammation is highly associated with frailty. This inflammatory state is measurable by elevated proinflammatory cytokines, such as interleukin-6, C-reactive protein (CRP),[17] elevated numbers of neutrophils and macrophages,[18] and activation of markers of clotting cascades, such as D-dimer, in frail older adults.[19] The inputs that are hypothesized to drive this multisystemic physiologic dysregulation and progression to frailty development include age-related biological changes (eg, proteostasis and mitochondrial function), genetics, and environmental exposures (see **Fig. 1**A).[20]

With such inputs, frail older adults enter an altered homeostatic state, which results in a reduced capacity to generate an appropriate stress response to both acute or chronic stressors, such as illness, hospitalization, and surgery. This inability to regain homeostasis, termed homeostenosis, causes an individual to spiral further into a cycle of frailty,[21] where each of the 5 frailty characteristics (ie, decreased mobility and activity, weight loss, weakness, and fatigue) can initiate a vicious cycle that perpetuates worsening of dysregulated energetics, sarcopenia, and an aggregate frailty syndrome.[22] Ultimately, frailty in older adults increases the risk for other common geriatric syndromes or outcomes, such as falls, delirium, cognitive impairment,[23,24] long-term care placement, and mortality (see **Fig. 1**C).[25,26]

SEX DIFFERENCES IN FRAILTY PHENOTYPE AND THE SEX-FRAILTY PARADOX
Sex Differences in Frailty Prevalence, Adverse Outcomes, and Mortality

Community-dwelling women ages 65 years or older have a higher prevalence and greater burden of frailty compared with men of the same age (**Table 1**). In a study of 3079 community-dwelling older adults from the 2007 to 2010 National Health and Nutrition Examination Survey database, frailty has been found more prevalent in women (8.8% in women vs 5.4% in men).[27] Moreover, a similar sex-specific trend has been observed in prefrail older adults as determined in a recent meta-analysis of 240 studies spanning across 62 countries worldwide.[28] Moreover, although there is great variability in frailty assessment depending on the tool used,[29] women were

Table 1
Sex-specific associations in prefrailty, frailty, and frailty-associated adverse outcomes

		Finding	Reference
	Prefrailty prevalence	Women > men Women: 15% (95% CI, 14%–17%; n= 143; I^2 = 99%; $P<.005$) Men: 11% (95% CI, 10%–12%; n = 145; I^2 = 97%; $P<.005$)	Meta-analysis (O'Caoimh et al.,[28] 2020)
		Women: 39.0% (95% CI, 38.1%–39.9%) Men: 37.3% (95% CI, 36.6%–38.0%; x^2 = 8629; df = 1; P = .003)	Systematic review (Collard et al.,[35] 2012)
	Frailty prevalence	Women > men Women: 9.6% (95% CI, 9.2%–10%) Men: 5.2% (95% CI, 4.9%–5.5%; $P<.001$)	Systematic review (Collard et al.,[35] 2012)
		Women: 49% (95% CI, 14%–17%; $P<.005$) Men: 45% (95% CI, 44%–47%; n = 119; I^2 = 97%; $P<.005$)	Meta-analysis (O'Caoimh et al.,[28] 2020)
Frailty-associated adverse outcomes	Survival	1. HR 0.43 (95% CI, 0.299–0.561); $P<0001$ 2. Survival rate of women > men independent of frailty status	1. Observational, 10-y longitudinal study (Corbi et al., 2019) 2. Secondary analysis of SHARE (Theou et al.,[30] 2014)
	Mortality	Mortality rate lower in women vs men (up to age 90, after which mortality rate increases to above 30% in women).	Meta-analysis (Gordon et al.,[10] 2017)

Please note that other adverse outcomes, including readmission rate, emergency department visits, and hospital admissions, are not shown because those outcomes have not yet been shown to have sex-specific associations.
Abbreviations: I2 = Higgins I2 statistic; Df = Degrees of freedom.

found to have higher frailty scores than men regardless.[30] Additionally, frail women are at increased risk of developing deficits in activities of daily living (ADLs) and/or instrumental ADLs and institutionalization.[31] Frail older adults also are at risk of associated adverse outcomes, including hospitalizations, emergency room visits,[32] readmissions, disability, and overall reduced survival[33] and increased mortality rates[34] but, thus far, sex-specific differences have been noted only in frailty prevalence, survival, and mortality rates (see **Table 1**).[28,30,35]

Regardless of age or level of frailty, older frail women have better survival compared with men. In a meta-analysis of 2 large cohort studies (Survey of Health, Ageing, and Retirement in Europe [SHARE][36] and Mexican Health and Aging Study[37]) that used the FI to determine frailty, men have higher rates of mortality compared with women until age 90.[10] In another study of older adults, the mortality rate in frail men (22.5%) is much higher compared with women (8.5%). In this study, sex-specific differences in the causes of death also are found. In men, the predominant causes for death are heart disease (41%) and chronic lower respiratory disease (23%), compared with nephritis/nephrosis in women (32.3%).[27]

The Sex-Frailty Paradox

The sex-associated divergence in frailty prevalence and mortality has been referred to as the sex-frailty paradox.[11] This is consistent with the long-recognized observation that women have longer life span than men despite having higher chronic disease burden and disability.[11] The sex-frailty paradox is best illustrated by a meta-analysis of 7 large studies of community-dwelling older adults showing that mortality rate is lower in women irrespective of their age or frailty severity.[10] Although the reasons for this phenomenon are yet to be elucidated, some investigators have hypothesized that this may be due to men having more life-threatening chronic conditions (eg, stroke and ischemic heart disease), whereas women may experience more non–life-threatening chronic conditions that are associated with higher morbidity (eg, fractures, depression, constipation, and headaches).[11,25]

Sex Differences in Frailty-Associated Contributing Factors

Frailty and its progression are driven by multi-domain inputs (see **Fig. 1**), which may have differential impact, depending on the sex of the individual. Based on growing evidence focusing on these sex-specific differences in frailty and their contributing factors, it has been hypothesized that sex-specific differences in frailty likely is due to a combined effect of biological, psychosocial, and behavioral differences between women and men.[12] This article conceptually categorizes contributing factors for sex-differences in frailty in older adults into biological, social and behavioral domains (**Fig. 2**). Although some of these contributing factors are common between both sexes, others have a more sex-specific contribution.

Biological factors that may contribute to sex-differences in frailty include chronic disease, changes in immunity, and endocrinologic changes, which occur in part, due to aging. As noted by Gordon and Hubbard,[11] although certain chronic medical conditions such as cardiac disease, congestive heart failure, diabetes mellitus, osteoarthritis, and glaucoma are similarly prevalent in older adults regardless of sex, differences do exist in other chronic conditions. For example, in men, a higher prevalence of hearing impairment, peripheral vascular disease, and gastrointestinal disease are reported, whereas in women, dementia, hip fracture, depression, headache, urinary incontinence, and thyroid disease are more prevalent.

Sex-specific differences in immune response and inflammatory signaling may partially stem from differences in sex chromosomes. Women have 2 copies of X

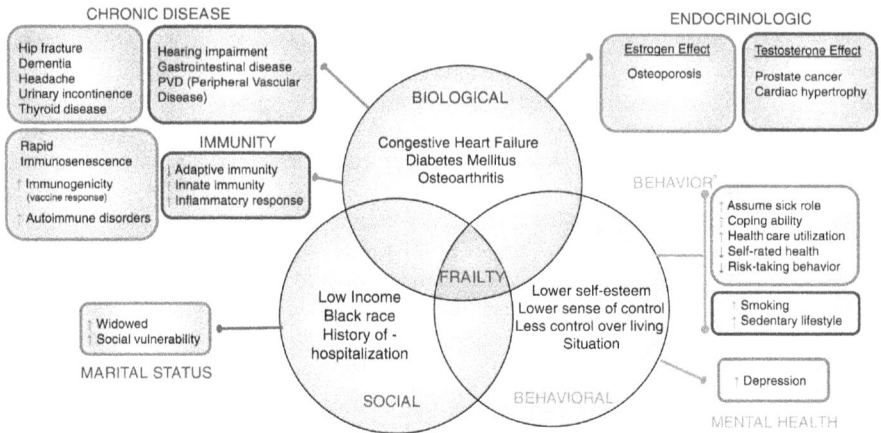

Fig. 2. Contributory domains and factors for frailty and sex-specific associations. Depicted within each circle of the Venn diagram are the contributing factor domains (biological, social, and behavioral) that are color-coded as blue, orange, and yellow shading. For each domain, contributing factors common to both genders (or are of equal prevalence) are listed inside the circle, and those that have gender-specific associations are depicted outside the circle in boxes that are outlined in pink (female-specific) or blue (male-specific). Note: for behavioral, only female-specific associations are shown in the boxes ([a]men have the opposite characteristics that are not shown).

chromosome, which carries genes that encode Toll-like receptor and multiple cytokine receptors and genes involved in T-cell and B-cell activity. In comparison, men carry 1 copy each of X chromosome and Y chromosome, which encodes some inflammatory pathway genes that are expressed exclusively in men.[38,39] Consequently, progression to immunosenescence, which contributes to age-related decline in immune function, is known to occur at a faster rate in men than in women.[40,41] Epigenomic and genomic changes regulate innate and humoral immunity in a sex-specific manner.[38] These genomic differences between sexes increase after age 65, with men having higher innate and proinflammatory activity, while having lower adaptive immunity, compared with women.[42]

Differences in levels and regulation of hormones also differentially contribute to frailty in a sex-specific manner. For example, estrogen reduces hepatic sensitivity to GH. In contrast, testosterone enhances the effect of GH, which increases the risk of some age-related diseases, such as prostate cancer and cardiac hypertrophy.[43] Additionally, several autoimmune disorders, including multiple sclerosis, rheumatoid arthritis, Sjögren syndrome, and systemic lupus erythematosus, are known to be more prevalent in women. This increase in susceptibility in women may be due to the reduced protective effect of some autoimmune regulatory genes that are down-regulated by estrogen.[44,45] COVID-19 is another example of how the regulatory role of sex hormones may affect disease pathogenesis. In COVID-19, the severe acute respiratory syndrome coronavirus 2 binds to the angiotensin-converting enzyme (ACE)-2 receptor, which serves as viral entry point.[46] Because testosterone up-regulates, whereas estrogen inhibits ACE-2 receptor expression, sex hormone differences may partially explain the increased risk of disease severity and mortality in men.[47]

Skeletal muscle changes with age, both in its overall architecture (ie, skeletal muscle remodeling, including increased intramyocellular lipid accumulation and fibrosis) as well as in its macronutrient (eg, fat, protein, and glucose) metabolism.[48] As a result, the absolute and relative loss of contractile skeletal muscle tissue is a shared feature in both aging men and women.[48,49] The decline in resting energy expenditure, however, in both skeletal muscle and overall adipose tissue occurs at a faster rate in women compared with men. This may partially explain why women are more prone to frailty than men.[50]

Apart from biological contributory factors, differences in the social and behavioral domains may contribute to sex-specific differences in frailty (see **Fig. 2**). Within the social domain, social vulnerability is a significant contributory factor. Marital status is 1 important determinant of social vulnerability, and studies have found that widowhood is associated more frequently with frailty,[51] as well as being socially frail, and thereby increases risk of mortality (hazard ratio [HR] 2.69; 95% CI, 1.01–7.25; $P<.05$).[52] Women may be able to better cope with social vulnerability, however, due to greater support networks, whereas men may be subject to increased mortality[53] due to a relative lack of coping mechanisms. Despite better coping mechanisms in women, widowhood is a known risk factor for the development of persistent depressive symptoms,[54] and this in turn may increase the risk of frailty.[55] It currently is unclear whether depression can increase the risk of frailty in a sex-specific manner.

In the behavioral domain, several contributory factors may contribute to sex-specific differences in frailty. For instance, coping mechanisms may differ between men and women, perhaps by activating different brain areas, thereby using different problem-solving strategies. Specifically, when exposed to an acute stressor, men are found to engage the prefrontal cortex regions, whereas women have more responses in the limbic/striatal regions, and these stress responses are associated with distinct neural networks.[56] Furthermore, it has been proposed that the psychological phenomenon of stress, such as life stressors from surgery or illness; emotional, physical or sexual abuse; divorce; or death of a loved one, may be related to microstructural changes in the corpus callosum of the brain.[57] Accordingly, these sex-specific differences in stress perception potentially may explain differences in women's behavior around health issues, including illness perception, self-rated health, and health care utilization. Women also are more sensitive to small physical changes and more likely to assume the sick role.[58] Although women have poorer self-rated health,[59] they are more likely to report either minor or major health issues.[60] A cautious reminder is that the perception of self-rated health is influenced by other social determinants of health as well, including occupation, marital status, household income, area of residence (rural/urban), and work environment.[61] When it comes to risky behavior, such as cigarette smoking or alcohol consumption, women also tend to be risk-averse compared with men.[62]

Other independent frailty-associated factors that are unique to, or shared between, men and women have been described[27,63] (see **Fig. 2**). Zhang and colleagues[27] showed that independent frailty-associated factors common to both men and women include sedentary lifestyle (physical inactivity) and prior history of hospitalizations. In contrast, higher family income to poverty ratio is protective against frailty in both sexes. In men, frailty is associated with additional risk factors, including being widowed, divorced, or separated; sleeping more than 9 hours a day; and smoking. In women, additional risk factors for frailty include obesity (body mass index ≥ 30 kg/m^2); elevated inflammatory markers, such as CRP; sleeping less than 6 hours a day; and family history of diabetes or myocardial infarction.

INTERVENTION FOR FRAILTY INCORPORATING THE 5 MS OF GERIATRICS

The overall approach to caring for an older adult with frailty should aim at diagnosing frailty using validated screening tools, followed by implementing individually tailored intervention plans.[64] A diagnosis of frailty can be made with tools, such as the Fried phenotype (ie, Hopkins frailty tool) or the FI as determined by a comprehensive geriatric assessment. Rapid screening tools, such as the FRAIL scale or the Study of Osteoporotic Fractures frailty tool, that allows quicker screening also may be used.[65,66] Although there currently is insufficient evidence to differentiate treatment interventions for frailty in a sex-specific manner, the 5 Ms (multicomplexity, mind, mobility, medications, and matters most) of geriatric care can be incorporated to augment frailty intervention.[67]

Intervention modalities, including exercise, nutrition management, and interdisciplinary geriatric models of care, have been found to improve clinical features of frailty or reduce adverse outcomes. For example, Travers and colleagues[68] have noted, in their systematic review of 925 studies, that a combination of muscle strength training and protein supplementation are the most effective and easiest interventions to implement, and to delay or reverse frailty. Multicomponent intervention is also imperative for preventing frailty-associated adverse outcomes. Marcucci and colleagues have proposed guidelines, as a part of the Frailty Management Optimisation through European Innovation Partnership on Active and Healthy Ageing (EIP-AHA) Commitments and Utilisation of Stakeholders' Input (FOCUS) project, that interventions, including exercise, nutritional management, and their combination, should be implemented to prevent or delay the progression of frailty.[64] Lastly, geriatric-focused interdisciplinary care programs, such as Geriatric Evaluation and Management (GEM), Acute Care for the Elders Unit (ACE), Program for All-Inclusive Care for the Elderly (PACE), and hospice care (**Fig. 3**) and their impact on the health of vulnerable older adults have been extensively studied in both outpatient and inpatient settings. As an example, a meta-analysis of 7 studies, including 1009 comprehensive geriatric assessment unit interventions are found effective in managing physical and psychological frailty, readmission, mortality, and patient satisfaction in hospitalized older adults.[69] Thus, geriatric interdisciplinary models of care should be integrated whenever feasible and take an active role in the clinical care of frail older adults.

Multicomplexity

The complex health care needs of frail older adults necessitate utilizing multimodal interventions that encompass management of chronic comorbidities, behavioral and psychosocial needs, and lifestyle modification that may be of benefit to reduce or prevent frailty. In a recent prospective cohort study of 6357 adults followed longitudinally

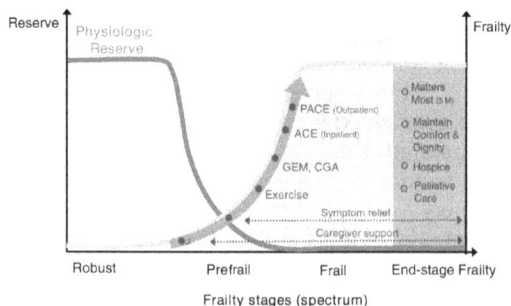

Fig. 3. Interventions for older adults along the frailty spectrum. Shaded areas depict possible interventions for the frail older adults (purple: early-stage/midstage frailty; and green: end-stage frailty). CGA, comprehensive geriatric assessment.

for 20 years, healthy habits exercised at age 50 are associated with a lower risk of frailty later in life. These habits include not smoking (HR 0.68; 95% CI, 0.52–0.89; $P = .01$), moderate alcohol consumption (HR 0.76; 95% CI, 0.59–0.98; $P<.001$), physical activity of at least 2.5 hours per week (HR 0.66; 95% CI, 0.48–0.88; $P = .0001$), and consuming fruits and vegetables more than twice daily (HR 0.70; 95% CI, 0.53–0.92; $P = .01$).[70] Frailty risk is reduced by 70% if all 4 healthy habits are present. Additionally, in this same study, the cumulative effect of multiple healthy habits and behavioral modification implemented at or before age 50 are shown to help prevent frailty later in life with a 31% reduction in frailty incidence for each additional healthy behavior. These findings indicate that early intervention with modification of risk factors can indeed prevent frailty.

Mind

As introduced briefly in the previous sections, frailty is impacted by multifaceted inputs, which include psychosocial variables, such as cognition and mood (eg, psychological wellness). First, frailty is associated with cognitive impairment[24] and dementia,[71] and cognitive training has been associated with improved frailty score and reduced frailty prevalence.[72] Second, older adults with depression are at risk of frailty,[73] and specifically in women, depressive symptoms increase the likelihood for frailty.[74] In men, more traumatic life events and perceived level of posttraumatic psychological stress are associated with increased likelihood of frailty. Thus, providers need to remain cognizant of these sex-specific differences in psychosocial correlates of frailty for both assessment and intervention, in order to better address the mind component of the 5 Ms–oriented geriatric care.

Mobility

Many single-component and multicomponent physical activity programs improve gait speed, muscle strength, mobility, and physical performance in frail older adults,[75] although modalities in which exercise interventions are implemented in frailty studies vary significantly.[76] In 1 study, a home-based video exercise program for frail older women greater than 75 years of age has shown to improve overall quality of life as measured by EuroQoL–5 Dimension,[77] including measures of mobility, self-care, usual activities, pain or discomfort, and anxiety or depression as well as self-rated health.[78] Thus, providers should consider the exercise training options that may be available to a frail older adult and prescribe an exercise intervention that best meet the individual's need and ability.

Medications

The impact of polypharmacy, and its associated adverse outcomes, on frail older adults, needs to be considered when devising a care plan. In a systematic review of 25 studies, polypharmacy is associated with frailty. Significant associations are found with every medication added to the treatment (odds ratio [OR] 1.13–1.20), with polypharmacy (OR 1.77–2.55), and with hyperpolypharmacy ($\geq$10 drugs [OR 4.47–5.8]).[79] Frail older adults subjected to polypharmacy also have a 13-fold longer hospital stay and a 5-fold greater risk for hospital readmission.[80] Furthermore, providers should be cognizant of how sex-specific differences in drug metabolism[81] can affect pharmacokinetics. Thus, extra efforts should be made to address polypharmacy in frail older adults.

Matters Most

The routine assessment of a frail older adult's priorities and goals of care, including treatment preferences and quality of life as well as psychosocial resources,[74] has become exceedingly important when aiming to provide improved 5 Ms–focused patient-centered care. This approach allows providers to recommend the most appropriate intervention strategy along the spectrum of frailty.[82,83] Specifically, it enables timely integration of the management of distressing symptoms as well as ensuring appropriate caregiver support. Moreover, multicomponent interventions, such as exercise training tailored toward the need and ability of the patient, as well as geriatric interdisciplinary models of care corresponding to the level of a patient's need, should be integrated into patient care in order to optimize outcomes.[64,69] Finally, older adults who are severely frail should be provided with necessary access to palliative and hospice care and related resources.[84]

SUMMARY AND FUTURE DIRECTIONS

Frailty is a clinical syndrome that leads to a progressive, multisystem decline in function and physiologic reserve and increased vulnerability to adverse outcomes. Various biological, psychosocial, and behavioral inputs contribute to the development of frailty. Moreover, some of these inputs may contribute to sex-specific differences in frailty and associated adverse outcomes. Future research efforts should focus on development of screening tools and therapeutic interventions that best incorporate sex-specific differences in frailty in order to reduce mortality and optimize outcomes in frail older adults.

CLINICS CARE POINTS

- Exercise, nutrition management, and interdisciplinary geriatric models of care have been found to improve clinical features of frailty or reduce adverse outcomes.
- The 5 Ms of geriatric medicine can be integrated in the clinical care of frail older adults.

DISCLOSURE

Primary funder of research is provided by grant K08 AG050808, National Institute on Aging.

REFERENCES

1. Fried LP, Tangen CM, Walston J, et al. Frailty in older adults: evidence for a phenotype. J Gerontol A Biol Sci Med Sci 2001;56(3):M146–56.
2. Rockwood K, Mitnitski A. Frailty in relation to the accumulation of deficits. J Gerontol A Biol Sci Med Sci 2007;62(7):722–7.
3. Rockwood K, Mitnitski A. Frailty defined by deficit accumulation and geriatric medicine defined by frailty. Clin Geriatr Med 2011;27(1):17–26.
4. Clegg A, Young J, Iliffe S, et al. Frailty in elderly people. Lancet 2013;381(9868): 752–62.
5. Keeble E, Parker SG, Arora S, et al. Frailty, hospital use and mortality in the older population: findings from the Newcastle 85+ study. Age Ageing 2019;48(6):797–802.
6. Hajek A, Bock JO, Saum KU, et al. Frailty and healthcare costs-longitudinal results of a prospective cohort study. Age Ageing 2018;47(2):233–41.
7. Nations U. World Population Ageing 2019: Highlights (ST/ESA/SER.A/430s). In: 2019, editor. United Nations, Department of Economic and Social Affairs, Population Division.

8. Kojima G, Liljas AEM, Iliffe S. Frailty syndrome: implications and challenges for health care policy. Risk Manag Healthc Policy 2019;12:23–30.

9. Ofori-Asenso R, Chin KL, Mazidi M, et al. Global incidence of frailty and Prefrailty among community-dwelling older adults: a systematic review and meta-analysis. JAMA Netw Open 2019;2(8):e198398.

10. Gordon EH, Peel NM, Samanta M, et al. Sex differences in frailty: a systematic review and meta-analysis. Exp Gerontol 2017;89:30–40.

11. Gordon EH, Hubbard RE. Do sex differences in chronic disease underpin the sex-frailty paradox? Mech Ageing Dev 2019;179:44–50.

12. Gordon EH, Hubbard RE. Differences in frailty in older men and women. Med J Aust 2020;212(4):183–8.

13. Leng SX, Cappola AR, Andersen RE, et al. Serum levels of insulin-like growth factor-I (IGF-I) and dehydroepiandrosterone sulfate (DHEA-S), and their relationships with serum interleukin-6, in the geriatric syndrome of frailty. Aging Clin Exp Res 2004;16(2):153–7.

14. Varadhan R, Walston J, Cappola AR, et al. Higher levels and blunted diurnal variation of cortisol in frail older women. J Gerontol A Biol Sci Med Sci 2008;63(2):190–5.

15. Kalyani RR, Varadhan R, Weiss CO, et al. Frailty status and altered glucose-insulin dynamics. J Gerontol A Biol Sci Med Sci 2012;67(12):1300–6.

16. Diamanti-Kandarakis E, Dattilo M, Macut D, et al. Mechanisms IN ENDOCRINOLOGY: aging and anti-aging: a Combo-Endocrinology overview. Eur J Endocrinol 2017;176(6):R283–308.

17. Puts MT, Visser M, Twisk JW, et al. Endocrine and inflammatory markers as predictors of frailty. Clin Endocrinol (Oxf) 2005;63(4):403–11.

18. Leng SX, Xue QL, Tian J, et al. Inflammation and frailty in older women. J Am Geriatr Soc 2007;55(6):864–71.

19. Walston J, McBurnie MA, Newman A, et al. Frailty and activation of the inflammation and coagulation systems with and without clinical comorbidities: results from the Cardiovascular Health Study. Arch Intern Med 2002;162(20):2333–41.

20. Walston J, Hadley EC, Ferrucci L, et al. Research agenda for frailty in older adults: toward a better understanding of physiology and etiology: summary from the American geriatrics society/National Institute on aging research Conference on frailty in older adults. J Am Geriatr Soc 2006;54(6):991–1001.

21. Xue QL, Bandeen-Roche K, Varadhan R, et al. Initial manifestations of frailty criteria and the development of frailty phenotype in the Women's Health and Aging Study II. J Gerontol A Biol Sci Med Sci 2008;63(9):984–90.

22. Xue QL. The frailty syndrome: definition and natural history. Clin Geriatr Med 2011;27(1):1–15.

23. Morley JE, Vellas B, van Kan GA, et al. Frailty consensus: a call to action. J Am Med Dir Assoc 2013;14(6):392–7.

24. Robertson DA, Savva GM, Kenny RA. Frailty and cognitive impairment–a review of the evidence and causal mechanisms. Ageing Res Rev 2013;12(4):840–51.

25. Case A, Paxson C. Sex differences in morbidity and mortality. Demography 2005;42(2):189–214.

26. Hessey E, Montgomery C, Zuege DJ, et al. Sex-specific prevalence and outcomes of frailty in critically ill patients. J Intensive Care 2020;8:75.

27. Zhang Q, Guo H, Gu H, et al. Gender-associated factors for frailty and their impact on hospitalization and mortality among community-dwelling older adults: a cross-sectional population-based study. PeerJ 2018;6:e4326.

28. O'Caoimh R, Sezgin D, O'Donovan MR, et al. Prevalence of frailty in 62 countries across the world: a systematic review and meta-analysis of population-level studies. Age Ageing 2020. https://doi.org/10.1093/ageing/afaa219.

29. Theou O, Brothers TD, Mitnitski A, et al. Operationalization of frailty using eight commonly used scales and comparison of their ability to predict all-cause mortality. J Am Geriatr Soc 2013;61(9):1537–51.

30. Theou O, Brothers TD, Peña FG, et al. Identifying common characteristics of frailty across seven scales. J Am Geriatr Soc 2014;62(5):901–6.

31. Bandeen-Roche K, Xue QL, Ferrucci L, et al. Phenotype of frailty: characterization in the women's health and aging studies. J Gerontol A Biol Sci Med Sci 2006; 61(3):262–6.

32. Kojima G. Frailty as a predictor of emergency Department utilization among community-dwelling older people: a systematic review and meta-analysis. J Am Med Dir Assoc 2019;20(1):103–5.

33. Corbi G, Cacciatore F, Komici K, et al. Inter-relationships between gender, frailty and 10-year survival in older Italian adults: an observational longitudinal study. Sci Rep 2019;9(1):18416.

34. Nguyen AT, Nguyen TX, Nguyen TN, et al. The impact of frailty on prolonged hospitalization and mortality in elderly inpatients in Vietnam: a comparison between the frailty phenotype and the Reported Edmonton Frail Scale. Clin Interv Aging 2019;14:381–8.

35. Collard RM, Boter H, Schoevers RA, et al. Prevalence of frailty in community-dwelling older persons: a systematic review. J Am Geriatr Soc 2012;60(8): 1487–92.

36. Romero-Ortuno R, Kenny RA. The frailty index in Europeans: association with age and mortality. Age Ageing 2012;41(5):684–9.

37. García-González JJ, García-Peña C, Franco-Marina F, et al. A frailty index to predict the mortality risk in a population of senior Mexican adults. BMC Geriatr 2009; 9:47.

38. Giefing-Kröll C, Berger P, Lepperdinger G, et al. How sex and age affect immune responses, susceptibility to infections, and response to vaccination. Aging Cell 2015;14(3):309–21.

39. Charchar FJ, Bloomer LD, Barnes TA, et al. Inheritance of coronary artery disease in men: an analysis of the role of the Y chromosome. Lancet 2012;379(9819): 915–22.

40. Kryspin-Exner I, Lamplmayr E, Felnhofer A. Geropsychology: the gender gap in human aging–a mini-review. Gerontology 2011;57(6):539–48.

41. Hirokawa K, Utsuyama M, Hayashi Y, et al. Slower immune system aging in women versus men in the Japanese population. Immun Ageing 2013;10(1):19.

42. Márquez EJ, Chung CH, Marches R, et al. Sexual-dimorphism in human immune system aging. Nat Commun 2020;11(1):751.

43. Ostan R, Monti D, Gueresi P, et al. Gender, aging and longevity in humans: an update of an intriguing/neglected scenario paving the way to a gender-specific medicine. Clin Sci (Lond) 2016;130(19):1711–25.

44. Kivity S, Ehrenfeld M. Can we explain the higher prevalence of autoimmune disease in women? Expert Rev Clin Immunol 2010;6(5):691–4.

45. Moulton VR. Sex hormones in Acquired immunity and autoimmune disease. Front Immunol 2018;9:2279.

46. Wang Q, Zhang Y, Wu L, et al. Structural and functional Basis of SARS-CoV-2 entry by using human ACE2. Cell 2020;181(4):894–904.e9.

47. Gadi N, Wu SC, Spihlman AP, et al. What's sex got to do with COVID-19? Gender-based differences in the host immune response to Coronaviruses. Front Immunol 2020;11:2147.

48. Gheller BJ, Riddle ES, Lem MR, et al. Understanding age-related changes in skeletal muscle metabolism: differences between females and males. Annu Rev Nutr 2016;36:129–56.

49. Kent-Braun JA, Ng AV, Young K. Skeletal muscle contractile and noncontractile components in young and older women and men. J Appl Physiol (1985) 2000; 88(2):662–8.

50. Geisler C, Braun W, Pourhassan M, et al. Gender-specific associations in age-related changes in resting energy expenditure (REE) and MRI measured body Composition in healthy Caucasians. J Gerontol A Biol Sci Med Sci 2016;71(7): 941–6.

51. Maciel G, da Silva H, Goncalves R, et al. Frailty assessment and its association with sociodemographic and health characteristics in community elderly. International Archives of Medicine, Section: Geriatrics 2017;10(134):1-7.

52. Andrew MK, Keefe JM. Social vulnerability from a social ecology perspective: a cohort study of older adults from the National Population Health Survey of Canada. BMC Geriatr 2014;14:90.

53. Shor E, Roelfs DJ, Curreli M, et al. Widowhood and mortality: a meta-analysis and meta-regression. Demography 2012;49(2):575–606.

54. Buigues C, Padilla-Sánchez C, Garrido JF, et al. The relationship between depression and frailty syndrome: a systematic review. Aging Ment Health 2015; 19(9):762–72.

55. Lee GR and DeMaris A. Widowhood, Gender and Depression. A Longitudinal analysis. Research On Aging 2007;29(1):56-72.

56. Goldfarb EV, Seo D, Sinha R. Sex differences in neural stress responses and correlation with subjective stress and stress regulation. Neurobiol Stress 2019;11: 100177.

57. Seckfort DL, Paul R, Grieve SM, et al. Early life stress on brain Structure and function across the lifespan: a Preliminary study. Brain Imaging Behav 2008;2(1):49.

58. Hibbard JH, Pope CR. Another look at sex differences in the use of medical care: illness orientation and the types of morbidities for which services are used. Women Health 1986;11(2):21–36.

59. Boerma T, Hosseinpoor AR, Verdes E, et al. A global assessment of the gender gap in self-reported health with survey data from 59 countries. BMC Public Health 2016;16:675.

60. Verbrugge LM. Gender and health: an update on hypotheses and evidence. J Health Soc Behav 1985;26(3):156–82.

61. Hosseinpoor AR, Stewart Williams J, Amin A, et al. Social determinants of self-reported health in women and men: understanding the role of gender in population health. PLoS One 2012;7(4):e34799.

62. Oksuzyan A, Juel K, Vaupel JW, et al. Men: good health and high mortality. Sex differences in health and aging. Aging Clin Exp Res 2008;20(2):91–102.

63. Zheng Z, Guan S, Ding H, et al. Prevalence and incidence of frailty in community-dwelling older people: Beijing longitudinal study of aging II. J Am Geriatr Soc 2016;64(6):1281–6.

64. Marcucci M, Damanti S, Germini F, et al. Interventions to prevent, delay or reverse frailty in older people: a journey towards clinical guidelines. BMC Med 2019; 17(1):193.

65. Morley JE, Malmstrom TK, Miller DK. A simple frailty questionnaire (FRAIL) predicts outcomes in middle aged African Americans. J Nutr Health Aging 2012; 16(7):601–8.

66. Ensrud KE, Ewing SK, Taylor BC, et al. Comparison of 2 frailty indexes for prediction of falls, disability, fractures, and death in older women. Arch Intern Med 2008; 168(4):382–9.

67. Molnar F, Frank CC. Optimizing geriatric care with the GERIATRIC 5. Can Fam Physician 2019;65(1):39.

68. Travers J, Romero-Ortuno R, Bailey J, et al. Delaying and reversing frailty: a systematic review of primary care interventions. Br J Gen Pract 2019;69(678):e61–9.

69. Rezaei-Shahsavarloo Z, Atashzadeh-Shoorideh F, Gobbens RJJ, et al. The impact of interventions on management of frailty in hospitalized frail older adults: a systematic review and meta-analysis. BMC Geriatr 2020;20(1):526.

70. Gil-Salcedo A, Dugravot A, Fayosse A, et al. Healthy behaviors at age 50 years and frailty at older ages in a 20-year follow-up of the UK Whitehall II cohort: a longitudinal study. Plos Med 2020;17(7):e1003147.

71. Solfrizzi V, Scafato E, Frisardi V, et al. Frailty syndrome and the risk of vascular dementia: the Italian Longitudinal Study on Aging. Alzheimers Dement 2013; 9(2):113–22.

72. Ng TP, Feng L, Nyunt MS, et al. Nutritional, physical, cognitive, and combination interventions and frailty reversal among older adults: a randomized controlled trial. Am J Med 2015;128(11):1225–36.e1.

73. Pegorari MS, Tavares DM. Factors associated with the frailty syndrome in elderly individuals living in the urban area. Rev Lat Am Enfermagem 2014;22(5):874–82.

74. Freitag S, Schmidt S. Psychosocial correlates of frailty in older adults. Geriatrics (Basel) 2016;1(4). https://doi.org/10.3390/geriatrics1040026.

75. Kidd T, Mold F, Jones C, et al. What are the most effective interventions to improve physical performance in pre-frail and frail adults? A systematic review of randomised control trials. BMC Geriatr 2019;19(1):184.

76. Negm AM, Kennedy CC, Thabane L, et al. Management of frailty: a systematic review and network meta-analysis of randomized controlled trials. J Am Med Dir Assoc 2019;20(10):1190–8.

77. Balestroni G, Bertolotti G. [EuroQol-5D (EQ-5D): an instrument for measuring quality of life]. Monaldi Arch Chest Dis 2012;78(3):155–9.

78. Vestergaard S, Kronborg C, Puggaard L. Home-based video exercise intervention for community-dwelling frail older women: a randomized controlled trial. Aging Clin Exp Res 2008;20(5):479–86.

79. Gutiérrez-Valencia M, Izquierdo M, Cesari M, et al. The relationship between frailty and polypharmacy in older people: a systematic review. Br J Clin Pharmacol 2018;84(7):1432–44.

80. Rosted E, Schultz M, Sanders S. Frailty and polypharmacy in elderly patients are associated with a high readmission risk. Dan Med J 2016;63(9).

81. Shapiro BH, Agrawal AK, Pampori NA. Gender differences in drug metabolism regulated by growth hormone. Int J Biochem Cell Biol 1995;27(1):9–20.

82. Ko FC. The clinical care of frail, older adults. Clin Geriatr Med 2011;27(1):89–100.

83. Walston J, Buta B, Xue QL. Frailty screening and interventions: Considerations for clinical Practice. Clin Geriatr Med 2018;34(1):25–38.

84. Stow D, Spiers G, Matthews FE, et al. What is the evidence that people with frailty have needs for palliative care at the end of life? A systematic review and narrative synthesis. Palliat Med 2019;33(4):399–414.

Exercise as Medicine for Older Women

Carole B. Lewis, PT, DPT, GCS, GTCCS, MPA, MSG, PhD, FSOAE, FAPTA[a],*,
Molly Laflin, PhD, FSOAE[b], Debra L. Gray, PT, DPT, DHS, MEd[c]

KEYWORDS

- Exercise • Women • Aged • Fitness

KEY POINTS

- Exercise for older women is not generic.
- Physical therapists can decrease injury risk and increase functional independence and quality of life among older women by comprehensively assessing and treating deficits in posture, balance, flexibility, strength, and endurance.
- Physicians play a key role in prescribing and motivating exercise for older women.

INTRODUCTION

Evidence for the health benefits of physical activity among older women is robust.[1] Regular exercise has been associated with protective effects for cognitive decline and mortality; decreased anxiety, depression, inflammation, falls, and frailty; better weight management, physical functioning, and hormone regulation; and decreased risk of heart disease, type 2 diabetes, metabolic syndrome, some cancers, and osteoporosis.[2]

Despite the many benefits, most adults in this country do not meet the physical activity recommendations set forth in the Physical Activity Guidelines for Americans.[2] Older adults have been slowly increasing activity levels over time, but adherence to aerobic and strength training guidelines remains low in this population.[3]

Older Americans, especially older women, are less physically active than any other age group and generate the highest expenditures for medical care.[4] More than 30 million adults aged 50 years or older are physically inactive (ie, no activity beyond the needs of daily living).[5] Only 16% of individuals aged 65 to 74 years report participating in the recommended 30 minutes or more of moderate physical activity 5 or more days per week.[6]

[a] Topics in Geriatric Rehabilitation, George Washington University College of Medicine and Health Sciences; [b] Health Promotion, Bowling Green State University, 221 Baldwin Avenue, Bowling Green, OH 43402, USA; [c] University of St Augustine for Health Sciences, Gray Therapy Education Consulting LLC, 3434 Blanding Boulevard #225, Jacksonville, FL 32210, USA
* Corresponding author. 5343 43rd Street Northwest, Washington, DC 20015.
E-mail address: Clewis@greatseminarsonline.com

Clin Geriatr Med 37 (2021) 639–650
https://doi.org/10.1016/j.cger.2021.05.009
0749-0690/21/© 2021 Elsevier Inc. All rights reserved.

geriatric.theclinics.com

Of particular concern,

- 8.3% of deaths have been attributed to inadequate levels of physical activity.[7]
- Low levels of physical activity are associated with an estimated $117 billion annually in health care costs.[8]
- 11.1% of aggregate health care expenditures are associated with inadequate physical activity (ie, inactive and insufficiently active levels).[8]
- 8.7% of aggregate health care expenditures have been associated with inadequate physical activity when adults with any reported difficulty walking due to a health problem are excluded.[8]

Exercise has a positive impact with few, if any, side effects, thus it is a concern as to why it is not more frequently prescribed by physicians. This article discusses how exercise affects disease and prevents functional decline. It will also clarify why exercise is not a generic cure-all but is instead a tool physicians can use with precision to affect a myriad of health issues. Specifics will be provided regarding physical fitness assessments and comprehensive treatments and how physicians can be more involved in using physical fitness to keep their older female patients healthy.

EXERCISE IMPACTS ON COMMON CONDITIONS

Although women have a longer life expectancy than men, in adults 55 years of age and older, women are more likely than men to have chronic medical conditions. Diseases and conditions that are more prevalent in older women include breast cancer, osteoporosis, diabetes, arthritis, cardiovascular disease, depression, and urinary incontinence.[9]

Exercise has been shown to help prevent breast cancer in postmenopausal women[10] and to reduce recurrence.[11] Many patients with breast cancer reduce their level of physical activity during active therapy and remain inactive despite the evidence that regular exercise can have positive effects on many of the acute and chronic symptoms associated with breast cancer such as reductions in physical, psychological, and social impairments.[11] No specific exercise protocol has been identified; however, a program of 150 minutes of moderate activity per week that includes both aerobic exercise and strength training has been found to be beneficial.[12] Individualized rehabilitation assessment and exercise prescription that focuses on patient goals are recommended to improve quality of life in patients with breast cancer and survivors.[11]

Although childhood and adolescence are the prime years to build bone strength, research has shown that bone mineral density can be maintained or increased through exercise in postmenopausal women.[13,14] Physical activity and exercise reduce the risk of osteoporosis-related fractures.[15,16] Therapeutic exercises to strengthen back muscles can reduce the risk of vertebral fractures.[17] There seems to be a dose-response relationship between exercise and bone density. A higher dose of exercise, particularly weight-bearing, affects forms of exercise, was shown to slow the age-related declines in bone density in postmenopausal women, and the effect persisted 12 months after the intervention ended.[18]

The risk of developing type 2 diabetes increases with age and is the highest in older women. Type 2 diabetes in turn increases their risk for physical disability and frailty.[19] Exercise is widely considered to be a key preventive and therapeutic component in the care of persons with diabetes including older adults. Moderate activity and limited sedentary behaviors should be encouraged. A 1 hour 3 times per week for 16 weeks monitored aerobic exercise program yielded improved body composition, glycemic control, Vo_{2max}, and physical capacity in 25 women aged 60 to 69 years, with no injuries or hypoglycemic events.[20] Moderate resistance exercise and high-intensity power training have been shown to improve physical function and attenuate the loss of muscle and bone mass in older adults with type 2 diabetes and chronic comorbidities.[21]

Based on the 2015 US Census Bureau National Population Projections, 31.3 million adult women and 18.3 older women have arthritis.[22] The risk of functional decline in patients with arthritis is greater in older women and in ethnic minorities; however, a highly prevalent but modifiable risk factor for functional decline in persons with arthritis is regular vigorous physical activity.[23] A study comparing Tai-chi and resistance exercise in older women with knee arthritis found both forms of exercise improved physical function and reduced pain and mobility disability.[24] Physical therapist–guided moderate- to high-intensity exercise decreased fatigue and improved symptoms of depression in older patients with rheumatoid arthritis.[25]

Cardiovascular disease (CVD) is the leading cause of death for women in the United States with associated conditions of heart disease, hypertension, and stroke being major causes of disability in that group.[26] The significant role of regular moderate physical activity in the prevention and treatment of CVD is widely accepted. A randomized controlled trial (RCT) of untrained older women performing one set of resistance exercise to fatigue 3 times per week for 15 weeks was sufficient to improve some biochemical markers and reduce CVD risk.[27]

Depression is another condition associated with greater prevalence in women. A meta-analysis of RCTs of the effects of exercise on depression symptoms in midlife and older women concluded that moderate exercise programs reduce depressive symptoms and improve perceived quality of life and stress.[28]

Urinary incontinence (UI) is a significant health and quality of life concern for aging women. Pelvic floor muscle training has been shown to increase muscle strength and endurance and improve quality of life in postmenopausal women with stress UI.[29] A 12-week RCT of bladder training and a physical activity program of walking and strengthening exercises for frail older women resulted in improved UI symptoms, balance, and gait.[30] A twice a week multidimensional exercise program including walking along with general and pelvic floor muscle strengthening reduced UI symptoms and improved function in community-dwelling older women.[31]

EXERCISE PREVENTS FUNCTIONAL DECLINE

Fitness is not unidimensional, and exercise programs that successfully address functional movement and disease prevention and treatment are not generic. Telling an older woman to exercise is like telling every patient to take simvastatin for every problem. One remedy does not work for every situation.

Promoting physical activity in general is a good start, but it does not go far enough. For optimal health and disease prevention, a physical therapist is required. Physical therapists are exercise specialists who can comprehensively assess and intervene in all 5 domains of fitness (posture, balance, flexibility, strength, and endurance). What follows are brief reviews of research for each domain, how each domain affects function, an example of how each may be assessed, and an example of a domain-specific exercise protocol.

Posture

Using a cross-sectional analysis of a cohort study, Ryan and Fried[32] found kyphosis to be associated with diminished function, especially in the performance of mobility tasks. There are several tools a therapist can use to assess posture ranging from incli-nometer to wall-occiput distance and more (**Fig. 1**). Several proven exercise protocols to improve posture in older women are now published. One example is the Bautmans protocol (**Box 1**), which involves manual therapy, elastic therapeutic tape, and pro-gressive exercises.[33]

Balance

Each year, approximately 30% of adults aged 65 years and older experience falls, often resulting in serious injuries, decreased mobility, and loss of independence. In 2015, medical costs for falls totaled more than $50 billion.[34] Medicare and Medicaid shouldered 75% of these costs.[35]

Most falls are caused by multiple risk factors. The following conditions, many of which can be modified, have been identified as contributing to fall risk: lower body weakness, vitamin D deficiency, walking and balance difficulties, prescription and over-the-counter medications that affect balance, vestibular hypofunction, vision problems, foot pain, poor footwear, and home hazards.[36]

There is no assessment that captures all aspects of balance; therefore, using mul-tiple measures is necessary to provide a more comprehensive picture of an older women's balance. For static balance, the authors suggest measures of vestibular hypofunction[37] and the 1-legged standing test.[38] For dynamic balance, they recom-mend the timed up and go[39] and the tandem walk test.[40–42]

Depending on the examination results, the intervention protocols selected by ther-apists will vary. Examples include the Otago program[43] as well as the exercises sug-gested by the Adult Functional Independence Test (formerly known as the MTS).[44]

Strength

Strength is essential for the proper functioning of every muscle. But grip strength, measured by a dynamometer, is additionally noteworthy because it is associated with functional decline and is often used as a proxy for overall body strength. Grip strength scores that are less than the norm for age and gender have been found to be a powerful predictor of cause-specific and total mortality.[45] Given its predictive val-idity in identifying patients at increased risk of deteriorating health, dynamometrically measured grip strength has been promoted as a vital sign useful for screening middle-aged and older adults.[46]

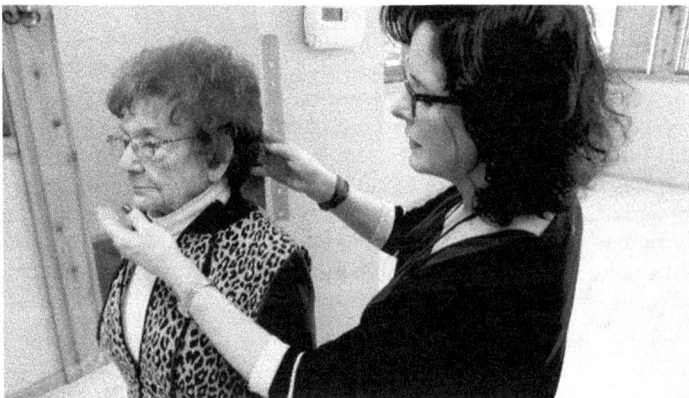

Fig. 1. Wall-occiput distance.

Box 1
Bautmans protocol

- 18 sessions over 3 months with decreasing frequency
- Thoracic spine mobilizations and taping
- Build to 3 sets of 15 exercises
  - Seated lift hands above head—add weights for progression
  - Straightening against wall—30 second hold
  - Seated thoracic arch
  - Wall arm reach
  - Supine, knees bent, towel roll at T6—30 seconds to 3 minutes

Data from Bautmans I, Van Arken J, Van Mackelenberg M, Mets T. Rehabilitation using manual mobilization for thoracic kyphosis in elderly postmenopausal patients with osteoporosis. J Rehabil Med. 2010;42(2):129-135.

To examine whether hand grip strength measured during midlife could predict later functional limitations and disability in initially healthy men, Rantanen and colleagues[47] used a 25-year prospective cohort study. The maximal hand grip strength of 6089 men aged 45 to 68 years who were healthy at baseline was measured from 1965 through 1970. A total of 2259 men died over the follow-up period and 3218 survivors participated in the follow-up from 1991 through 1993. The risk of self-care disability in the lowest group (one-third) was more than twice the highest grip strength tertile.

The relationship between handgrip strength and mortality was established when a 5-year prospective population-based cohort of 1919 moderately to severely disabled women aged 65 to 101 years found a significant association between muscle strength and total cause mortality.[48]

Grip strength is just one example of strength's predictive ability regarding function. Decreased shoulder external rotation has been found to predict current and future rotator cuff issues, and lower body strength can predict fall risk.[49–51]

Most effective strength training programs are based on a therapist's calculation of the patient's percentage of a one-repetition maximum (1RM) followed by a series of exercises designed to keep the person within 60% to 80% of a 1RM. **Box 2** is an example of a 1RM calculation for an individual muscle group. In addition, there are protocols that can be used for specific populations. **Box 3** is an example of a popular program called "exercise snacking."[52]

Flexibility

Flexibility is often overlooked when assessing physical fitness. Yet lack of adequate flexibility is a key factor in injurious falls and functional disabilities. Badley and colleagues[53] found a significant relationship between limitations in range of joint movement and the number and type of disabilities. Mecagni and colleagues[54] sampled community-dwelling women between the ages of 64 and 87 years and found that decreased ankle range of motion as measured by goniometry (**Fig. 2**) was a risk factor for falls.[55,56]

Interventions for flexibility focus on specific evidence-based stretches for identified limitations in range of motion. Stretches must be held for a minimum of 60 seconds, 4 times, 5 days a week.[57]

Endurance

As women age, particularly after menopause, unhealthy changes in abdominal obesity, insulin resistance, glucose tolerance, and dyslipidemia become increasingly

---

Box 2
Sample calculation of 1-repetition maximum

Calculating One-Repetition Maximum (1RM)
  Formula = weight of the repetition divided by the percentage (decimal) at number of repetitions

Sample Calculations
- Left knee extension: 15#, 25 repetitions
  - 25 repetitions = 65% of the 1RM
  - Weight of the repetition/percentage (decimal) at number of repetitions
  - 15/0.65 = 23# (1RM)
- Heel raises: 40#, 30 repetitions
  - 30 repetitions = 60% of the 1RM
  - Weight of the repetition/percentage (decimal) at number of repetitions
  - 40/0.60 = 66.67# (1RM)
- Weighted mini-squats: 20#, 20 repetitions
  - 20 repetitions = 71% of the 1RM
  - Weight of the repetition/percentage (decimal) at number of repetitions

Intensity of Strength Training
- "Normal" strength training = 80%
- "Moderate" strength training = 70%
- "Light" strength training = 60%

---

common.[58] Although insulin resistance is associated with aging, it is primarily the result of reduced physical activity, decreased muscle mass, and the accumulation of fat.[59] Insulin resistance is fundamental in the development of type 2 diabetes and metabolic syndrome, both of which are important risk factors for cardiovascular disease.[60]

Endurance training has been shown to improve glucose uptake and insulin sensitivity in both healthy as well as insulin-resistant individuals.[59,61] It also decreases blood pressure[62] and improves blood lipid profiles.[63]

Therapists use several tools to evaluate endurance. Common assessments include the 6-minute walk test[64] and the 2-minute step test[65] and the movement ability measure, which unlike the previous 2, is a paper and pencil test.[66]

Physical therapy interventions to address endurance deficits are designed and progress based on the patient's preferences. The options are limitless, but often include walking, jogging, biking, rowing, aerobic classes, or swimming. The nuances of setting up an individualized program include determining interest, motivation, safety

---

Box 3
Exercise snacking

- Exercise snack twice a day for 5 minutes.

- 5 activities were sit-to-stand, long arc quads, heel raises, standing knee flexion, marching

- Participants were instructed to do as many as they could of each exercise for 1 minute, twice a day.

- The experimental group improved in quadricep cross-sectional area and leg extension strength and sit-to-stand test.

Data from Perkin OJ, McGuigan PM, Stokes KA. Exercise Snacking to Improve Muscle Function in Healthy Older Adults: A Pilot Study. J Aging Res. 2019;2019:7516939. Published 2019 Oct 3.

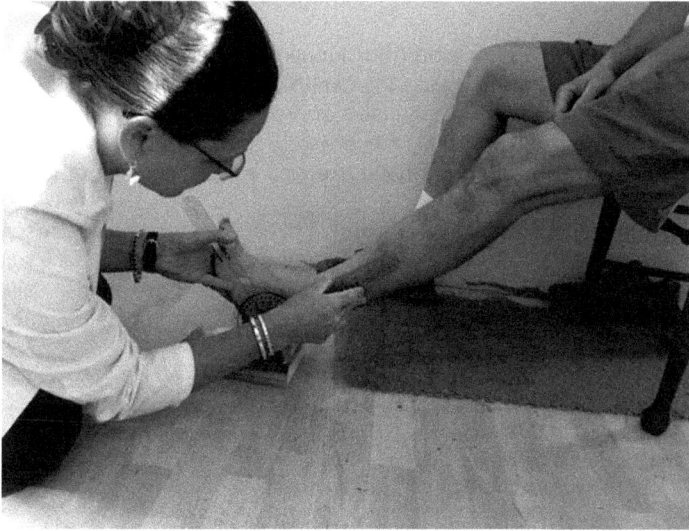

Fig. 2. Goniometry of the ankle.

concerns, appropriate dosage, and modulating the program by using techniques such as interval training. A skilled analysis and intermittently updated prescription is required for optimum benefit.

What can a physician do?

In 2007, the American Medical Association and the American College of Sports Medicine teamed up to endorse Exercise Is Medicine, which promotes assessing physical activity levels of each patient at every physician clinic visit, providing individual exercise prescriptions and referrals to activity programs.[67] Exercise Is Medicine's assessment, prescription, and referral goals are designed to be completed by physicians within as little as 20 to 30 seconds. Patients who seem to have no significant health deficits should be referred to "programs, places or professionals, or recommend active transportation and self-directed resources (websites, phone apps, activity trackers) that will best support their needs and interests."[68] Patients with compromised health conditions or functional deficits should be referred to "physical therapy, cardiac or disease-specific rehabilitation programs prior to participation in community-based options."[68]

Referring patients, especially middle-aged and older women, to physical therapists, the only members of the medical team specifically trained in exercise, is a prudent choice because if an exercise program is incorrectly applied, the patient may experience injury, lack of motivation, or lack of results.

Physicians encouraging their patients to exercise is not new. How to make that advice more effective has been the subject of research for every 2 decades. The 1998 Green Study found that when general practitioners wrote prescriptions for patients to exercise, they exercised more than when merely told to exercise.[69] This simple yet powerful motivational tool can help patients get started. Progress reports from physical therapists can be reviewed as blood work panels. Follow-up with patients should include either positive feedback and encouragement or open-ended questions to find out why progress is not being made.

SUMMARY

This article presents a new paradigm for functional wellness and demonstrates the importance of exercise for improving the health and function of our older female patients. A case is made for a comprehensive approach to exercise provided by the exercise expert on the medical team, the physical therapist. By referring patients to physical therapists, physicians can make exercise a crucial piece of the health package for our older female patients.

Just as prescribing statins for the prevention of CVD, so too should prescriptions be written for effective exercise intervention before as well as when our patients have problems. Once you prescribe, encourage your patients to exercise. Take steps to use this powerful part of medicine to keep your older adult female patients healthy.

CLINICS CARE POINTS

- Regular exercise for older women has been associated with protective effects for cognitive decline and mortality; decreased anxiety, depression, inflammation, falls, and frailty; better weight management, physical functioning, and hormone regulation; and decreased risk of heart disease, type 2 diabetes, metabolic syndrome, some cancers, and osteoporosis.

- Older Americans, especially older women, are less physically active than any other age group and generate the highest expenditures for medical care.

- Postural, balance, strength, endurance, and flexibility deficits in older women are tied to functional decline, and there are evidence-based tools and interventions to improve these deficits.

- Given its predictive validity in identifying patients at increased risk of deteriorating health, measured grip strength by dynamometry has been promoted as a vital sign useful for screening middle-aged and older adults.

- In 2007, the American Medical Association and the American College of Sports Medicine teamed up to endorse Exercise Is Medicine, which promotes assessing physical activity levels of each patient at every physician clinic visit, providing individual exercise prescriptions and referrals to activity programs.

- When general practitioners wrote prescriptions for patients to exercise, they exercised more than when merely told to exercise.

- Patients with compromised health conditions or functional deficits should be referred to "physical therapy, cardiac or disease-specific rehabilitation programs prior to participation in community-based options."

DISCLOSURE

The authors have no commercial or financial conflicts of interest.

REFERENCES

1. Senter C, Appelle N, Behera SK. Prescribing exercise for women. Curr Rev Musculoskelet Med 2013;6(2):164–72.
2. U.S. Department of Health and Human Services. Physical activity guidelines for Americans. 2nd edition. Washington, DC: U.S. Department of Health and Human Services; 2018. Available at: https://health.gov/sites/default/files/2019-09/Physical_Activity_Guidelines_2nd_edition.pdf. Accessed August 21, 2020.
3. Keadle SK, McKinnon R, Graubard BI, et al. Prevalence and trends in physical activity among older adults in the United States: a comparison across three national surveys. Prev Med 2016;89:37–43.

4. Nelson ME, Rejeski WJ, Blair SN, et al. Physical activity and public health in older adults: recommendation from the American College of Sports Medicine and the American Heart Association. Med Sci Sports Exerc 2007;39(8):1435–45.

5. National Center for chronic disease prevention and health promotion (NCCDPHP). Lack of physical activity. Page last reviewed September 25, 2019. Available at: https://www.cdc.gov/chronicdisease/resources/publications/fact sheets/physical-activity.htm. Accessed August 21, 2020.

6. Lee PG, Jackson EA, Richardson CR. Exercise prescriptions in older adults. Am Fam Physician 2017;95(7):425–32.

7. Carlson SA, Adams EK, Yang Z, et al. Percentage of deaths associated with inadequate physical activity in the United States. Prev Chronic Dis 2018;15:E38.

8. Carlson SA, Fulton JE, Pratt M, et al. Inadequate physical activity and health care expenditures in the United States. Prog Cardiovasc Dis 2015;57(4):315–23.

9. A Beard JR, Officer A, de Carvalho IA, et al. The World report on ageing and health: a policy framework for healthy ageing. Lancet 2016;387(10033):2145–54.

10. Gonçalves A, Florêncio G, de Atayde Silva M, et al. Effects of physical activity on breast cancer prevention: a systematic review. J Phys Act Health 2014;11(2):445–54.

11. Wirtz P, Baumann FT. Physical activity, exercise and breast cancer – what is the evidence for rehabilitation, aftercare, and survival: a review. Breast Care 2018;13:93–101.

12. Runowicz CD, Leach CR, Henry NL, et al. American cancer Society/American Society of clinical Oncology breast cancer survivorship care guideline. J Clin Oncol 2016;34:611–35.

13. Kemmler W, Lauber D, Weineck J, et al. Benefits of 2 years of intense exercise on bone density, physical fitness, and blood lipids in early postmenopausal osteopenic women: results of the Erlangen Fitness Osteoporosis Prevention Study (EFOPS). Arch Intern Med 2004;64(10):1084–91.

14. Asikainen TM, Kukkonen-Harjula K, Miilunpalo S. Exercise for health for early postmenopausal women: a systematic review of randomised controlled trials. Sports Med 2004;34(11):753–78.

15. Bonaiuti D, Shea B, Iovine R, et al. Exercise for preventing and treating osteoporosis in postmenopausal women. Cochrane Database Syst Rev 2002;3:CD000333.

16. Karlsson M. Has exercise an antifracture efficacy in women? Scand J Med Sci Sports 2004;14(1):2–15.

17. Sinaki M. Critical appraisal of physical rehabilitation measures after osteoporotic vertebral fracture. Osteoporos Int 2006;17(11):1702.

18. Gonzalo-Encabo P, McNeil J, Boyne DJ, et al. Dose-response effects of exercise on bone mineral density and content in post-menopausal women. Scand J Med Sci Sports 2019;29(8):1121–9.

19. Kautzky-Willer A, Harreiter J, Pacini G. Sex and gender differences in risk, pathophysiology and complications of type 2 diabetes mellitus. Endocr Rev 2016;37(3):278–316.

20. Jiang Y, Tan S, Wang Z, et al. Aerobic exercise training at maximal fat oxidation intensity improves body composition, glycemic control, and physical capacity in older people with type 2 diabetes. J Exer Sci Fitness 2020;18(1):7–13.

21. Simpson KA, Mavros Y, Kay S, et al. Graded resistance exercise and type 2 diabetes in older adults (The GREAT2DO study): methods and baseline cohort characteristics of a randomized controlled trial. Trials 2015;16(504).

22. Colby SL, Ortman JM. Projections of the size and composition of the U.S. population: 2014 to 2060 2015. Available at: https://www.census.gov/library/publications/2015/demo/p25-1143.html. Accessed August 31, 2020.

23. Dunlop DD, Semanik P, Song J, et al. Risk factors for functional decline in older adults with arthritis. Arthritis Rheum 2005;52:1274–82.

24. Kim SM, Song JM. The efficacy of community-based rehabilitation exercise to improve physical function in old women with knee arthritis. J Kor Soc Phys Ther 2010;22(1):9–17.

25. Kucharski D, Lange E, Ross AB, et al. Moderate-to-high intensity exercise with person-centered guidance influences fatigue in older adults with rheumatoid arthritis. Rheumatol Int 2019;39:1585–94.

26. Mozaffarian D, Benjamin EJ, Go AS, et al. Heart disease and stroke statistics—2015 update: a report from the American Heart Association. Circulation 2015;131(4):e29–322.

27. Cunha PM, Ribeiro AS, Nunes JP. Resistance training performed with single-set is sufficient to reduce cardiovascular risk factors in untrained older women: the randomized clinical trial. Arch Gerontol Geriatr 2019;81:171–5.

28. Pérez-López FR, Martínez-Domínguez SJ, Lajusticia H, et al. Effects of programmed exercise on depressive symptoms in midlife and older women: a meta-analysis of randomized controlled trials. Maturitas 2017;106:38–47.

29. Bertotto A, Schvartzman R, Uchoa S, et al. Effect of electromyographic biofeedback as an add-on to pelvic floor muscle exercises on neuromuscular outcomes and quality of life in postmenopausal women with stress urinary incontinence: a randomized controlled trial. Neurourol Urodynamics 2017;36:2142–7.

30. Talley KMC, Wyman JF, Bronas U, et al. Defeating urinary incontinence with exercise training: results of a pilot study in frail older women. J Am Geriatr Soc 2017;65(6):1321–7.

31. Hunkyung K, Hideyo Y, Takao S. The effects of multidimensional exercise on functional decline, urinary incontinence, and fear of falling in community-dwelling elderly women with multiple symptoms of geriatric syndrome: a randomized controlled and 6-month follow-up trial. Arch Gerontol Geriatr 2011;52(1):99–105.

32. Ryan SD, Fried LP. The impact of kyphosis on daily functioning. J Am Geriatr Soc 1997;45(12):1479–86.

33. Bautmans I, Van Arken J, Van Mackelenberg M, et al. Rehabilitation using manual mobilization for thoracic kyphosis in elderly postmenopausal patients with osteoporosis. J Rehabil Med 2010;42(2):129–35.

34. Florence CS, Bergen G, Atherly A, et al. Medical costs of fatal and Nonfatal falls in older adults. J Am Geriatr Soc 2018;66(4):693–8.

35. Centers for Disease Control and Prevention. Important Facts about falls. Available at: https://www.cdc.gov/homeandrecreationalsafety/falls/adultfalls.html. Accessed August 7, 2020.

36. Centers for disease control and prevention, important Facts about falls. Available at: https://www.cdc.gov/homeandrecreationalsafety/falls/adultfalls.html. Accessed October 21, 2020.

37. Bhattacharyya N, Gubbels SP, Schwartz SR, et al. Clinical Practice guideline: Benign Paroxysmal Positional Vertigo (update). Otolaryngol Head Neck Surg 2017;156(3_suppl):S1–47.

38. Vellas BJ, Wayne SJ, Romero L, et al. One-leg balance is an important predictor of injurious falls in older persons. J Am Geriatr Soc 1997;45(6):735–8.

39. Podsiadlo D, Richardson S. The timed "Up & Go": a test of basic functional mobility for frail elderly persons. J Am Geriatr Soc 1991;39(2):142–8.

40. Chu LW, Pei CK, Chiu A, et al. Risk factors for falls in hospitalized older medical patients. J Gerontol A Biol Sci Med Sci 1999;54(1):M38–43.
41. Cohen HS, Mulavara AP, Peters BT, et al. Sharpening the tandem walking test for screening peripheral neuropathy. South Med J 2013;106(10):565–9.
42. Cohen HS, Mulavara AP, Stitz J, et al. Screening for vestibular disorders using the modified clinical test of sensory interaction and balance and tandem walking with eyes closed. Otol Neurotol 2019;40(5):658–65.
43. Centers for Disease Control and Prevention, National Center for Injury Prevention and Control. Tools to Implement the Otago exercise program: a program to reduce falls. Available at: https://www.med.unc.edu/aging/cgwep/files/2018/09/ImplementationGuideforPT.pdf. Accessed August 21, 2020.
44. Laflin M, Lewis C. Functional Standards for optimal aging: the development of the moving Target screen (name later changed to the AFIT). J Geriatr Phys Ther 2017;33(4):224–30.
45. Malhotra R, Tareque MI, Tan NC, et al. Association of baseline hand grip strength and annual change in hand grip strength with mortality among older people. Arch Gerontol Geriatr 2020;86:103961.
46. Bohannon RW. Hand-grip dynamometry predicts future outcomes in aging adults. J Geriatr Phys Ther 2008;31(1):3–10.
47. Rantanen T, Guralnik JM, Foley D, et al. Midlife hand grip strength as a predictor of old age disability. JAMA 1999;281(6):558–60.
48. Rantanen T, Volpato S, Ferrucci L, et al. Handgrip strength and cause-specific and total mortality in older disabled women: exploring the mechanism. J Am Geriatr Soc 2003;51(5):636–41.
49. MacDermid JC, Ramos J, Drosdowech D, et al. The impact of rotator cuff pathology on isometric and isokinetic strength, function, and quality of life. J Shoulder Elbow Surg 2004;13(6):593–8.
50. Melzer I, Benjuya N, Kaplanski J, et al. Association between ankle muscle strength and limit of stability in older adults. Age Ageing 2009;38(1):119–23.
51. Herman S, Kiely DK, Leveille S, et al. Upper and lower limb muscle power relationships in mobility-limited older adults. J Gerontol A Biol Sci Med Sci 2005; 60(4):476–80.
52. Perkin OJ, McGuigan PM, Stokes KA. Exercise snacking to improve muscle function in healthy older adults: a pilot study. J Aging Res 2019;2019:7516939.
53. Badley EM, Wagstaff S, Wood PH. Measures of functional ability (disability) in arthritis in relation to impairment of range of joint movement. Ann Rheum Dis 1984;43(4):563–9.
54. Mecagni C, Smith JP, Roberts KE, et al. Balance and ankle range of motion in community-dwelling women aged 64 to 87 years: a correlational study. Phys Ther 2000;80(10):1004–11.
55. Martin RL, McPoil TG. Reliability of ankle goniometric measurements: a literature review. J Am Podiatr Med Assoc 2005;95(6):564–72.
56. Kang MH, Oh JS. Relationship between Weightbearing ankle Dorsiflexion Passive range of motion and ankle Kinematics during gait. J Am Podiatr Med Assoc 2017; 107(1):39–45.
57. Feland JB, Myrer JW, Schulthies SS, et al. The effect of duration of stretching of the hamstring muscle group for increasing range of motion in people aged 65 years or older. Phys Ther 2001;81(5):1110–7.
58. Sillanpää E, Laaksonen DE, Häkkinen A, et al. Body composition, fitness, and metabolic health during strength and endurance training and their combination in middle-aged and older women. Eur J Appl Physiol 2009;106(2):285–96.

59. Lakka TA, Laaksonen DE. Physical activity in prevention and treatment of the metabolic syndrome. Appl Physiol Nutr Metab 2007;32(1):76–88.

60. Laaksonen DE, Niskanen L, Lakka HM, et al. Epidemiology and treatment of the metabolic syndrome. Ann Med 2004;36(5):332–46.

61. Röckl KS, Witczak CA, Goodyear LJ. Signaling mechanisms in skeletal muscle: acute responses and chronic adaptations to exercise. IUBMB Life 2008;60(3): 145–53.

62. Cornelissen VA, Smart NA. Exercise training for blood pressure: a systematic review and meta-analysis. J Am Heart Assoc 2013;2(1):e004473.

63. Leon AS, Sanchez OA. Response of blood lipids to exercise training alone or combined with dietary intervention. Med Sci Sports Exerc 2001;33(6 Suppl): S502–29.

64. Shirley Ryan AbilityLab. 6 minute walk test. Available at: https://www.sralab.org/rehabilitation-measures/6-minute-walk-test. Accessed August 20, 2020.

65. Rossier P, Wade DT. Validity and reliability comparison of 4 mobility measures in patients presenting with neurologic impairment. Arch Phys Med Rehabil 2001; 82(1):9–13.

66. Allen DD, Wagner JM. Assessing the gap between current movement ability and preferred movement ability as a measure of disability. Phys Ther 2011;91(12): 1789–803.

67. Exercise is medicine. Available at: https://www.exerciseismedicine.org/support_page.php/eim-in-action/. Accessed August 21, 2020.

68. Exercise is medicine. Healthcare Providers' action Guide. Available at: https://www.exerciseismedicine.org/assets/page_documents/Complete%20HCP%20Action%20Guide.pdf. Accessed August 21, 2020.

69. Swinburn BA, Walter LG, Arroll B, et al. The green prescription study: a randomized controlled trial of written exercise advice provided by general practitioners. Am J Public Health 1998;88(2):288–91.

Cardiovascular Disease in Older Women

Essraa Bayoumi, MD[a], Pamela Karasik, MD[b],*

KEYWORDS

- Older women • Cardiovascular risk • CVD prevention and treatment

KEY POINTS

- Risk with aging, risk mitigation, better diagnosis, and treatment in women.
- Cardiovascular disease remains the most frequent cause of morbidity and mortality in women, despite recent advances in disease prevention, detection and treatment.
- Clinical presentation of cardiovascular disease can be variable and atypical in women, and clinicians need a high degree of sensitivity to make the diagnosis.
- Risk factors in women are in general similar to those in men, but do include non traditional clinical risks such as a history of auto immune disease, pregnancy related diabetes, and prior treatment of malignancy.
- Risk factor modification even in the older population can reduce future risk of cardiovascular events.

INTRODUCTION

Great strides have been made in the prevention, diagnosis, and treatment of cardiovascular disease (CVD) over the past 40 years. In the past decade, death attributable to coronary heart disease has declined by one-third.[1] Despite this, CVD, including cerebrovascular and atherosclerotic heart disease, remains the most frequent cause of death in women.[2,3] As women age, this burden of disease becomes an even greater threat to the quality and quantity of their lives.[2] In truth, the prevention of CVD starts early in life with adherence to a heart-healthy diet, regular exercise, avoidance of tobacco and excessive alcohol, and treatment of nonmodifiable risk factors, such as hypertension and hyperlipidemia. Mitigation of risk, however, is not age limited, and women at any age can adopt lifestyle changes and begin appropriate medical therapy that can have positive effects on future morbidity and mortality. The Framingham Heart Study showed that even those who are free from CVD at age 70 still have a 24% risk of developing coronary disease.[4] Women have often been underrepresented

No Financial Disclosures, No COI for either author.
[a] Medstar Washington Hospital Center, Georgetown University, VA Medical Center, 110 Irving Street Northwest, Washington, DC 20422, USA; [b] Medical Service VA Medical Center, 50 Irving Street Northwest 4A 154, Washington, DC 20422, USA
* Corresponding author.
E-mail address: Pamela.karasik@va.gov

in clinical trials, in part because of the erroneous notion that women were not at the same risk as men for CVD. It was also not recognized until recently that women may have more atypical presentation of disease, sometimes leading to underdiagnosis of CVD, which resulted in increased mortalities. In this article, the authors review the current state of CVD in older women with a view toward modifying risk, improving diagnosis, and accessing treatment. Although not the subject of this article, the presence of noncoronary atherosclerotic diseases, such as peripheral arterial disease, abdominal aortic aneurysm, and carotid artery disease, is associated with a more than 20% risk of developing CVD.[5,6]

INCIDENCE AND RISK

According to the American Heart Association (AHA) heart disease and stroke statistics 2019 update,[1] the leading cause of death in the United States is heart disease, and if hypertension is included, 48% of American adults over the age of 20 has CVD.[2] In men and women over the age of 60, as many as 75% may have CVD, with the number going up as the population ages.[7] With that as the background, it is important to consider what risks exist for the development of CVD, what are unique to women, which are modifiable, and which are not. Although this focus is on the older woman, in assessing any individual's risk, one should start with a focused history, and for women, that should include an understanding of their early years. For example, women who have experienced complications during pregnancy, such as gestational diabetes and preeclampsia, carry an increased risk of future CVD. These are some of the gender-specific risks that are addressed first (**Fig. 1**).

PREGNANCY RELATED

According to the American College of Obstetrics and Gynecology, preeclampsia is defined as hypertension and proteinuria after 20 weeks' gestation in a previously normotensive patient. It affects 5% to 7% of all pregnancies worldwide and is a leading cause of both maternal and fetal death in the United States and worldwide.[8] Rates of preeclampsia have increased 25% between 1987 and 2004 in the United States.[9] Although preeclampsia and CVD share many of the same risk factors, preeclampsia

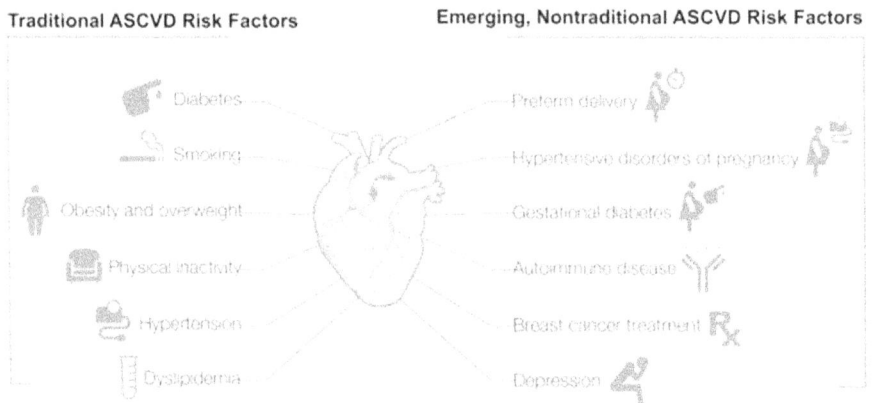

Fig. 1. Traditional versus new, emerging risk factors for CVD in women. ASCVD, atherosclerotic cardiovascular disease. (*From* Garcia M, Mulvagh SL, Merz CN, Buring JE, Manson JE. Cardiovascular Disease in Women: Clinical Perspectives. Circ Res. 2016;118(8):1273-1293. https://doi.org/10.1161/CIRCRESAHA.116.307547; with permission.)

itself is also a risk factor for the development of CVD later in life, presenting a vicious cycle.[8] Preeclampsia occurs in 2 stages, including abnormal placentation in the first and early second trimester followed by a maternal syndrome defined as excess anti-angiogenic factors, which antagonize vascular endothelial growth factor, causing a reduction in levels and leading to local and systemic endothelial dysfunction, which ultimately result in hypertension, coagulation disorders, and proteinuria.[8] Although delivery cures the woman of preeclampsia, the endothelial dysfunction persists, leading to future atherosclerotic disease.[10] Several months and years after pregnancy, women with preeclampsia have been shown to have decreased endothelium-dependent dilation as well as increased sensitivity to angiotensin II.[10–12] Studies have shown up to a 3- to 4-fold increased risk of hypertension in women with preeclampsia.[10,13] A history of preeclampsia confers up to a 2-fold increase in death from CVD.[10] Those with early preeclampsia, defined as occurring before 34 weeks' gestation, have up to a 4- to 8-fold increase of death from CVD.[10,13–15] Prepregnancy risk factors, such as hypertension, diabetes, and obesity, lead to an increased risk of preeclampsia as well as CVD.[10] There is also evidence of elevated levels of C-reactive protein (CRP) up to 30 years after pregnancy in patients with subclinical insulin resistance, increasing the risk of CVD.[10,16] Pregnancy may be a stressor that either unmasks subclinical disease or injures the endothelium and increases inflammation, thereby predisposing to later CVD.[10,17]

In addition, those women who develop gestational diabetes have a 7-fold increased risk for developing diabetes type 2, which is a risk factor for CVD.[18–20] They also have a 2- to 4-fold increased risk for the development of CVD risk independent of the development for diabetes type 2.[18–20]

AUTOIMMUNE DISEASES

Systemic lupus erythematosus (SLE), rheumatoid arthritis, and systemic sclerosis are autoimmune diseases that disproportionately affect women, with SLE affecting woman at a ratio of 7:1.[21] One theory for the gender discrepancy is the role of estrogen in the development of disease.[22] Some of these syndromes are marked by increased inflammation that may lead to atherosclerosis.[23] The multiorgan involvement and subsequent therapies may result in the development of CVD. In SLE, hypertension secondary to renal involvement and steroid use, insulin insensitivity and obesity from corticosteroid use, thrombosis from antiphospholipid antibody, atherosclerosis from immune dysregulation and inflammation as well as valvular damage from Libman-Sacks endocarditis all contribute to the development of CVD.[24,25] Those with SLE also have a 2- to 10-fold increase in stroke and myocardial infarction as well as death compared with others of the same age.[24,26] One study found that those with SLE have elevated risks of CVD that are well beyond those captured by Framingham Scoring metrics.[24]

BREAST CANCER

According to the Centers for Disease Control and Prevention, breast cancer is the second most common cancer among women in the United States. Many who now survive owing to improved screening, surveillance, and treatment develop CVD from chemotherapy and radiation.[18] Studies have shown that women receiving radiation to the left breast developed coronary artery disease (CAD) at higher rates than those receiving radiation to the right breast.[18,27] Furthermore, the risk of CAD increased by 7.8% for every increase in Gray delivered.[18,27] Women may also develop valvular disease as well as cardiomyopathies from radiation.[18] Anthracycline-based chemotherapy is also implicated in the development of cardiomyopathies. Experts recommend surveillance for cardiomyopathy with an echocardiogram (ECHO) every 2 years for asymptomatic patients, and for valvular disease within 10 years of radiation and repeated in 5-year intervals. For CAD, they recommend noninvasive stress testing within 10 years of radiation and repeated in 5-year intervals.[28]

POLYCYSTIC OVARY SYNDROME

Polycystic ovary syndrome (PCOS) is defined by oligomenorrhea, infertility, acne, and hirsutism with polycystic ovaries. Although patients with PCOS have been shown to have a higher risk for other CVD risk factors, including hypertension, a negative lipid profile, obesity, and insulin resistance, it has not been shown to be an independent risk factor for CVD, especially in postmenopausal women.[29,30]

MENOPAUSE

Menopause is an inevitable transition that every woman who lives long enough will experience. Menopause confers an independent risk factor for CVD apart from the normal aging process.[31] The SWAN study demonstrated that within 1 year of the last menstrual period, total cholesterol, low-density lipoprotein (LDL), and apolipoprotein B levels all increased independent of ethnicity, weight, or age.[31] Early menopause has also been associated with increased risk for CVD, which has been postulated to be secondary to a drop in estrogen.[32] Large-scale trials (Women's Health Initiative and Heart and Estrogen-Progestin Replacement Study) looking at whether hormone replacement improved cardiovascular health in postmenopausal women failed to demonstrate a positive correlation.[32–34] This has led some to question whether early menopause confers an increased CVD risk or whether those with an increased risk for CVD have earlier menopause.[32] In either case, menopause and the age at which it occurs can lend important information regarding the possible risk of CVD in a woman.

TRADITIONAL RISK FACTORS

In addition to the gender-specific risk factors that all women should be asked about, traditional risk factors are common and require attention, especially as there are ample data that show women are underdiagnosed and undertreated.[35]

DIABETES

Approximately 13.4 million women in the United States have diabetes, and this appears to be a greater risk factor for the development of CVD in women as compared with men. In 1 study, women with diabetes type 2 had a higher adjusted hazard ratio (HR) of fatal CAD (HR = 14.74; 95% confidence interval [CI], 6.16–35.27) compared with men with diabetes (HR = 3.77; 95% CI, 2.52–5.65).[18,36] In another study, the relative risk for CVD in those with diabetes was 44% greater in women as compared with men.[18,37] The theory behind the gender discrepancy is that diabetes in women leads to greater hypercoagulability, dyslipidemia, and metabolic syndrome.[18]

SMOKING AND OBESITY

Although fewer adult women (15%) than men (19%) smoke, women over the age of 44 who smoke had a 25% increased risk for CVD compared with men.[18,38] Likewise, obesity has a greater impact on the development of CVD in women as compared with men, as demonstrated in the Framingham Heart Study, where the relative risk of CVD was increased by 64% in women, as opposed to 46% in men.[18,39]

HYPERLIPIDEMIA

Dyslipidemia confers the greatest risk for CVD compared with all other risk factors, which only becomes apparent after menopause even if levels are elevated before.[18] Statins are recommended for both men and women; however, the benefit of primary prevention in women is still unclear.[18] Despite the evidence for the benefit of statins, women continue to be prescribed these drugs less frequently than men for unknown reasons and demonstrate the need for physicians to be more vigilant in discovering and preventing CVD.[18]

HYPERTENSION

In women, hypertension develops on average 10 years later than men, as estrogen serves as an antihypertensive via vasodilation.[18] The incidence of hypertension is more in elderly women than elderly men.[18] Antihypertensive medications are recommended for a goal of systolic blood pressure less than 130 mm Hg.

Metabolic syndrome as defined by the National Cholesterol Education Program Adult Treatment Panel III is having 3 of the following 5 traits: elevated glucose, elevated blood pressure, low high-density lipoprotein (HDL), high triglycerides, and an increased waist circumference.[40] Although equally common in both men and women, African American and Mexican American women have twice the prevalence as compared with men.[41] The presence of metabolic syndrome is associated with a significant increase in the relative risk of developing CVD, as well as an increased mortality and thus requires early identification and aggressive treatment.[42] HIV is another disease that is associated with an increased risk for CVD because of a cascade of events that lead to increased inflammation and coagulation disorders. In addition, antiretrovirals have side effects similar to metabolic syndrome, including insulin resistance, dyslipidemia, and endothelial dysfunction.[43]

The foundation of preventing CVD begins with an assessment of the individual's personal risk for development of CVD. There are numerous tools available to the clinician to make that assessment. Perhaps the most well known is the Framingham Risk Score, first published in 1998, developed from the landmark Framingham Heart Study and last revised in 2008. This model incorporates well-known easily obtained information and laboratory test values and is gender specific. The variables include age, total cholesterol, smoking status, HDL cholesterol, and systolic blood pressure. The Reynolds Risk Score calculator is another simple system used to calculate CVD risk over 10 years. It adds CRP and family history to the algorithm, and it also shows how modifying these factors can reduce the risk of future CVD. The AHA recommends using a pooled risk assessment tool available at http://tools.acc.org/ASCVD-Risk-Estimator-plus, every three to five years.

The AHA guidelines for primary prevention of CVD aligns risk as follows, based on atherosclerotic risk factor estimators: low risk is less than 5%; borderline risk is 5% to less than 7.5%; intermediate risk is 7.5% to less than 20%; and greater than 20% is identified as being at high risk. These assessments should be used to engage the patient in discussions regarding risk-factor modification and mitigation. As clinicians, the goal is to match the intensity of the therapy with the absolute risk to the patient.

Once risk has been estimated, appropriate efforts should be made with a patient-centered approach, to lower the risk of development or progression of CVD. The 2019 American College of Cardiology (ACC)/AHA guidelines state that initial recommendations for risk reduction begin with following a diet high in vegetables, fruit, whole grains, and fish, along with reduction in saturated fats and cholesterol. Second, there is ample evidence to support encouragement of regular exercise and other types of physical activity, of at least 150 minutes per week. If the person is overweight or obese, then weight loss, especially if diabetic, is a critical nonpharmacologic intervention. Smoking cessation is an equally important recommendation, and it has been suggested that tobacco status should be treated as a vital sign.[1] Once these behavioral risk modifications have been initiated, if blood pressure and cholesterol remain uncontrolled (blood pressure >130/90 mm Hg and CVD risk >7.5%), then there is class 1a support for initiation of medical therapy. Current guidelines suggest that patients with CVD risk greater than 7.5% and less than 20% who choose to start medication should aim for a 30% reduction in LDL levels. In women at high risk (>20%), an early conversation about initiation of high-intensity statins is indicated. Patients with diabetes should be started on a moderate-intensity statin regardless of risk. For women with hypertension, despite adoption of appropriate lifestyle modification and CVD risk more than 10%, it is recommended in the ACC/AHA guidelines that treatment with blood pressure–lowering medication is indicated. Unfortunately, women have historically been undertreated with both antihypertensive and lipid-lowering medications. In 2010, it was reported that the proportion of women receiving lipid-lowering medication was 5.7% versus 7.3% in men.[44] Although aspirin use is supported by numerous randomized clinical trials for secondary prevention of myocardial infarction, its use in primary prevention in women remains controversial. It is not recommended that adults over the age of 70 take primary-prevention aspirin, as this group has an elevated bleeding risk. In response to several recent trials of primary-prevention low-dose aspirin in adults with high CVD risk, the use of 81-mg aspirin is now a class 2b recommendation.[45]

TESTING

For those patients who need diagnostic testing, either for symptoms or for enhanced risk stratification, there are numerous diagnostic strategies available. Some have better sensitivity and specificity in women than others, and there are pros and cons to all of them. Decisions regarding what testing or imaging to pursue will depend on the age of the patient, the desire to avoid ionizing radiation exposure, and the differential diagnosis under consideration. All patients regardless of gender should have a baseline 12-lead electrocardiogram (ECG) obtained at the time of initial evaluation. Although a full discussion of the ECG and CVD is beyond the scope of this article, the ECG is critical for guiding the next step in evaluating a patients' symptoms (after history and physical examination).

EXERCISE TREADMILL STRESS TEST

Exercise stress testing is the oldest and first-line diagnostic tool for the evaluation of ischemic heart disease. The ACC/AHA 2002 guidelines recommend exercise stress test with ECG as the initial noninvasive test for symptomatic, intermediate-risk women with a normal baseline ECG who are able to exercise.[46] ECG stress testing has excellent negative predictive value; however, positive results are less diagnostic in women. In 1 study, it was found that the positive predictive value in women as compared with men was 47% versus 77%, respectively.[47] There are gender differences in ST segment changes during exercise, which have been hypothesized to be due to more baseline ST-T segment changes in women, greater ST depressions, and estrogen, causing digitalis-like changes.[48,49] It has also been shown that postmenopausal women on estrogen replacement therapy have greater ST segment depressions than other women, thus affecting results.[50–52] Therefore, ST segment changes, although helpful for diagnostic purposes, have less prognostic value in regards to cardiovascular mortality in women.[49,52] In addition to informing about ischemic disease, exercise stress testing also gives prognostic information regarding functional capacity, chronotropic and blood pressure response, and heart rate recovery and thus remains a useful tool.[49,53]

ECHOCARDIOGRAM

Stress echocardiography is often used when there are baseline ECG changes, inability to exercise, and nondiagnostic ECG stress tests.[53] Adding imaging to stress testing results in increased sensitivity in the hands of experienced sonographers and cardiologists.[54] The level of sensitivity, however, has been shown to be different among men and women. In the Women's Ischemia Syndrome Evaluation study, dobutamine stress echo (DSE) was shown to have a sensitivity of about 40%.[55] One reason is that DSE has a lower sensitivity in identifying single-vessel disease, and women tend to have more single-vessel disease than men.[56] Nonetheless, stress ECHO still remains an excellent option for stress testing, given the lack of radiation, high negative predictive value, and ability to assess ventricular and valvular function.

MYOCARDIAL PERFUSION IMAGING

Like ECHO, myocardial perfusion imaging (MPI) with either single-photon emission computed tomography (SPECT) or PET, is another method of imaging used in stress testing that has a higher sensitivity than exercise stress test.[53] Despite breast attenuation lowering specificity of MPI with SPECT to 74% in women as compared with 94% in men, it still remains an important tool with a sensitivity of about 81%.[53] PET offers even more sensitivity and specificity even in obese patients.[53] PET also offers the ability to better detect severe multivessel disease that may be missed on SPECT because of balanced ischemia.[53] As with computed tomography (CT), MPI carries the risk of radiation and is important to consider in women when choosing a modality of stress imaging.

CARDIAC MRI

Cardiac MRI is the newest imaging technique in cardiology. It is used for its ability to combine high-quality images to evaluate both cardiac structure and function. It is also preferred for women in the premenopausal stage of life and is safe for pregnant women because of its lack of ionizing radiation.[55,57] Unfortunately, the available literature is lacking regarding female-specific reference values and diseases. Several publications have shown that women in general have smaller absolute and indexed right and left mass and volume.[58] There are also several disease states that primarily affect women and for which MRI functions as an important tool for diagnosis and prognostication for diseases like nonischemic heart failure and SLE.[58]

Another area for which cardiac MRI is an emerging and important diagnostic tool is diagnosing myocardial infarction with nonobstructive coronary artery disease. In a systematic review, it was found that in women presenting with a myocardial infarction, 43% had nonobstructive disease versus 24% of women who had obstructive coronary disease.[59] In those with elevated troponins, but nonobstructive disease, cardiac MRI was able to identify the cause in 74% to 87% of patients.[60,61] Diagnosis is important, as it informs prognosis.[61] Although the incidence of obstructive disease increases with age (approximately 48% of women between the ages of 55 and 64 years, 65% of women between the ages of 65 and 74 years, and 79% of women ≥75 years), women's diagnosis is often missed or delayed, leading to excess morbidity and mortality as compared with men.[62] Not only are women more likely to present with atypical features but also traditional methods of diagnosing CAD are oftentimes less sensitive in women.[62] In addition, many women have microvascular disease that will not be picked up with traditional stress testing and for which stress cardiac MRI can be useful.[58,62] Cardiac MRI demonstrated subendocardial hypoperfusion in women with nonobstructive disease presenting with symptoms.[63] The AHA recommends cardiac MRI in symptomatic women with intermediate risk of CAD and resting ST-segment abnormalities or inability to exercise.[54]

For women who require serial monitoring of cardiac function after cardiotoxic therapy, ECHO is the recommended modality. However, this can be problematic, as the ejection fraction (EF) estimation with transthoracic ECHO is reader dependent, and changes as small as 10% in ejection fraction may result in yearly cardiac evaluation after completion of therapy.[64] One study found that as compared with TTE, cardiac MRI was able to capture more patients with an EF less than 50%.[65] Furthermore, TTE may be difficult to do as frequently in women who have completed surgery because of pain.[58]

CARDIAC COMPUTED TOMOGRAPHY

Cardiac CT, both coronary artery calcium (CAC) and coronary CT angiography (CCTA), are noninvasive methods to detect CAD. In 2018, the ACC/AHA Cholesterol Guidelines suggested that "coronary artery calcium (CAC) testing may be considered in adults 40-75 years of age without diabetes mellitus and with LDL-C levels ≥70 mg/dl-189 mg/dl at a 10-year atherosclerotic cardiovascular disease (ASCVD) risk of ≥7.5% to <20% (i.e., intermediate risk group) if a decision about statin therapy is uncertain."[66,67] If CAC is ≥1, statin therapy is recommended especially in those ≥55 years of age.

For symptomatic, intermediate-risk patients, CCTA is often a good alternative for those with poor exercise capacity, baseline ECG abnormalities, or an intermediate-risk stress test.[53] In referring patients for these tests, be aware that a slower heart rate can help with obtaining better images, and patients should have normal renal function, as the test requires administration of contrast. Radiation, especially the cumulative risk, is a growing concern within medicine and specifically in cardiology. One study estimated that the absolute risk for cancer from 1 CCTA was 0.35% (1 in 284) for a 40-year-old woman, 0.22% (1 in 466) for a 60-year-old woman, and 0.075% (1 in 1338) for an 80-year-old woman.[67] One possible obstacle for CT imaging in women is the poor image quality of mid to distal segments of the coronaries because of smaller-caliber vessels.[68] In the ACCURACY (Assessment by Coronary Computed Tomographic Angiography of Individuals Undergoing Invasive Coronary Angiography) trial, CCTA was found to have a sensitivity of 90% and specificity of 88% in women and thus did not differ in its diagnostic accuracy between men and women, rendering it a great tool for the evaluation of ischemic heart disease in women.[69]

THERAPEUTICS

Improvements in clinical outcomes in women with CVD have lagged those metrics in men.[70] There are many reasons for this disturbing trend, which includes women underreporting their symptoms and not seeking necessary health care, health care providers underestimating a woman's risk of heart disease and misdiagnosing symptoms as noncardiac, and the lack of women in clinical trials. In fact, a recent report from AHA noted that women's awareness that CVD is the leading cause of death has declined over the decade from 2009 to 2019, especially among women of color and in younger women.[71,72]

In the United States, acute coronary syndrome (ACS) affects more than 250,000 women per year.[70] More women will present with non-ST elevation myocardial infarction than men and are more likely to have unusual manifestations of heart disease, such as spontaneous coronary artery dissection and Takatsubo cardiomyopathy.[70] Women are also older than men at the first presentation (71.8 years old as compared with men at 65 years of age).[70]

There are many reasons women have a poorer prognosis than men. In general, women present for evaluation of symptoms less often than men and with greater delay. Several studies have shown that women with ACS present up to 2 days later than men with similar symptoms. Symptoms of acute myocardial ischemia/infarction can be different in women as compared with men. The classic complaint of squeezing substernal chest pressure, radiating to the arm and jaw may be present, but women often will present with more "atypical" symptoms. These symptoms may include marked fatigue, shortness of breath, nausea, palpitations, anxiety, and dizziness. Women may have more frequent complaints of shoulder and arm pain as compared with men. The combination of unusual symptoms and delay in presentation for evaluation may contribute to the undertreatment of women.

There are no gender-specific guidelines for the treatment of ACS, and as such, women should receive the same guideline-directed therapy as men, as reflected in the AHA/ACC ACS guidelines. Lytic therapy is indicated for patients without timely access to percutaneous intervention, but women have a higher likelihood of complications. This higher likelihood of complications may be due in part to their higher frequency of comorbidities, including older age at presentation. Early studies of lytic-based reperfusion strategies showed that women had higher rates of bleeding complications, both peripheral and intracranial, as well as heart failure and shock. Subsequent trials of PCI showed improvement in outcomes for women as compared

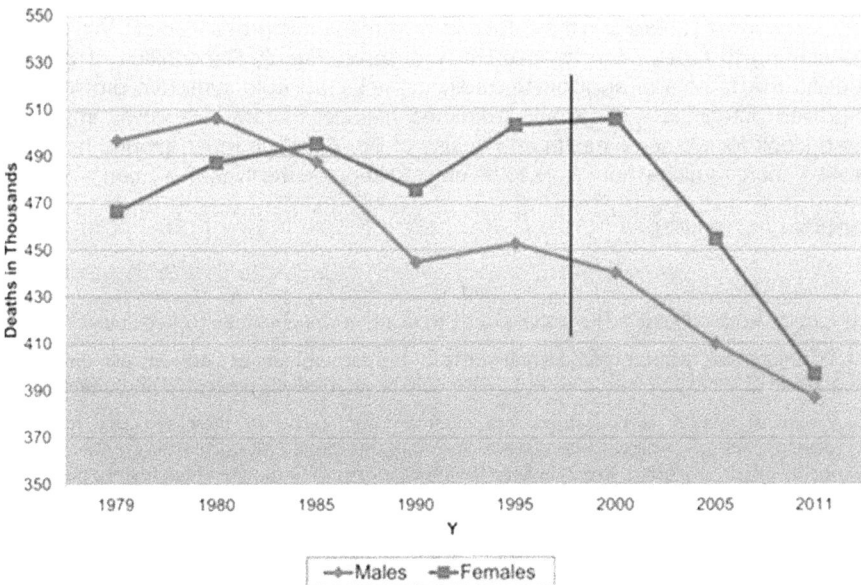

Fig. 2. CVD mortality trends for men and women in the United States from 1979 to 2011. *Reprinted with permission from* Mehta LS, Beckie TM, DeVon HA, et al. Acute Myocardial Infarction in Women: A Scientific Statement From the American Heart Association. Circulation. 2016;133(9):916-947. https://doi.org/10.1161/CIR.0000000000000351 ©2015 American Heart Association, Inc.

with lytic therapy.[73] In fact, several studies have confirmed that women with high-risk features in general fare better with an invasive strategy of percutaneous coronary intervention (PCI) for non-STEMI, as compared with a noninvasive strategy. In 2013, Stefanini and colleagues[74] performed a pooled analysis of 12 trials that included women, with a primary safety endpoint of death or myocardial infarction in patients who received drug-eluting stents (DES). When compared with bare metal stents and early-generation DES, women who received DES had better outcomes. Although they did not report on the outcomes in the male patients, the outcomes for women compare favorably with that reported for men who receive DES. Despite this and other similar reports, the AHA Scientific Statement on Acute Myocardial Infarction in women in 2016 still reports that women are less likely to receive appropriate intervention for ACS and are less likely to be discharged on evidence-based medication for established coronary disease.[70]

Early reviews of coronary artery bypass grafting (CABG) from the landmark CASS study (Coronary Artery Surgery Study) reported in 1982 showed marked difference in mortality between men and women. In men, operative mortality was 1.9%, and in women, operative mortality was 4.5%. In part, this was attributed to the smaller stature of women.[75] Two decades later, in a cohort study of more than 68,000 patients of which 15,000 were women, data again showed that women were older, were more often operated on urgently, and were less likely to receive arterial bypass grafts.[76] Others have reported that although women under 50 years of age may have higher adverse outcomes from CABG, the gender difference is reduced in older women as compared with men. Better use of arterial grafting and better attention to postoperative care may yield improved outcomes in women undergoing bypass surgery.[77]

SUMMARY

After decades of progress in the diagnosis, treatment, and prevention of CVD, women are starting to receive the attention they deserve (**Fig. 2**) Recognition of gender-specific risk factors in addition to traditional risks, variable symptom profiles, and improved outcomes with guideline-directed medical therapy are slowly improving the outlook for women's health and quality of life. Although much ground has been broken, there remains more work to be done to improve the lives of women with CVD.

CLINICS CARE POINTS

- Cardiovascular disease is the leading cause of death in women in the United States.
- Traditional risk factors portend a higher risk for the development of cardiovascular disease in women as compared with men and thus should be aggressively prevented and treated.
- Pregnancy-related complications are common and carry an increased risk for the development of cardiovascular disease. Although traditional risk calculators do not include them in scoring, every clinician should be incorporating these elements of a patient's history into their medical decisions.
- Testing for ischemic disease is the same for men and women; however, the ordering provider should be aware of certain limitations that are unique to women and how this will impact the results and plan of care.
- There are no gender-specific guidelines or treatments, yet women continue to be underdiagnosed and undertreated, and efforts should be made to make sure therapies, including statins and PCI, are done appropriately and timely.

REFERENCES

1. Arnett DK, Blumenthal RS, Albert MA, et al. 2019 ACC/AHA guideline on the primary prevention of cardiovascular disease: executive summary: a report of the American College of Cardiology/American Heart Association Task Force on Clinical Practice Guidelines. J Am Coll Cardiol 2019;74(10):1376.
2. Mosca L, Appel LJ, Benjamin EJ, et al. Evidence-based guidelines for cardiovascular disease prevention in women. J Am Coll Cardiol 2004;43(5):900–21.
3. Benjamin EJ, Muntner P, et al. Heart disease and stroke statistics-2019 update. A report from the American Heart Association. Circulation 2019.
4. Lloyd-Jones DM, Larson MG, Beiser A, et al. Lifetime risk of developing coronary heart disease. Lancet 1999;353(9147):89.
5. Golomb BA, Dang TT, Criqui MH. Peripheral arterial disease: morbidity and mortality implications. Circulation 2006;114(7):688–99.
6. Kallikazaros I, Tsioufis C, Sideris S, et al. Carotid artery disease as a marker for the presence of severe coronary artery disease in patients evaluated for chest pain. Stroke 1999;30(5):1002–7.
7. Lloyd-Jones D, Adams R, Carnethon M, et al. Heart disease and stroke statistics–2009 update: a report from the American Heart Association Statistics Committee and Stroke Statistics Subcommittee. Circulation 2009;119(3):e21–181.
8. Rana S, Lemoine E, Granger JP, et al. Preeclampsia: pathophysiology, challenges, and perspectives. Circ Res 2019;124(7):1094–112.
9. Wallis AB, Saftlas AF, Hsia J, et al. Secular trends in the rates of preeclampsia, eclampsia, and gestational hypertension, United States, 1987-2004. Am J Hypertens 2008;21(5):521–6.
10. Powe CE, Levine RJ, Karumanchi SA. Preeclampsia, a disease of the maternal endothelium: the role of antiangiogenic factors and implications for later cardiovascular disease. Circulation 2011;123(24):2856–69.
11. Chambers JC, Fusi L, Malik IS, et al. Association of maternal endothelial dysfunction with preeclampsia. JAMA 2001;285(12):1607–12.
12. Saxena AR, Karumanchi SA, Brown NJ, et al. Increased sensitivity to angiotensin II is present postpartum in women with a history of hypertensive pregnancy. Hypertension 2010;55(5):1239–45.
13. Bellamy L, Casas JP, Hingorani AD, et al. Pre-eclampsia and risk of cardiovascular disease and cancer in later life: systematic review and meta-analysis. BMJ 2007;335(7627):974.
14. Ray JG, Vermeulen MJ, Schull MJ, et al. Cardiovascular health after maternal placental syndromes (CHAMPS): population-based retrospective cohort study. Lancet 2005;366(9499):1797–803.
15. Lykke JA, Langhoff-Roos J, Sibai BM, et al. Hypertensive pregnancy disorders and subsequent cardiovascular morbidity and type 2 diabetes mellitus in the mother. Hypertension 2009;53(6):944–51.
16. Hubel CA, Powers RW, Snaedal S, et al. C-reactive protein is elevated 30 years after eclamptic pregnancy. Hypertension 2008;51(6):1499–505.
17. Wolf M, Kettyle E, Sandler L, et al. Obesity and preeclampsia: the potential role of inflammation. Obstet Gynecol 2001;98(5 Pt 1):757–62.
18. Garcia M, Mulvagh SL, Merz CN, et al. Cardiovascular disease in women: clinical perspectives. Circ Res 2016;118(8):1273–93.
19. Bellamy L, Casas JP, Hingorani AD, et al. Type 2 diabetes mellitus after gestational diabetes: a systematic review and meta-analysis. Lancet 2009;373(9677):1773–9.

20. Vrachnis N, Augoulea A, Iliodromiti Z, et al. Previous gestational diabetes mellitus and markers of cardiovascular risk. Int J Endocrinol 2012;2012:458610.
21. Chakravarty EF, Bush TM, Manzi S, et al. Prevalence of adult systemic lupus erythematosus in California and Pennsylvania in 2000: estimates obtained using hospitalization data. Arthritis Rheum 2007;56(6):2092–4.
22. Cunningham MA, Richard ML, Wirth JR, et al. Novel mechanism for estrogen receptor alpha modulation of murine lupus. J Autoimmun 2019;97:59–69.
23. Willerson J, Ridker P. Inflammation as a cardiovascular risk factor. Circulation 2004;109. https://doi.org/10.1161/01.CIR.0000129535.04194.38Circulation. II-2–II-10.
24. Esdaile JM, Abrahamowicz M, Grodzicky T, et al. Traditional Framingham risk factors fail to fully account for accelerated atherosclerosis in systemic lupus erythematosus. Arthritis Rheum 2001;44(10):2331–7.
25. Casey KA, Smith MA, Sinibaldi D, et al. Modulation of cardiometabolic disease markers by type I interferon inhibition in systemic lupus erythematosus. Arthritis Rheumatol 2021;73(3):459–71.
26. Yazdany J, Pooley N, Langham J, et al. Systemic lupus erythematosus; stroke and myocardial infarction risk: a systematic review and meta-analysis RMD. Open 2020;6:e001247.
27. Darby SC, Ewertz M, McGale P, et al. Risk of ischemic heart disease in women after radiotherapy for breast cancer. N Engl J Med 2013;368:987–98.
28. Lancellotti P, Nkomo VT, Badano LP, et al. Expert consensus for multi-modality imaging evaluation of cardiovascular complications of radiotherapy in adults: a report from the European Association of Cardiovascular Imaging and the American Society of Echocardiography. J Am Soc Echocardiogr 2013;26:1013–32.
29. Schmidt J, Landin-Wilhelmsen K, Brännström M, et al. Cardiovascular disease and risk factors in PCOS women of postmenopausal age: a 21-year controlled follow-up study. J Clin Endocrinol Metab 2011;96(12):3794–803.
30. Wild S, et al. Cardiovascular disease in women with polycystic ovary syndrome at long-term follow-up: a retrospective cohort study. Clin Endocrinol 2000;52: 595±600.
31. Matthews K, Crawford SL, Chae CU, et al. Are changes in cardiovascular disease risk factors in midlife women due to chronological aging or to the menopausal transition? J Am Coll Cardiol 2009;54(25):2366–73.
32. Kok H, van Asselt KM, van der Schouw YT, et al. Heart disease risk determines menopausal age rather than the reverse. J Am Coll Cardiol 2006;47(10):1976–83.
33. Hulley S, Grady D, Bush T, et al. Randomized trial of estrogen plus progestin for secondary prevention of coronary heart disease in postmenopausal women. Heart and Estrogen/Progestin Replacement Study (HERS) Research Group. JAMA 1998;280:605–13. 10.
34. Rossouw JE, Anderson GL, Prentice RL, et al. Risks and benefits of estrogen plus progestin in healthy postmenopausal women: principal results from the Women's Health Initiative randomized controlled trial. JAMA 2002;288(3):321–33.
35. Wengner N. Women and coronary heart disease: a century after Herrick; understudied, underdiagnosed, and undertreated. Circulation 2011;124:A612.
36. Juutilainen A, Kortelainen S, Lehto S, et al. Gender difference in the impact of type 2 diabetes on coronary heart disease risk. Diabetes Care 2004;27: 2898–904.
37. Huxley R, Barzi F, Woodward M. Excess risk of fatal coronary heart disease associated with diabetes in men and women: meta-analysis of 37 prospective cohort studies. Bmj 2006;332:73–8.

38. Huxley RR, Woodward M. Cigarette smoking as a risk factor for coronary heart disease in women compared with men: a systematic review and meta-analysis of prospective cohort studies. Lancet 2011;378:1297–305.

39. Wilson PW, D'Agostino RB, Sullivan L, et al. Overweight and obesity as determinants of cardiovascular risk: the Framingham experience. Arch Intern Med 2002; 162:1867–72.

40. Executive summary of the third report of the National Cholesterol Education Program (NCEP) expert panel on detection, evaluation, and treatment of high blood cholesterol in adults (Adult Treatment Panel III). JAMA 2001;285:2486–97.

41. Ford ES, Giles WH, Dietz WH, et al. Prevalence of the metabolic syndrome among US adults: findings from the third National Health and Nutrition Examination Survey. JAMA 2002;287:356–9.

42. Wilson PW, D'Agostino RB, Parise H, et al. Metabolic syndrome as a precursor of cardiovascular disease and type 2 diabetes mellitus. Circulation 2005;112(20): 3066–72.

43. Vachiat A, McCutcheon K, Tsabedze N, et al. HIV and ischemic heart disease. J Am Coll Cardiol 2017;69(1):73–82.

44. Koopman C, Vaartjes I, Heintjes, et al. Persisting gender differences and attenuating age differences in cardiovascular drug use for prevention and treatment of coronary heart disease, 1998-2010. Eur Heart J 2013;34:3198–205.

45. McNeil JJ, Woods RL, Tonkin AM, et al. Effect of aspirin on cardiovascular events and bleeding in the healthy elderly. N Engl J Med 2018;379:16.

46. Gibbons RJ, Balady GJ, Bricker JT, et al. Smith SCACC/AHA 2002 guideline update for exercise testing: summary article: a report of the American College of Cardiology/American Heart Association Task Force on Practice guidelines (committee to update the 1997 exercise testing guidelines). Circulation 2002;106: 1883–92.

47. Barolsky SM, Gilbert CA, Faruqui A, et al. Differences in electrocardiographic response to exercise of women and men: a non-Bayesian factor. Circulation 1979;60:1021–7.

48. Kohli P, Gulati M. Exercise stress testing in women: going back to the basics. Circulation 2010;122(24):2570–80.

49. Weiner DA, Ryan TJ, McCabe CH, et al. Exercise stress testing: correlations among history of angina, ST-segment response and prevalence of coronary-artery disease in the Coronary Artery Surgery Study (CASS). N Engl J Med 1979;301:230–5.

50. Morise AP, Beto R. The specificity of exercise electrocardiography in women grouped by estrogen status. Int J Cardiol 1997;60:55–65.

51. Henzlova MJ, Croft LB, Diamond JA. Effect of hormone replacement therapy on the electrocardiographic response to exercise. J Nucl Cardiol 2002;9(4):385–7.

52. Gulati M, Pandey DK, Arnsdorf MF, et al. Exercise capacity and the risk of death in women: the St James Women Take Heart Project. Circulation 2003;108:1554–9.

53. Mieres JH, Gulati M, Bairey Merz N, et al, American Heart Association Cardiac Imaging Committee of the Council on Clinical Cardiology; Cardiovascular Imaging and Intervention Committee of the Council on Cardiovascular Radiology and Intervention. Role of noninvasive testing in the clinical evaluation of women with suspected ischemic heart disease: a consensus statement from the American Heart Association. Circulation 2014;130(4):350–79 [Erratum in: Circulation. 2014;130(4):e86].

54. Picano E, Lattanzi F, Orlandini A, et al. Stress echocardiography and the human factor: the importance of being expert. J Am Coll Cardiol 1991;17(3):666–9.

55. Expert Panel on MRS, Kanal E, Barkovich AJ, et al. ACR guidance document on MR safe practices: 2013. J Magn Reson Imaging 2013;37:501–30, 183.

56. Lewis JF, Lin L, McGorray S, et al. Dobutamine stress echocardiography in women with chest pain. Pilot phase data from the National Heart, Lung and Blood Institute Women's Ischemia Syndrome Evaluation (WISE). J Am Coll Cardiol 1999; 33(6):1462–8.

57. Ray JG, Vermeulen MJ, Bharatha A, et al. Association between MRI exposure during pregnancy and fetal and childhood outcomes. JAMA 2016;316:952–61.

58. Bucciarelli-Ducci C, Ostenfeld E, Baldassarre LA, et al. Cardiovascular disease in women: insights from magnetic resonance imaging. J Cardiovasc Magn Reson 2020;22:71.

59. Pasupathy S, Air T, Dreyer RP, et al. Systematic review of patients presenting with suspected myocardial infarction and nonobstructive coronary arteries. Circulation 2015;131:861–70.

60. Pathik B, Raman B, Mohd Amin NH, et al. Troponin-positive chest pain with unobstructed coronary arteries: incremental diagnostic value of cardiovascular magnetic resonance imaging. Eur Heart J Cardiovasc Imaging 2016;17(10):1146–52.

61. Dastidar AG, Baritussio A, De Garate E, et al. Prognostic role of CMR and conventional risk factors in myocardial infarction with nonobstructed coronary arteries. JACC Cardiovasc Imaging 2019;12(10):1973–82.

62. Bairey Merz CN, Shaw LJ, Reis SE, et al, WISE Investigators. Insights from the NHLBI-Sponsored Women's Ischemia Syndrome Evaluation (WISE) Study: part II: gender differences in presentation, diagnosis, and outcome with regard to gender-based pathophysiology of atherosclerosis and macrovascular and microvascular coronary disease. J Am Coll Cardiol 2006;47(3 Suppl):S21–9.

63. Panting JR, Gatehouse PD, Yang GZ, et al. Abnormal subendocardial perfusion in cardiac syndrome X detected by cardiovascular magnetic resonance imaging. N Engl J Med 2002;346:1948–53.

64. Mackey JR, Clemons M, Côté MA, et al. Cardiac management during adjuvant trastuzumab therapy: recommendations of the Canadian Trastuzumab Working Group. Curr Oncol 2008;15(1):24–35.

65. Armstrong GT, Plana JC, Zhang N, et al. Screening adult survivors of childhood cancer for cardiomyopathy: comparison of echocardiography and cardiac magnetic resonance imaging. J Clin Oncol 2012;30(23):2876–84.

66. Grundy SM, Stone NJ, Bailey AL, et al. 2018 AHA/ACC/AACVPR/AAPA/ABC/ACPM/ADA/AGS/APhA/ASPC/NLA guideline on the management of blood cholesterol: a report of the American College of Cardiology/American Heart Association Task Force on Practice guidelines. J Am Coll Cardiol 2019;73(24):3234–7.

67. Einstein AJ, Henzlova MJ, Rajagopalan S. Estimating risk of cancer associated with radiation exposure from 64-slice computed tomography coronary angiography. JAMA 2007;298(3):317–23.

68. Pampolano M. Imaging of heart disease in women: an updated review. ACC 2018.

69. Tsang JC, Min JK, Lin FY, et al. Sex comparison of diagnostic accuracy of 64-multidetector row coronary computed tomographic angiography: results from the multicenter ACCURACY trial. J Cardiovasc Comput Tomogr 2012;6:246–51.

70. Mehta LS, Beckie TM, DeVon HA, et al. Acute myocardial infarction in women. Circulation 2016;133:916–47.

⬛ M, Shay CM, Howard VJ, et al. Ten-year differences in women's awareness ⌐ coronary heart disease: results of the 2019 American Heart Association nal Survey. Circulation 2020;142:e1–10.

72. Mozaffarian D, Benjamin EJ, Go AS, et al. Heart disease and stroke statistics—2015 update. A report from the American Heart Association. Circulation 2015;131(4):e29–322.
73. Boersma E, the PCAT Group. Does time matter? A pooled analysis of randomized clinical trials comparing primary PCI and in hospital fibrinolysis in acute myocardial infarction patients. Eur Heart J 2006;27:779–88.
74. Stefanini GG, Baber U, Windecker S, et al. Safety and efficacy of drug-eluting stents in women: a patient-level pooled analysis of randomised trials. Lancet 2013;382:1879–88.
75. Fisher L, Kennedy J, Davis K, et al. Association of sex, physical size, and operative mortality after CABG in the Coronary Artery Surgery Study (CASS). J Thorac Cardiovasc Surg 1982;84:334–41.
76. Guru V, Fremes S, Tu J. Time-related mortality for women after CABG surgery: a population-based study. J Thorac Cardiovasc Surg 2004;127:1158–65.
77. Nicolini F, Vezzani A, Fortuna D, et al. Gender differences in outcomes following isolated coronary artery bypass grafting: long-term results. J Thorac Cardiothorac Surg 2016;11:144.

Sleep Disorders and Aging in Women

Wahida Akberzie, MD[a], Lynn Kataria, MD[b],*

KEYWORDS

- Sleep • Elderly women • Insomnia • Sleep-disordered breathing

KEY POINTS

- Several sleep disorders increase as women age, such as insomnia and sleep-disordered breathing.
- RLS tends to have a female predominance, whereas OSA and RBD are more common in males; however, it is important to keep an open mind when evaluating older women.
- Disruptions in sleep leading up to menopause and thereafter can have a significant impact on women.
- If a patient is a limited historian, reliance on family and caregivers may be necessary along with diagnostic testing, such as actigraphy and PSG.

INTRODUCTION

It has been proposed by the US Census Bureau that 20% of the population will be 65 years old or older by 2030.[1] This is notable because more than half of older patients report difficulties with sleep.[2,3] Common sleep complaints in individuals aged 65 and older include trouble falling asleep, waking up in the middle of the night, awakening too early, needing to nap, and not feeling rested.[4] The Cardiovascular Health Study in older surveyed 4467 participants and found the incidence of trouble falling asleep was 2.8%, frequent awakenings was 12.3%, and excessive daytime sleepiness was 4.4%.[5] Women were specifically more likely to have trouble falling asleep.[5] The importance of these sleep complaints is significant because there is preliminary evidence that suggests poor sleep is associated with functional impairment and poor health in the older adults.[5–8] Not only have these sleep disturbances among older individuals been subjective in nature, but studies using polysomnography (PSG) objectively confirm that age-related changes in sleep predispose older individuals to increased

[a] Department of Neurology, George Washington University School of Medicine, Washington DC VA Medical Center, 3B-103, 50 Irving Street Northwest, Washington, DC 20422, USA; [b] Sleep Laboratory, Department of Neurology, George Washington University School of Medicine, Washington DC VA Medical Center, 3B-103, 50 Irving Street Northwest, Washington, DC 20422, USA
* Corresponding author.
E-mail address: Lynn.kataria@va.gov

Clin Geriatr Med 37 (2021) 667–682
https://doi.org/10.1016/j.cger.2021.05.011
0749-0690/21/Published by Elsevier Inc.
geriatric.theclinics.com

wakefulness at night and sleep fragmentation.[9] Therefore, it is vital for clinicians and scientists to understand sleep physiology and architectural changes as people age, particularly in older women where treatment strategies can be tailored.

In aging women, hormonal changes also play a large role in sleep. Steroid hormones, such as estrogen and progesterone, influence sleep patterns that are associated with hormonal cycles of women throughout lifespan including menopause.[10] Along with physiologic and hormonal changes that occur in the aging population, there is a higher prevalence of sleep disorders among older adults, including restless legs syndrome (RLS),[11,12] sleep-disordered breathing,[11–17] and insomnia.[11,12,18]

In recent years there is evolving evidence regarding sleep disorders and sleep disturbance and their effects on mortality and outcomes in women 65 years of age and above, particularly effects on cardiovascular health, obesity risk, and risk of developing depression.[19] However, there is still much to be learned regarding sleep disturbance and sleep disorders and their effects on aging women, such as the risk of developing dementia. Sleep complaints and disturbance in older adults has been associated with impairment in daily activities, mobility, and gait speed.[3,7,20] A prospective cohort study of 817 older women found that objective findings of shorter sleep duration, greater wake after sleep onset, and lower sleep efficiency are risk factors for functional or physical decline in aging women.[21] Some research even suggests a correlation between sleep disturbance and likelihood for nursing home placement.[22] However, many confounding factors may be playing a role, including comorbid conditions. This article reviews sleep disorders including insomnia, circadian rhythm sleep-wake disorder (CRSWD), RLS, disorders of hypersomnia, and sleep-disordered breathing in older women, prevalence, and recommended treatment options.

BACKGROUND
Sleep Across the Lifespan

Sleep is composed of two main states: rapid eye movement (REM) and non-REM (NREM) sleep. NREM sleep involves a synchronous cortical electroencephalogram, including sleep spindles, K-complexes, and slow waves.[23] It is associated with low muscle tone and minimal psychological activity. REM sleep has a desynchronized electroencephalogram, muscles are atonic, and dreaming occurs during this stage.[24] In adults the natural progression of sleep involves sleep beginning in NREM sleep and progressing into deeper NREM stages and then eventually REM sleep. As people age, the composition of sleep changes. Starting in preteenage years slow wave sleep (SWS; stage N3) starts declining by 40% and continues a slower decline into old age.[23] In the aging population, PSG studies of sleep architecture display decreases in total sleep time, sleep efficiency, and SWS with age.[25–29]

In women 65 years of age and older there is a greater association between declining total sleep time and aging.[9] Age-related changes on stage 1 sleep are more apparent in women including less percentage of stage 2 sleep and a greater percentage of SWS than age-matched men.[9] The SIESTA study found that men had a 1.7% decrease in SWS per decade of age compared with women who had no change in SWS with age.[30] This same study found that women had a smaller rate of increase in stage 1 sleep, a greater rate of increase in stage 2 sleep, and a greater rate of decline in REM, in comparison with men.[30] Changes in sleep architecture may be one reason why women are more likely to report sleep problems. Another important component that may be playing a role in sleep quality and contributing to changes sleep architecture are the hormonal changes that occur throughout a woman's lifespan.

Hormonal Changes and Sleep in Women

Women report more sleep disturbances and poor sleep quality around time of menses.[31] Despite subjective sleep complaints, PSG variables have shown that sleep continuity and sleep efficiency remain stable at different phases of the ovulatory menstrual cycle in young healthy women.[31] Percentages of SWS and slow wave activity in NREM sleep are unchanged across the menstrual cycle.[31]

As women transition into menopause, lower estradiol levels were associated with poorer sleep over time.[32] The decline of endogenous estrogen that occurs in menopause poses a great factor in sleep quality in this population.

In a community-based survey of women's health and menopausal symptoms, it was found that perimenopausal and postmenopausal women are more likely to report difficulty sleeping compared with premenopausal women.[33] During this time period, there is an increase in follicle-stimulating hormone (FSH) and luteinizing hormone, with a decline in estradiol levels.[34] Kravitz and Joffe[35] investigated the effects of estradiol and FSH on sleep disturbances and noticed that a reduction of estradiol levels correlated with trouble falling asleep and staying asleep. An increase in FSH levels was associated with reports of difficulty staying asleep.[35] Additionally, Sowers and colleagues[36] found that accelerated FSH changes correlated with poor sleep quality. Although the specific effects of estrogen, FSH, and luteinizing hormone on sleep as women go through menopause is controversial their contribution to sleep disruption cannot be ignored and may have lasting effects as women age.

Sleep Requirements

According to the National Sleep Foundation, sleep time duration recommended is 7 to 8 hours for healthy older adults.[37] As individuals age the ability to sleep becomes more difficult and older individuals tend to show an increase in disturbed sleep.[6] Some research suggests that the quantity of sleep differs by age not because of changes in the necessity, but more that the ability to obtain needed sleep decreases with age.[38] The ability to sleep declines and may be related to medical and/or psychiatric illness and circadian changes.[38]

Ohayon and Vecchierini[6] looked at 1000 older French adults who reported approximately 7 hours of sleep with men sleeping slightly more than women. On average, total sleep time declined by 10 minutes per decade; however, this decline was more prominent in women than in men.[6] Empana and colleagues[39] included 9294 subjects aged greater than or equal to 65 years (60% of them being women), and found that 18.7% of the participants had regular or frequent excessive daytime sleepiness. A decline in the quantity and quality of sleep in elderly women are contributors to sleep disorders in this population.

Patient Evaluation

Older women patients can suffer from an array of sleep disorders. Women 65 years of age and older may present with sleep disturbances resulting in hypersomnolence, delirium, and disturbed cognition, which can contribute to increased risk of accidents and injury. Obtaining a thorough history is imperative and may often involve family members, caregivers, and/or a bed partner. Secondary collateral Information can provide useful information regarding any unusual nocturnal events, such as acting out dreams, leg movements, snoring, and witnessed apneic events. When obtaining a history of present illness and sleep history (**Box 1**), it is important to ask about sleep/wake schedules, weekend routines, the sleep environment, typical sleep habits, and substance use (caffeine, alcohol, illicit drugs, and herbals).

Box 1
Sleep questionnaire for geriatric women and caretakers

Focused Sleep Questionnaire for Geriatric Women and Caretakers

What time do you wake up in the morning?

What time do you fall asleep at night?

Where do you sleep?

Do you have a bed partner?

How long does it take you to fall asleep?

How many hours do you sleep per night?

How many times do you wake up during a typical night?

Do you feel that you are excessively sleepy during the daytime and take naps?

Do you have difficulties falling asleep or staying asleep?

Do you take medications or use alcohol to help you sleep?

Does pain bother you during sleep?

Do you snore, gasp, or stop breathing at night?

Do you have uncomfortable sensations in your legs at night or unusual movements at night?

Do you have symptoms of sleep paralysis, hallucinations at sleep onset or waking, or cataplexy?

Are there any environmental noises or disturbances, such as TV, bright lights, pets, or noises that disturb your sleep?

When did you reach menopause?

Do you have any other medical, neurologic, or psychiatric conditions that interfere with sleep?

Sleep-disordered breathing is common in older women.[40,41] There are several sleep questionnaires used to screen for sleep-disordered breathing. Excessive daytime sleepiness is a symptom of sleep apnea and a commonly used survey to assess this is the Epworth Sleepiness Scale.[42] This is an eight-item questionnaire that quantifies likelihood of dozing off with the scale of zero chance of dozing off (0), slight (1), moderate (2), and high (3), with scores of 10 or higher suggesting pathologic daytime sleepiness.[42] Another helpful tool for screening patients for sleep-disordered breathing is the STOP-BANG questionnaire, which is based on eight yes/no questions related to clinical features of sleep apnea (snoring, tired, observed apneas, hypertension, body mass index greater than >35 kg/m^2, age >50, neck size >40 cm, male).[43] The questionnaire has shown to have a high sensitivity when using a cutoff score of three or more, with a sensitivity of 84% in detecting any sleep apnea, 93% in detecting moderate to severe sleep apnea, and 100% in detecting severe sleep apnea.[44] Another commonly used questionnaire is the Insomnia Severity Index.[45] It consists of seven items assessing the subjective symptoms and consequences of insomnia and the severity of concerns.[45] A score of 15 or greater suggests moderate to severe insomnia, with a specificity of 98.3% to 100% and sensitivity of 47.7% to 78.1%.[46]

A simplistic approach can be adopted when considering the sleep complaints in older women (**Figs. 1** and **2**). Clinical providers can evaluate whether sleep complaints are focused around excessive daytime sleepiness versus difficulty falling or staying asleep at night. There is certainly overlap between the two; however, this approach can help determine possible etiologies and appropriate next steps with respect to screening and testing.

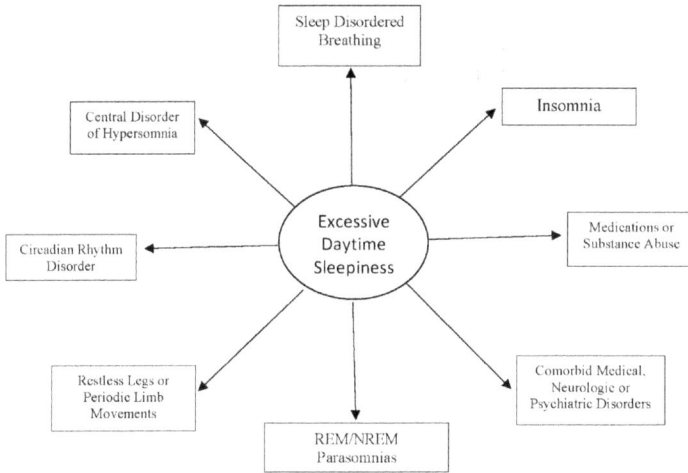

Fig. 1. Etiologies for complaints of excessive daytime sleepiness in women ages 65 and older. This figure provides a simplistic approach for possible differential diagnoses to clinical providers when considering complaints of excessive daytime sleepiness.

CLINICAL CARE POINTS: SLEEP DISORDERS IN WOMEN AGES 65 AND ABOVE
Insomnia

Women have high rates of insomnia.[47,48] Several epidemiologic studies have found that prevalence of insomnia symptoms reaches close to 40% in individuals 65 years of age and older.[49–51] Also, women older than age 45 are 1.7 times more likely to have insomnia than men.[49] Patients may present with symptoms of difficulty initiating or maintaining sleep. According to the International Classification of Sleep Disorders-3, insomnia is defined as "a persistent difficulty with sleep initiation, duration, consolidation, or quality that occurs despite adequate opportunity and circumstances for sleep, and results in some form of daytime impairment."[52] Chronic insomnia consists of symptoms for at least 3 months at least three times per week, and short-term as

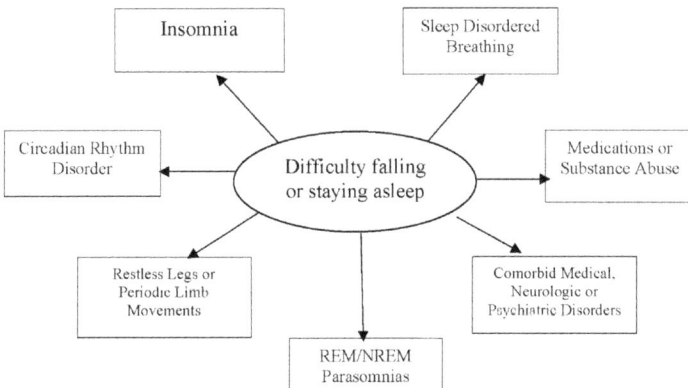

Fig. 2. Etiologies for complaints of difficulty falling and staying asleep in geriatric women. This figure provides a simplistic approach for possible differential diagnoses to clinical providers when considering complaints of falling asleep and staying asleep in elderly women.

being less than 3 months.[52] Performing a thorough sleep history and past medical history is needed, paying attention to medical, neurologic, and psychiatric comorbidities. Substances and medications that may disturb sleep are over-the-counter decongestants, β-agonists, corticosteroids, selective serotonin reuptake inhibitors, antipsychotics, diuretics, anticholinergics, alcohol, caffeine, and stimulants.[53] Obtaining information regarding sleep hygiene, including sleep time, wake time, and use of electronics before bed, is necessary. A sleep diary is used to further assess sleep patterns and actigraphy may also provide more information regarding the regular sleep-wake schedule and disturbances.

Regardless of medical history, the treatment of insomnia in adults ages 65 and above includes maintaining a regular sleep-wake schedule.[54] Cognitive behavioral therapy-insomnia (CBT-I) is first-line treatment of insomnia in older adults.[55] Several prospective studies have compared the efficacy of CBT-I, medications, and combination of CBT-I with medication.[56–58] Extending CBT-I may also prove to be beneficial in this patient population to maintain short-term gains.[56–59] CBT-I consists of cognitive and behavioral techniques, such as stimulus control therapy, sleep restriction therapy, cognitive restructuring, relaxation techniques, and sleep hygiene education.[60] There are several risks with pharmacotherapy because of changing pharmacodynamics and pharmacokinetics in older adults. Therefore, the discussion of risks should occur with patients and caregivers, which include falls, oversedation, confusion, and cognitive impairment. Long-acting benzodiazepines should be avoided because of the previously mentioned risks. Nonbenzodiazepines, such as zolpidem and eszopiclone, are considered shorter acting, although they are not completely devoid of significant side effects.[61] Ramelteon and other melatonin receptor agonists are Food and Drug Administration approved for insomnia and have been shown to be effective with sleep initiation insomnia.[62] Other medications that are often used for the treatment of insomnia include trazodone, mirtazapine, tricyclic antidepressants, gabapentin, and first-generation antihistamines; however, several of these medications may cause significant side effects including orthostatic hypotension and increased risk of falls and caution should be exercised in older individuals. Antidepressants should only be considered for insomnia when there is underlying depression.

There are evolving data regarding alternative nonpharmacologic therapies in women and randomized controlled trials are warranted. Small studies have found that yoga may produce a reduction in insomnia severity in perimenopausal and postmenopausal women.[63,64] There are limited data regarding therapeutic massage. However, one small study looked at 44 postmenopausal volunteers that were randomly distributed into three groups of therapeutic massage, passive movements, and control.[65] The individuals in the therapeutic massage group demonstrated improvement in Insomnia Severity Index and the menopause quality of life questionnaire.[65]

Sleep-Disordered Breathing: Obstructive Sleep Apnea

Sleep-related breathing disorders include disorders of abnormal respiration during sleep. These include obstructive sleep apnea (OSA) disorders, central sleep apnea (CSA) disorders, sleep-related hypoventilation disorders, and sleep-related hypoxemia disorder.[52] OSA is characterized by repeated episodes of partial or complete obstruction of the respiratory passages during sleep while respiratory effort continues.[52] OSA is estimated to be double the prevalence compared with the younger population.[66] It has been shown that the prevalence of OSA increases with increasing age and has been estimated to be as high as 90% in men and 78% in women ages 60 to 85 years.[40,41] Also, postmenopausal women have a higher prevalence of OSA than premenopausal women, and estrogen may play a protective role in premenopausal women.[67–69] Given the greater association in postmenopausal women, a diagnosis of OSA should be appropriately considered as part of the evaluation of older women presenting with sleep disruption.

Symptoms of sleep-disordered breathing include excessive daytime sleepiness, snoring, witnessed apneic events, choking or gasping in sleep, and morning headaches. PSG is indicated for the confirmation of the diagnosis of OSA. Home sleep apnea testing that is technically adequate may also be used to diagnose OSA in a patient with no significant cardiopulmonary disease, neuromuscular disease, history of stroke, chronic opiate use, or concerns of hypoventilation.[70] OSA is diagnosed in a patient who is experiencing symptoms or a comorbid condition and has at least five obstructive respiratory events on PSG or out of center sleep test. When discussing treatment once the diagnosis of OSA has been confirmed, first-line therapy is continuous positive airway pressure (CPAP).[71] Other treatment options include oral appliances or positional devices. Another treatment modality, called upper airway stimulation or hypoglossal nerve stimulation, has been developed for use in individuals with moderate to severe OSA who are unable to use CPAP therapy.[72] Hypoglossal nerve stimulation is an implantable device that acts as a pacemaker and delivers stimulation to the hypoglossal nerve.[72] This treatment option includes drug-induced sleep endoscopy and surgery, and risks and benefits should be discussed when evaluating an older patient for this type of therapy. There are also more invasive surgical options for the treatment of OSA.[73] These options may not normalize apnea-hypopnea index and require the patient to be a good surgical candidate.[74] Careful consideration should be exercised before proceeding with surgical treatment modalities in the older adult patient population.

Sleep-Disordered Breathing: Central Sleep Apnea

CSA syndromes are described as having a reduction or cessation of airflow caused by absent or reduced respiratory effort.[52] Data from the Sleep Heart Health Study show the prevalence of CSA and Cheyne-Stokes respiration to be 0.9% and predominant OSA with a CSA component has been found to be 2.7% in adults aged 40 and older.[75] However, the prevalence has been found to be 7.5% in men 65 years of age and older in another cohort.[76] Individuals with CSA tend to be older and men.[75] While evaluating a patient, it is important to keep in mind that a patient may have both CSA and OSA, especially because the prevalence of both increases with age. Patients may present with excessive daytime sleepiness, insomnia, or nocturnal dyspnea. It is important to keep in mind that CSA, specifically with CSA/Cheyne-Stokes breathing, is associated with heart failure, and a patient's symptoms of frequent awakenings or disturbed sleep may be falsely assumed to be caused by their heart failure.[52] CSA has been found to be associated with such conditions as heart failure, atrial fibrillation, renal failure, and chronic use of opiates.[77–80] These are all conditions that are commonly seen in older adults and likely exist in aging women presenting with sleep complaints. Gold standard testing is PSG for the confirmation of the diagnosis of CSA. CSA is diagnosed in individuals with symptoms or comorbid conditions, at least five central respiratory events on PSG, and most respiratory events are central in nature. Treatment needs to be tailored to the type of CSA, comorbid conditions, and underlying cause. The different options may include CPAP, bilevel PAP in a spontaneous timed mode, and adaptive servoventilation.

Restless Legs Syndrome

RLS is a sensorimotor disorder characterized by a complaint of a strong, nearly irresistible urge to move the limbs.[52] Population-based studies for RLS report a prevalence of 5% to 10% in western industrial countries.[81] Both prevalence and severity increase with age.[82] In a study evaluating 369 individuals 65 to 83 years of age, women had a higher prevalence of RLS at 13.9% compared with the overall prevalence of 9.8%.[83] The prevalence of restless legs in women has been reported to be twice as high as in men.[81] More research in determining prevalence specific to older women is warranted.

RLS symptoms include creeping or crawling sensation in the lower legs and an urge to move the legs at night that is worse at rest and improved with movement. RLS can cause sleep disruption and reduce sleep time and be a source of distress and morbidity. It is diagnosed through focused questioning rather than diagnostic testing.[84] Five clinical criteria must be met to establish the diagnosis of RLS that were developed by the International Restless Legs Syndrome Study Group.[85] When evaluating the diagnosis and approaching the discussion of treatment, it is essential to review medications because several medications may cause sleep-related leg cramps and may present as RLS. Some of these medications that are commonly used in older individuals include diuretics, raloxifene, and statins. Because it has been shown to be associated with iron deficiency anemia, if RLS is suspected, initial work-up includes obtaining ferritin levels. Iron supplementation is recommended if levels are less than or equal to 75 µg/L or whose transferrin saturation is less than 20%.[86] Nonpharmacologic therapy includes regular exercise, reducing intake of caffeine and other stimulants, proper sleep hygiene, avoiding sleep deprivation, cold water massages or leg baths, vibratory stimulation device, yoga, or acupuncture.[82]

If symptoms continue to be bothersome and a patient does not respond to nonpharmacologic therapy, some of the medications commonly used in the initial symptomatic treatment in RLS include dopaminergic agonists (ie, pramipexole and ropinirole) and the $\alpha2\delta$ ligands (ie, gabapentin or pregabalin) can be considered. Common side effects of dopamine agonists include nausea, headache, sleepiness, and impulse control disorders.[82] Impulse control disorders have been reported to develop in 6% to 17% of patients with RLS who are being treated with dopamine agonists.[87] Therefore, a patient should be evaluated regarding a history of impulse control and risks should be discussed with the family and patient. There is also a long-term risk of augmentation of symptoms with dopamine agonists. $\alpha2\delta$ ligands (ie, gabapentin or pregabalin) have been proven to be effective for RLS. Some side effects include somnolence, dizziness, fatigue, weight gain, and headache.[82] Therefore, because of sedation effects, it is important to use caution in any patient that may be a fall risk.

Parasomnias

Parasomnias are undesirable physical events or experiences that occur during entry into sleep, within sleep, or during arousal from sleep.[52] Parasomnias are divided as NREM-related, REM-related, or other parasomnias. NREM parasomnias tend to be more common in the pediatric population. However REM parasomnias, particularly REM sleep behavior disorder (RBD), occurs more commonly in men and patients older than the age of 50 years.[88] Overall prevalence is 0.5% but has increased prevalence in older individuals as high as 2%.[89–91] Data are lacking in terms of prevalence among aging women. Patients with RBD experience lack of muscle atonia in REM sleep, resulting in vivid dreams with dream enactment. Although RBD may be more common in men, it can have significant effects on patients and bed partners resulting in injuries, sleep disruption, and adverse health effects and therefore, need to be evaluated for in older women presenting with similar sleep complaints.

Individuals often present with caregivers or bed partners who are noticing dramatic and intense motor activity during sleep as the individual is acting out dreams, and some movements may be violent in nature. RBD is common in patients with movement disorders and RBD symptoms present itself years before the diagnosis of the movement disorder. RBD has been shown to have an association with α-synucleinopathy neurodegenerative diseases including Parkinson disease, multiple system atrophy, and Lewy body dementia.[92] There are also medications that can precipitate and exacerbate symptoms of RBD, such as selective serotonin reuptake inhibitors, tricyclic antidepressants, and monoamine oxidase inhibitors. Medication-associated RBD may occur in 6% of patients using them.[91,92] Obtaining a PSG with four-limb electromyography may be helpful to identify REM sleep without atonia and dream enactment. Also, PSG is helpful ruling out other possible underlying sleep disorders that may mimic RBD, such as OSA causing pseudo-RBD.

First steps of treatment include ensuring a safe bedroom environment. Removal of firearms or other weapons, sharp objects, and even lamps or alarm clocks should be discussed. Because of the high risk of falling, the height of the bed should be lowered.[93] Bed partners should be advised to sleep in a separate room. Once safety measures have been implemented, additional pharmacotherapy may be necessary if the patient is leaving the bed or standing up in it.[93] Initial therapy can include melatonin or clonazepam. Melatonin can decrease dream enactment and sleep-related injury.[93] Common side effects include abdominal discomfort, vivid dreams, and sleep fragmentation. Clonazepam decreases dream enactment and sleep-related injury.[93] Common side effects include sedation, imbalance, and cognitive disturbances, which may be even more detrimental to older adults given impairments in drug metabolism. Therefore, clonazepam should be used with much caution and risks and benefits thoroughly discussed with patient and caregivers.

Circadian Rhythm Sleep-Wake Disorders

CRSWD is defined by the alterations of the circadian time-keeping system, its entrainment mechanisms, or a misalignment of the endogenous circadian rhythm and the external environment.[52] There are different types of CRSWD, but one commonly seen disorder in older individuals is advanced sleep-wake phase disorder. The patient has features of early or advanced timing of the major sleep episode in relation to the desired sleep time and wake-up time. There are limited data regarding prevalence of CRSWD among older women and even the general population. It is estimated that prevalence of CRSWD in the general population is less than 3%; however, these disorders may be underestimated because they are often confused with insomnia.[94] A 2014 population survey evaluating advanced sleep-wake phase disorder demonstrated a prevalence of 0.25% to 7%.[95]

Advanced sleep-wake phase disorder is found more frequently in older adults; however, it is difficult to determine the prevalence because many of these individuals have depression, pain, physical limitations, and respiratory symptoms that may contribute or cause symptoms of advanced sleep-wake phase disorder, such as early morning awakenings.[94] Also, if the elderly female patient is a shift-worker, it is important to keep in mind that older individuals are more prone to developing shift-work sleep disorder.[94] When evaluating a patient for a CRSWD, in addition to history and obtaining daily timing of social activities and meals, such tools as a sleep log and actigraphy can help assess sleep-wake patterns more thoroughly. It is recommended to obtain at least 7 days of data, but preferably 14 days.[52] The primary recommendation for the treatment of advanced sleep-wake phase disorder is the implementation of evening bright light to delay circadian rhythms.[96]

Another CRSWD that is seen in aging women is irregular sleep-wake rhythm disorder. It is especially common in individuals with neurodegenerative disorders. The patient may present with irregular bouts of sleep and wake without a clear sleep-wake schedule. The diagnosis requires a documentation of irregular rest activity pattern.[97] Patients may not be able to provide sleep logs, therefore caregiver documentation or actigraphy may be used. Therapy mostly focuses on using cues to regularize sleep-wake schedule.[97] Melatonin, which is commonly used in children, may cause depression or worsen cognitive impairment in dementia patients. Therefore, it is recommended to increase activity and light exposure during the day, regularize the rest-activity schedule, and maintain regular sleep-wake timing.[97]

CENTRAL DISORDERS OF HYPERSOMNIA EVALUATION

A patient may present with hypersomnia that is not caused by disturbed nocturnal sleep or misaligned circadian rhythm. Some examples of central disorders of hypersomnia include narcolepsy type 1 or 2, idiopathic hypersomnia, Kleine-Levin syndrome, hypersomnia caused by a medical disorder or medication, and insufficient sleep syndrome. There are lacking data of hypersomnia confirmed by diagnostic testing in aging women. However, in an Australian study the prevalence of patient-reported hypersomnia among older women was 13.2% (ages 70–79 years) and 17.0% (ages $\geq$80 years).[98]

Hypersomnias are not generally diagnosed in patients ages 65 and above as they tend to present with symptoms at a younger age. However, if a patient has persisting hypersomnolence, it is important to take into account these disorders. This is especially important in patients who are obtaining recommended hours of sleep, have appropriate sleep hygiene, and do not have a contributing comorbid condition or take a medication that would be a cause of the existing symptoms. To evaluate for a disorder of hypersomnolence, overnight PSG is recommended with next day Multiple Sleep Latency Test. Actigraphy before the PSG/Multiple Sleep Latency Test is recommended to evaluate for sleep-wake cycle disturbance or insufficient sleep. Nonpharmacologic treatment consists of frequent scheduled naps. Medications that are used to treat sleepiness of narcolepsy or idiopathic hypersomnolence include modafinil/armodafinil, traditional stimulants, sodium oxybate, solriamfetol, and pitolisant.[99] However, there are several serious side effects to these medications, such as psychosis or suicidal ideation; cardiac arrythmias; and increases in blood pressure, QT prolongation, or sedation. Therefore, when discussing pharmacologic therapy, it is important to consider comorbid conditions, interactions with other medications, and overall risks of therapy.

SUMMARY

When evaluating an older woman regarding sleep concerns, obtaining a complete sleep history, past medical history, and reviewing medications are great sources of information. Caregiver and family involvement are most likely needed in situations where the individual has underlying dementia or even mild cognitive decline. A focused history may be necessary depending on the level of functioning. Reviewing symptoms and timing of menopause, medications, and comorbid conditions are of great importance when evaluating for sleep disorders in older women. Other contributing factors, such as socioeconomic status and individual independence, play large roles in this population group and play a role in choosing further testing modalities, ability to have close follow-up, and success of treatment.

CLINICS CARE POINTS

- There is an association between a decline in total sleep time and increasing age.
- Average recommended sleep time in older adults is 7 to 8 hours, however, the ability to sleep may decline not only due to ageing but also due to medical/psychiatric illness or circadian changes.
- Some key information to obtain in the sleep history includes unusual nocturnal events, witnessed apneic events, daytime somnolence, sleep-wake schedule, sleep habits, and sleep environment.
- The Epworth Sleepiness Scale can be used to help gauge severity of daytime sleepiness.
- The STOP-BANG questionnaire is a helpful screening tool for obstructive sleep apnea and if there is a moderate or high suspicion, polysomnography testing is recommended.
- First-line treatment of insomnia in older adults is cognitive behavioral therapy-insomnia.
- Women have a higher prevalence of Restless Leg Syndrome and severity increases with age.
- Restless leg syndrome is commonly associated with iron deficiency anemia and if suspected, ferritin and transferrin levels are recommended.
- Although REM sleep behavior disorder is more common in men, it is important to appropriately evaluate older women as this condition can result in injuries.
- A common circadian rhythm sleep-wake disorder in ageing adults is advanced sleep-wake phase disorder and results in early timing of sleep compared to desired sleep time and implementing evening bright light to delay circadian rhythm is the primary recommended treatment.
- Central disorders of hypersomnias typically present at a younger age; however in a patient with persistent hypersomnolence without sleep deprivation, other sleep disorders, or contributing comorbid conditions or medications, it is important to consider this diagnosis.

DISCLOSURE

The authors have nothing to disclose.

REFERENCES

1. Hamidi M, Joseph B. Changing epidemiology of the American population. Clin Geriatr Med 2019;35(1):1–12.
2. Yaremchuk K. Sleep disorders in the elderly. Clin Geriatr Med 2018;34(2):205–16.
3. Foley DJ, Monjan AA, Brown SL, et al. Sleep complaints among elderly persons: an epidemiologic study of three communities. Sleep 1995;18(6):425–32.
4. Cornoni-Huntley J, Ostfeld AM, Taylor JO, et al. Established populations for epidemiologic studies of the elderly: study design and methodology. Aging Milan Italy 1993;5(1):27–37.
5. Quan SF, Katz R, Olson J, et al. Factors associated with incidence and persistence of symptoms of disturbed sleep in an elderly cohort: the Cardiovascular Health Study. Am J Med Sci 2005;329(4):163–72.
6. Ohayon MM, Vecchierini M-F. Normative sleep data, cognitive function and daily living activities in older adults in the community. Sleep 2005;28(8):981–9.
7. Goldman SE, Stone KL, Ancoli-Israel S, et al. Poor sleep is associated with poorer physical performance and greater functional limitations in older women. Sleep 2007;30(10):1317–24.

8. Newman AB, Enright PL, Manolio TA, et al. Sleep disturbance, psychosocial correlates, and cardiovascular disease in 5201 older adults: the Cardiovascular Health Study. J Am Geriatr Soc 1997 Jan;45(1):1–7.

9. Ohayon MM, Carskadon MA, Guilleminault C, et al. Meta-analysis of quantitative sleep parameters from childhood to old age in healthy individuals: developing normative sleep values across the human lifespan. Sleep 2004;27(7):1255–73.

10. Teran-Perez G, Arana-Lechuga Y, Esqueda-Leon E, et al. Steroid hormones and sleep regulation. Mini Rev Med Chem 2012;12(11):1040–8.

11. Gulia KK, Kumar VM. Sleep disorders in the elderly: a growing challenge: sleep in elderly. Psychogeriatrics 2018;18(3):155–65.

12. Rediehs MH, Reis JS, Creason NS. Sleep in old age: focus on gender differences. Sleep 1990;13(5):410–24.

13. Zalai D, Bingeliene A, Shapiro C. Sleepiness in the elderly. Sleep Med Clin 2017; 12(3):429–41.

14. Ancoli-Israel S, Kripke DF, Klauber MR, et al. Sleep-disordered breathing in community-dwelling elderly. Sleep 1991;14(6):486–95.

15. Predictors of sleep-disordered breathing in community-dwelling adults: the Sleep Heart Health Study - PubMed [Internet]. . Available at: https://pubmed.ncbi.nlm.nih.gov/11966340/. Accessed: November 20, 2020.

16. Hoch CC, Reynolds CF, Monk TH, et al. Comparison of sleep-disordered breathing among healthy elderly in the seventh, eighth, and ninth decades of life. Sleep 1990;13(6):502–11.

17. Bixler EO, Vgontzas AN, Ten Have T, et al. Effects of age on sleep apnea in men: I. Prevalence and severity. Am J Respir Crit Care Med 1998;157(1):144–8.

18. Alessi C, Vitiello MV. Insomnia (primary) in older people: non-drug treatments. BMJ Clin Evid 2015;2015.

19. Stone KL, Xiao Q. Impact of poor sleep on physical and mental health in older women. Sleep Med Clin 2018;13(3):457–65.

20. Stenholm S, Kronholm E, Sainio P, et al. Sleep-related factors and mobility in older men and women. J Gerontol A Biol Sci Med Sci 2010;65A(6):649–57.

21. Spira AP, Covinsky K, Rebok GW, et al. Poor sleep quality and functional decline in older women. J Am Geriatr Soc 2012;60(6):1092–8.

22. Spira AP, Covinsky K, Rebok GW, et al. Objectively measured sleep quality and nursing home placement in older women. J Am Geriatr Soc 2012;60(7):1237–43.

23. Carskadon MA, Dement WC. Principles and practice of sleep medicine. In: Chapter 2, normal Human Sleep : an Overview. 5th edition. St. Louis: Elsevier Saunders; 2011. p. 16–26.

24. Fuller PM, Gooley JJ, Saper CB. Neurobiology of the sleep-wake cycle: sleep architecture, circadian regulation, and regulatory feedback. J Biol Rhythms 2006; 21(6):482–93.

25. Landolt HP, Dijk DJ, Achermann P, et al. Effect of age on the sleep EEG: slow-wave activity and spindle frequency activity in young and middle-aged men. Brain Res 1996;738(2):205–12.

26. Carrier J, Land S, Buysse DJ, et al. The effects of age and gender on sleep EEG power spectral density in the middle years of life (ages 20-60 years old). Psychophysiology 2001;38(2):232–42.

27. Gaudreau H, Carrier J, Montplaisir J. Age-related modifications of NREM sleep EEG: from childhood to middle age. J Sleep Res 2001;10(3):165–72.

28. Crowley K, Trinder J, Kim Y, et al. The effects of normal aging on sleep spindle and K-complex production. Clin Neurophysiol 2002;113(10):1615–22.

29. Parrino L, Boselli M, Spaggiari MC, et al. Cyclic alternating pattern (CAP) in normal sleep: polysomnographic parameters in different age groups. Electroencephalogr Clin Neurophysiol 1998;107(6):439–50.
30. Dorffner G, Vitr M, Anderer P. The effects of aging on sleep architecture in healthy subjects. Adv Exp Med Biol 2015;821:93–100.
31. Baker FC, Driver HS. Circadian rhythms, sleep, and the menstrual cycle. Sleep Med 2007;8(6):613–22.
32. Hollander LE, Freeman EW, Sammel MD, et al. Sleep quality, estradiol levels, and behavioral factors in late reproductive age women. Obstet Gynecol 2001;98(3): 391–7.
33. Kravitz HM, Ganz PA, Bromberger J, et al. Sleep difficulty in women at midlife: a community survey of sleep and the menopausal transition. Menopause N Y N 2003;10(1):19–28.
34. Moline ML, Broch L, Zak R. Sleep in women across the life cycle from adulthood through menopause. Med Clin North Am 2004;88(3):705–36.
35. Kravitz HM, Joffe H. Sleep during the perimenopause: a SWAN story. Obstet Gynecol Clin North Am 2011;38(3):567–86.
36. Sowers MF, Zheng H, Kravitz HM, et al. Sex steroid hormone profiles are related to sleep measures from polysomnography and the Pittsburgh Sleep Quality Index. Sleep 2008;31(10):1339–49.
37. Hirshkowitz M, Whiton K, Albert SM, et al. National Sleep Foundation's sleep time duration recommendations: methodology and results summary. Sleep Health 2015;1(1):40–3.
38. Ancoli-Israel S, Alessi C. Sleep and aging. Am J Geriatr Psychiatry Off J Am Assoc Geriatr Psychiatry 2005 May;13(5):341–3.
39. Empana J-P, Dauvilliers Y, Dartigues J-F, et al. Excessive daytime sleepiness is an independent risk indicator for cardiovascular mortality in community-dwelling elderly. Stroke 2009;40(4):1219–24.
40. Heinzer R, Vat S, Marques-Vidal P, et al. Prevalence of sleep-disordered breathing in the general population: the HypnoLaus study. Lancet Respir Med 2015; 3(4):310–8.
41. Senaratna CV, Perret JL, Lodge CJ, et al. Prevalence of obstructive sleep apnea in the general population: a systematic review. Sleep Med Rev 2017;34:70–81.
42. Johns MW. A new method for measuring daytime sleepiness: the Epworth sleepiness scale. Sleep 1991;14(6):540–5.
43. Chung F, Abdullah HR, Liao P. STOP-bang questionnaire: a practical approach to screen for obstructive sleep apnea. CHEST 2016;149(3):631–8.
44. Chung F, Yegneswaran B, Liao P, et al. STOP questionnaire: a tool to screen patients for obstructive sleep apnea. Anesthesiology 2008;108(5):812–21.
45. Bastien C. Validation of the Insomnia Severity Index as an outcome measure for insomnia research. Sleep Med 2001;2(4):297–307.
46. Morin CM, Belleville G, Bélanger L, et al. The insomnia severity index: psychometric indicators to detect insomnia cases and evaluate treatment response. Sleep 2011;34(5):601–8.
47. Hall MH, Kline CE, Nowakowski S. Insomnia and sleep apnea in midlife women: prevalence and consequences to health and functioning. F1000prime Rep [Internet] 2015;7. Available at: https://www.ncbi.nlm.nih.gov/pmc/articles/PMC4447062/. Accessed December 30, 2020.
48. Martin JL, Schweizer CA, Hughes JM, et al. Estimated prevalence of insomnia among women veterans: results of a postal survey. Womens Health Issues 2017;27(3):366–73.

49. Ohayon MM. Epidemiology of insomnia: what we know and what we still need to learn. Sleep Med Rev 2002;6(2):97–111.

50. Crowley K. Sleep and sleep disorders in older adults. Neuropsychol Rev 2011; 21(1):41–53.

51. Foley D, Ancoli-Israel S, Britz P, et al. Sleep disturbances and chronic disease in older adults: results of the 2003 National Sleep Foundation sleep in America survey. J Psychosom Res 2004;56(5):497–502.

52. American Academy of Sleep Medicine. International classification of sleep disorders. 3rd ed. Darien, IL: American Academy of Sleep Medicine; 2014.

53. Misra S, Malow BA. Evaluation of sleep disturbances in older adults. Clin Geriatr Med 2008;24(1):15–26.

54. Tatineny P, Shafi F, Gohar A, et al. Sleep in the elderly. Mol Med 2020;117(5): 490–5.

55. Morgenthaler T, Kramer M, Alessi C, et al. Practice parameters for the psychological and behavioral treatment of insomnia: an update. An American Academy of Sleep Medicine report. Sleep 2006;29(11):1415–9.

56. Morin CM, Colecchi C, Stone J, et al. Behavioral and pharmacological therapies for late-life insomnia: a randomized controlled trial. J Am Med Assoc 1999; 281(11):991.

57. Jacobs GD, Pace-Schott EF, Stickgold R, et al. Cognitive behavior therapy and pharmacotherapy for insomnia: a randomized controlled trial and direct comparison. Arch Intern Med 2004;164(17):1888.

58. Morin CM, Vallières A, Guay B, et al. Cognitive-behavior therapy, singly and combined with medication, for persistent insomnia: acute and maintenance therapeutic effects. J Am Med Assoc 2009;301(19):2005–15.

59. Beaulieu-Bonneau S, Ivers H, Guay B, et al. Long-term maintenance of therapeutic gains associated with cognitive-behavioral therapy for insomnia delivered alone or combined with zolpidem. Sleep 2017;40(3).

60. Morin CM, Bootzin RR, Buysse DJ, et al. Psychological and behavioral treatment of insomnia: update of the recent evidence (1998-2004). Sleep 2006;29(11): 1398–414.

61. McCall WV. Sleep in the elderly: burden, diagnosis, and treatment. Prim Care Companion J Clin Psychiatry 2004;6(1):9–20.

62. Roth T, Seiden D, Sainati S, et al. Effects of ramelteon on patient-reported sleep latency in older adults with chronic insomnia. Sleep Med 2006;7(4):312–8.

63. Afonso RF, Hachul H, Kozasa EH, et al. Yoga decreases insomnia in postmenopausal women: a randomized clinical trial. Menopause N Y N 2012;19(2):186–93.

64. Guthrie KA, Larson JC, Ensrud KE, et al. Effects of pharmacologic and nonpharmacologic interventions on insomnia symptoms and self-reported sleep quality in women with hot flashes: a pooled analysis of individual participant data from four MsFLASH trials. Sleep 2018;41(1).

65. Oliveira DS, Hachul H, Goto V, et al. Effect of therapeutic massage on insomnia and climacteric symptoms in postmenopausal women. Climacteric J Int Menopause Soc 2012;15(1):21–9.

66. McMillan A, Morrell MJ. Sleep disordered breathing at the extremes of age: the elderly. Breathe 2016;12(1):50–60.

67. Block AJ, Wynne JW, Boysen PG. Sleep-disordered breathing and nocturnal oxygen desaturation in postmenopausal women. Am J Med 1980;69(1):75–9.

68. Bixler EO, Vgontzas AN, Lin H-M, et al. Prevalence of sleep-disordered breathing in women: effects of gender. Am J Respir Crit Care Med 2001;163(3 Pt 1):608–13.

69. Gislason T, Benediktsdóttir B, Björnsson JK, et al. Snoring, hypertension, and the sleep apnea syndrome. An epidemiologic survey of middle-aged women. Chest 1993;103(4):1147–51.

70. Kapur VK, Auckley DH, Chowdhuri S, et al. Clinical practice guideline for diagnostic testing for adult obstructive sleep apnea: an American Academy of Sleep Medicine clinical practice guideline. J Clin Sleep Med 2017;13(3):479–504.

71. Patil Susheel P, Ayappa Indu A, Caples Sean M, et al. Treatment of adult obstructive sleep apnea with positive airway pressure: an American Academy of Sleep Medicine clinical practice guideline. J Clin Sleep Med 2019;15(02):335–43.

72. Costantino A, Rinaldi V, Moffa A, et al. Hypoglossal nerve stimulation long-term clinical outcomes: a systematic review and meta-analysis. Sleep Breath 2020; 24(2):399–411.

73. Caples SM, Rowley JA, Prinsell JR, et al. Surgical modifications of the upper airway for obstructive sleep apnea in adults: a systematic review and meta-analysis. Sleep 2010;33(10):1396–407.

74. Aurora RN, Casey KR, Kristo D, et al. Practice parameters for the surgical modifications of the upper airway for obstructive sleep apnea in adults. Sleep 2010; 33(10):1408–13.

75. Donovan LM, Kapur VK. Prevalence and characteristics of central compared to obstructive sleep apnea: analyses from the sleep heart health study cohort. Sleep 2016;39(7):1353–9.

76. Mehra R, Stone KL, Blackwell T, et al. Prevalence and correlates of sleep-disordered breathing in older men: osteoporotic fractures in men sleep study. J Am Geriatr Soc 2007;55(9):1356–64.

77. Javaheri S, Parker TJ, Liming JD, et al. Sleep apnea in 81 ambulatory male patients with stable heart failure. Types and their prevalences, consequences, and presentations. Circulation 1998;97(21):2154–9.

78. Hanly PJ, Pierratos A. Improvement of sleep apnea in patients with chronic renal failure who undergo nocturnal hemodialysis. N Engl J Med 2001;344(2):102–7.

79. Leung RST, Huber MA, Rogge T, et al. Association between atrial fibrillation and central sleep apnea. Sleep 2005;28(12):1543–6.

80. Wang D, Teichtahl H, Drummer O, et al. Central sleep apnea in stable methadone maintenance treatment patients. Chest 2005;128(3):1348–56.

81. Allen RP, Walters AS, Montplaisir J, et al. Restless legs syndrome prevalence and impact: REST general population study. Arch Intern Med 2005;165(11):1286.

82. Garcia-Malo C, Peralta SR, Garcia-Borreguero D. Restless legs syndrome and other common sleep-related movement disorders. Contin Lifelong Learn Neurol 2020;26(4):963–87.

83. Rothdach A, Trenkwalder C, Haberstock J, et al. Prevalence and risk factors of RLS in an elderly population: the MEMO study. Memory and Morbidity in Augsburg Elderly. Neurology 2000;54(5):1064–8.

84. Becker PM. Diagnosis of restless leg syndrome (Willis-Ekbom disease). Sleep Med Clin 2015;10(3):235–40.

85. Allen RP, Picchietti DL, Garcia-Borreguero D, et al. Restless legs syndrome/Willis–Ekbom disease diagnostic criteria: updated International Restless Legs Syndrome Study Group (IRLSSG) consensus criteria – history, rationale, description, and significance. Sleep Med 2014;15(8):860–73.

86. Wijemanne S, Ondo W. Restless legs syndrome: clinical features, diagnosis and a practical approach to management. Pract Neurol 2017;17(6):444–52.

87. Cornelius JR, Tippmann-Peikert M, Slocumb NL, et al. Impulse control disorders with the use of dopaminergic agents in restless legs syndrome: a case-control study. Sleep 2010;33(1):81–7.

88. Singh S, Kaur H, Singh S, et al. Parasomnias: a comprehensive review. Cureus 2018;10(12):e3807.

89. Poryazova R, Oberholzer M, Baumann CR, et al. REM sleep behavior disorder in Parkinson's disease: a questionnaire-based survey. J Clin Sleep Med JCSM Off Publ Am Acad Sleep Med 2013;9(1):55–9.

90. Kang S-H, Yoon I-Y, Lee SD, et al. REM sleep behavior disorder in the Korean elderly population: prevalence and clinical characteristics. Sleep 2013;36(8): 1147–52.

91. Boeve BF. REM sleep behavior disorder: updated review of the core features, the RBD-neurodegenerative disease association, evolving concepts, controversies, and future directions. Ann N Y Acad Sci 2010;1184:15–54.

92. Olson EJ, Boeve BF, Silber MH. Rapid eye movement sleep behaviour disorder: demographic, clinical and laboratory findings in 93 cases. Brain J Neurol 2000; 123(Pt 2):331–9.

93. Howell MJ. Rapid eye movement sleep behavior disorder and other rapid eye movement parasomnias. Contin Lifelong Learn Neurol 2020;26(4):929–45.

94. Kim JH, Duffy JF. Circadian rhythm sleep-wake disorders in older adults. Sleep Med Clin 2018;13(1):39–50.

95. Paine S-J, Fink J, Gander PH, et al. Identifying advanced and delayed sleep phase disorders in the general population: a national survey of New Zealand adults. Chronobiol Int 2014;31(5):627–36.

96. Auger RR, Burgess HJ, Emens JS, et al. Clinical practice guideline for the treatment of intrinsic circadian rhythm sleep-wake disorders: advanced sleep-wake phase disorder (ASWPD), delayed sleep-wake phase disorder (DSWPD), non-24-hour sleep-wake rhythm disorder (N24SWD), and irregular sleep-wake rhythm disorder (ISWRD). An update for 2015. J Clin Sleep Med JCSM Off Publ Am Acad Sleep Med 2015;11(10):1199–236.

97. Abbott SM, Reid KJ, Zee PC. Circadian rhythm sleep-wake disorders. Psychiatr Clin North Am 2015;38(4):805–23.

98. Hayley AC, Williams LJ, Kennedy GA, et al. Prevalence of excessive daytime sleepiness in a sample of the Australian adult population. Sleep Med 2014; 15(3):348–54.

99. Khan Z, Trotti LM. Central disorders of hypersomnolence. Chest 2015;148(1): 262–73.

Bone Health

Ivy Akid, MD[a],*, Danielle J. Doberman, MD, MPH, HMDC[b]

KEYWORDS

- Bone mineral density • Osteoporosis • Fragility fracture
- Dual-energy x-ray absorptiometry

KEY POINTS

- Osteoporosis is highly prevalent among the female geriatric and palliative cohort.
- Historically, osteoporosis has been underdiagnosed and undertreated in women, for whom prevention and treatment is both beneficial and cost-effective.
- Being aware of the downstream effects of osteoporosis will compel the astute physician to diagnose and treat osteoporosis in a timely manner. Complications of osteoporosis include, but are not limited to, hip fractures, vertebral compression fractures, depression from chronic pain, spinal deformities, restrictive lung disease, and decreased global functional status. In addition, some may experience dysphagia and malnutrition from either the impact of their kyphoscoliosis or adverse effects of some forms of osteoporosis treatment itself.
- Options for treatment of osteoporosis include oral and intravenous agents with a wide range of dosing intervals from daily to annually.

---

*CASE: You are a palliative medicine physician at a large tertiary care hospital. You are asked to consult for "feeding options" on a previously independent, cognitively intact, 89-year-old female named Martha with osteoporosis, osteoarthritis and visual impairment from macular degeneration who was admitted with profound weight loss due to dysphagia. She was noted in the Emergency Department to have hypoxia, and a right lower lobe infiltrate was additionally detected. Physical exam demonstrates severe kyphotic curvature of the spine. In the previous few months, she has experienced several falls which have begun limiting her mobility and served as a catalyst for overall functional decline (**Fig. 1**).*

DEFINITIONS
Osteoporosis vs Osteopenia

Osteoporosis is a disorder of the bone characterized by low bone mass, disruption, and weakening of the skeletal structure, which can lead to increased risk of fracture.

---

[a] Department of Medicine, Division of General Internal Medicine, Section of Palliative Medicine, JHUSOM, Johns Hopkins Hospital, 600 North Wolfe Street Blalock 371, Baltimore, MD 21287, USA; [b] Department of Medicine, Division of General Internal Medicine, Section of Palliative Medicine, Palliative Medicine Program, JHUSOM, Johns Hopkins Hospital, 600 North Wolfe Street Blalock 371, Baltimore, MD 21287, USA
* Corresponding author.
E-mail address: iakid1@jh.edu

Clin Geriatr Med 37 (2021) 683–696
https://doi.org/10.1016/j.cger.2021.05.012
0749-0690/21/© 2021 Elsevier Inc. All rights reserved.

geriatric.theclinics.com

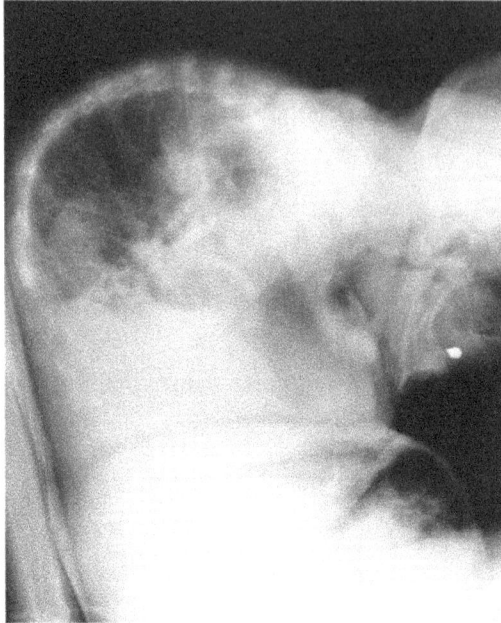

Fig. 1. Chest film; lateral view. (*From* [New England Journal of Medicine, Blechacz, Severe Kyphosis, 358;24. Copyright © (2008) Massachusetts Medical Society. Reprinted with permission.])

It can be defined by the presence of a fragility fracture: fracture following a fall from standing height. In the absence of a fragility fracture, osteoporosis is diagnosed when an individual's bone mineral density on dual-energy x-ray absorptiometry (DEXA) scan is less than or equal to 2.5 standard deviations less than that of an adult female reference population, typically cited as aged 30 to 40 years.[1] This is often referred to a T-score of −2.5, and because bone mineral density decreases the older a person is, a greater proportion of people become osteoporotic as they age. Bone mineral density assessment by DEXA scan is considered the gold standard for diagnosis of osteoporosis and is also used to define osteopenia or a less severe form of low bone mass characterized by some degree of skeletal structural impairment with T scores ranging from −1.0 to −2.5.[1]

EPIDEMIOLOGY

Worldwide it was estimated that 9 million new osteoporotic fractures occurred in the year 2000, with 1.6 million hip fractures and 1.4 million vertebral fractures.[2] In western countries the risk a women will have an osteoporotic fracture during her lifetime is 40% to 50%, whereas men have a risk between 13% and 22%.[2] The United States alone averages more than 2 million new fractures a year, which are attributed to osteoporosis, with 550,000 vertebral and 300,000 hip fractures among those.[2] In elderly patients, a fracture is often followed by the sequelae of hospitalization, impaired quality of life, need for long-term care, disability, and even death,[2] which helps illustrate why osteoporosis and osteoporotic fractures are significant public health problems in the United States and worldwide.[2]

By 2020, approximately 12.3 million individuals in the United States older than 50 years are expected to have osteoporosis.[3] Osteoporotic fractures, particularly hip fractures, are associated with limitations in ambulation, chronic pain and disability, loss of independence, and decreased quality of life, and 21% to 30% of patients who experience a hip fracture die within 1 year.[3] Virtually all hip fractures may be attributed to either primary or secondary osteoporosis, with falls as the primary event leading to fracture.[4] Annually, hip fracture cases occur approximately 0.3 million in the United States and 1.7 million in Europe.[4] The female-to-male ratio attributed to hip fractures is 2:1.[4] By 2050, the number of hip fractures worldwide is expected to increase to 6 million due to the increase in aging population.[5] Furthermore, according to the World Health Organization the cost burden of hip fractures weighs heavily on the health care system due to increased hospitalizations and permanently disabling half of the patients who have hip fracture.[5]

The risk factors for osteoporosis include age, sex, race, low estrogen levels, low body mass index, smoking, excess alcohol intake, low calcium intake, and an array of medications. With age, bone mineral density decreases, and the skeletal structure weakens becoming more porous.[2] Thus, the rate of osteoporotic fractures, including hip and vertebral fractures, increases with age.[2]

Along with age, 2 other important risk factors influencing the incidence of osteoporotic fractures are ethnicity and race.[6] An article in 2009 showed a decline in the number of white women with hip fractures; however, other studies have showed an increase in the number of hip fractures in Hispanic women.[6] Data in 2005 showed that only 12% of all fractures occurred in nonwhites, and predictive models suggest that this number will increase to 21% by 2025.[6] The frequency of hip fractures varies greatly based on race and ethnicity. In the United States, in people older than 50 years, the lifetime risk of hip fracture is 15.8% in women and 6.0% in men, whereas in China these numbers are 2.4% for women and 1.9% in men. The lifetime risk of hip fracture for Hispanic women is 8.5%, whereas it is 3.8% in Hispanic men. Rates of hip fractures are highest in northern Europe.[6] Unlike hip fractures, vertebral fractures show much less variability based on ethnic or racial factors.[6] The prevalence of vertebral fractures in women older than 65 years is 70% for white women, 68% for Japanese, 55% for Mexican, and 50% for African American women.[6] Depending on your ethnicity, one of the biggest factors in developing osteoporotic fractures is sex, for example, white women generally experience twice as many hip fractures as white men; however, the sex difference in hip fracture risk is negligible between men and women of African American and Asian descent.[6] Annual hip fracture rates in the United States are highest in white women (140.7 per 100,000) compared with Asian women (85.4 per 100,000) versus African American women (57.3 per 100,000) and Hispanic women (49.7 per 100,000).[6] Despite the lower relative risk of fractures in minority women compared with white women, the absolute risk of fractures is still quite substantial, and fractures are more common than the combined number of myocardial infarctions, coronary heart disease deaths, and breast cancer in minority women.[6] Despite the high lifetime prevalence across all women, disparities in treatment unfortunately do exist. Historically, osteoporosis is underdiagnosed and undertreated, especially in patients older than 75 years, for whom treatment is both most beneficial and most cost-effective.[7] In addition, Blacks have the lowest treatment rates among all racial/ethnic groups.[8]

RISK FACTORS

As women age, their risk for osteoporosis increases over time, especially after menopause, due to decreasing estrogen levels.[9] Estrogen influences bone metabolism and remodeling.[9] (See pathogenesis section below for further details.) Just as osteoporosis risk increases with the reduction in circulating estrogens at menopause, another important risk factor for osteoporotic fracture is the therapeutic reduction in serum endogenous estrogen levels secondary to breast cancer treatment.[9] Invasive breast cancer is one of the most common cancer types in women.[10] Antihormone therapy that blocks the aromatase enzyme is a very common treatment of breast cancer and leads to a decrease in circulating serum estrogens. Although this decrease in estrogen improves disease-free survival following breast cancer, it also leads to increased bone turnover, bone loss, and increased fracture risk in patients.[9]

Antiestrogen medications, such as the aromatase inhibitors anastrozole and letrozole, are known for causing osteoporosis.[9] Similarly, therapies used to treat breast cancer often accelerate bone loss due to the mechanism of action of the chemotherapy, which can affect bone loss by disrupting ovarian function and causing premature menopause.[11] In addition, endocrine therapies such as androgen and estrogen deprivation therapy in cancer treatment decreases bone formation, as deficiency in hormone levels regulate bone resorption and radiation can directly affect bone turnover.[9] Survivors of breast cancer have a 15% increased risk of fractures compared with cancer-free women.[9] Interestingly, data have shown that postmenopausal women have decreased hip fracture rates as well as decreased overall fracture rates with use of tamoxifen, a selective estrogen receptor modulator,[9] and this highlights the large role that hormones, and estrogen, play in bone health.

Frailty is another risk factor that has been linked to poor bone health and osteoporotic fractures.[12] Frailty has been defined as a clinical condition that results from aging-related changes and degeneration in patients' psychological, physical, and social functioning, thus leading to increased vulnerability to illness (refer to chapters 5 and 11 for additional information on frailty).[2] As people age, frailty plays a larger role in health status, including what is believed to be those factors contributing to illness resiliency or precipitous declines in vitality leading to death.[12] Importantly, studies suggest an association between osteoporosis and frailty.[12] Worldwide, frailty has been increasing in aged patients, and a prevalence of 10.7% has been noted in community-dwelling elders aged greater than 65 years, and in those older than 85 years, it is estimated that 25% to 50% are frail.[2] Fundamentally, it is understood the more frail a person is, the more likely they are to fall and have an osteoporotic fracture and the higher their risk is of having a fracture in the future,[2] and therefore, the increase in frailty is concerning for a possible increase in osteoporosis-related morbidity and mortality, if prevention efforts are not undertaken.

PREVENTION/SCREENING

The United States Preventive Services Task Force (USPSTF) recommends baseline screening for osteoporosis in all women age 65 years and older with bone mineral density (BMD) testing to prevent osteoporotic fractures.[3] The USPSTF also recommends screening for osteoporosis with BMD testing in postmenopausal women younger than 65 years with risk factors that place them at increased risk of osteoporosis, as determined by a formal clinical risk assessment tool.[3] These are both grade B recommendations by the USPSTF suggesting there is high certainty that the net benefit is moderate, or there is moderate certainty that the net benefit is moderate to substantial.[3] Risk factors for osteoporotic fractures include history of hip fracture in a parent, smoking status, excessive alcohol intake, and low body mass. In addition, menopausal status, specifically being postmenopausal, or other low estrogen states are also key considerations. For postmenopausal women younger than 65 years who have at least one risk factor; the USPSTF suggests determining who should be screened with bone measurement testing by using a clinical risk assessment tool.[3] Several tools are available to assess osteoporosis risk, such as the OST (Osteoporosis Self-assessment Tool), ORAI (Osteoporosis Risk Assessment Instrument), OSIRIS (Osteoporosis Index of Risk), SCORE (Simple Calculated Osteoporosis Risk Estimation Tool), or the FRAX (Fracture Risk Assessment Tool).[3]

In addition to those risks factors outlined earlier, certain medications are known to increase risk for osteoporosis, chiefly glucocorticoids, excess thyroid replacement, androgen deprivation therapy in men, antihormone therapy in women, long-term use of proton pump inhibitors (PPIs), and antiepileptic agents.[13,14] It is further recommended that all postmenopausal women who begin treatment with aromatase inhibitors undergo a detailed baseline evaluation for osteoporosis assessing their risk of fracture; premenopausal women with early breast cancer are also recommended to undergo fracture risk evaluation.[15]

PATHOGENESIS

The pathogenesis for the regulation of bone formation and resorption is complex with multiple mechanisms regulated by several factors, including osteoblasts, osteoclasts, other marrow cell lines, hormones such as estrogen, cytokines of interleukins and prostaglandins, growth factors, and other functional proteins.[16]

Estrogen regulates bone turnover, playing a critical role during puberty for bone formation through anabolic and anticatabolic mechanisms. Studies in mice models indicate distinct estrogen receptors lie in marrow cells and that deficiency creates higher bone resorption.[16] Another risk factor for osteoporosis is calcium deficiency, which is common in the elderly, either due to poor nutritional intake, impaired intestinal absorption, or both.[16] PPIs interrupt calcium absorption and are believed to affect bone density via this mechanism.[14] Secondary hyperparathyroidism and vitamin D deficiency from calcium deficiency can lead to neuromuscular impairment and subsequent increased risk for falls, as well as accelerate fragility and bone loss.[16]

> CASE: Over 5 years ago, Martha was seen by her primary care provider (PCP) and had a FRAX analysis done. She was found to have a 10-year hip fracture probability of 2.3%. Her PCP also went through a thorough medication reconciliation before prescribing medications to help treat her osteoporosis. Despite this, at her last physical, she was noted to have lost four pounds of weight and a half inch of height from the previous year and was otherwise asymptomatic with slight dyspepsia. Martha's kyphosis is likely caused by her underlying osteoporosis. With each of her falls, she is at risk of a fracture: vertebral, hip, or other bone. Following her third fall in a month, she was brought into the emergency department for severe back pain which travels like a band around her neck and back. Imaging indicated that she had a compression fracture in her cervical spine at C8.

SIGNS AND SYMPTOMS

Osteoporosis itself is asymptomatic. However, the consequences and impact of osteoporosis on the body can be quite significant. For example, individuals with vertebral compression fractures may not only lose height but some may also experience chronic pain or reduced mobility. It is therefore important to be mindful of prompt diagnosis of osteoporosis, as the downstream effects carry significant morbidity and mortality.

DOWNSTREAM EFFECTS OF OSTEOPOROSIS
Fractures: a Tumultuous Pattern

Regardless of the bone fractured, once an osteoporotic fracture occurs, a sequence of hospitalization, an impaired quality of life with increased prefracture pain and depression, possible disability with increased dependence on others for daily care or the need for long-term care facility placement, and eventual death often follows.[2] Hip fractures are the complication with the highest morbidity and mortality, and estimates indicate that 50% of women older than 50 years and 20% of men will experience an osteoporosis-related hip fracture. Of all osteoporosis-related fractures, a hip fracture is the most devastating due to the disability it causes, the eventual mortality, and the costs, both to the individual and to society for recovery and support from the time of the fracture onwards.[7] For example, in the United States an estimated annual hospitalization cost of $9.2 billion are from hip fracture admissions alone.[17] Vertebral compression fractures may have similar implications, with the injury leading to pain and immobility. Population estimates suggest a doubling of the number of people with osteoporosis in the next 20 years, which could lead to an exponential increase in the expected number of fractures and thus, an increased burden on health care systems.[7]

Kyphosis/Restrictive Lung Diseases

The weight-bearing part of the vertebral spine resides within the vertebral body. With osteoporotic disease, the bone becomes increasingly porous and unstable, creating accentuation of the spine and bone deformity. When this happens within the thoracic cavity, this is known as hyperkyphosis (**Fig. 2**). In addition, chest wall compliance decreases with age, leading to decline in forced vital capacity and in turn restrictive lung disease, which is further worsened if kyphosis is present.[18] The degree of kyphosis correlates with the degree of decline in vital capacity. In a prospective study of several hundred individuals aged 50 to 79 years, observed for more than 16 years, baseline kyphosis severity was associated with a greater decline in forced expiratory volume in the first second.[19]

CASE: Our patient now suffers with hypoxic respiratory failure for which she was now hospitalized for the third time in the past 12 months. Her multiple hospitalizations have indebted her to decreased global functional status resulting in physical and emotional isolation. Standardized screening tools, such as PHQ-9, used to assess psychological health may be helpful. This can be part of a full geriatric assessment as a guide and framework for understanding geriatric patients with complex disease. Does the patient have a well-structured support network? It is important to understand the patient's psychosocial element, a key component of the geriatric scaffold in order to ensure appropriate disposition level of care.

DYSPHAGIA/MALNUTRITION

The mainstay of long-term therapy for osteoporosis remains bisphosphonate therapy. Although this is a very effective and safe class of drugs, they do have some important side effects, chiefly a risk for gastrointestinal (GI) discomfort and more significantly osteonecrosis of the jaw. Both adverse effects may affect oral intake chronically. GI side effects include, but are not limited to, gastroesophageal reflux disease (GERD),

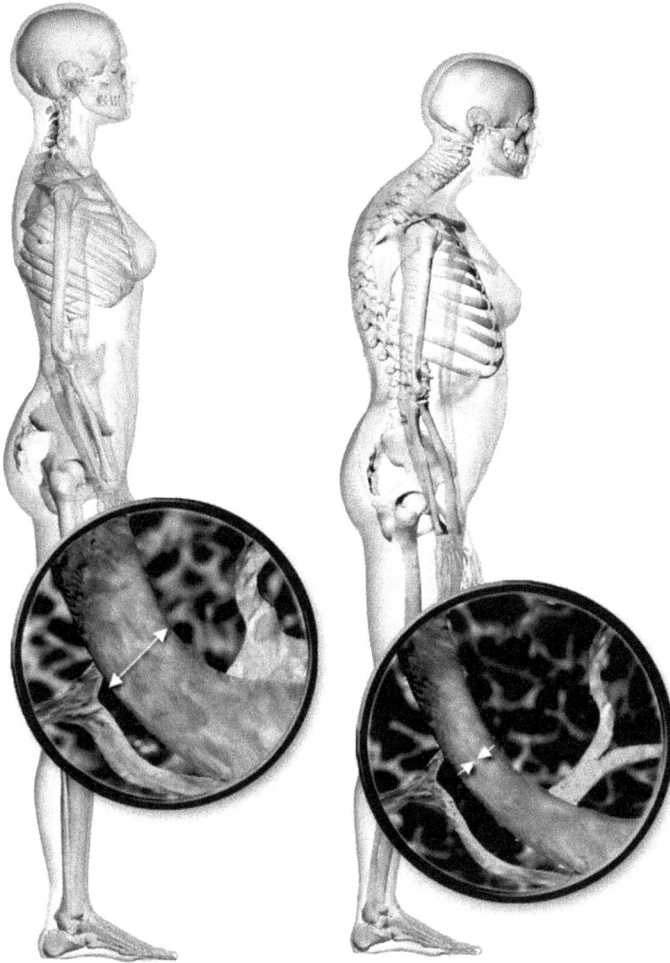

Fig. 2. (*Left*) Normal; (*right*) kyphosis. (*From* Blausen.com staff (2014). "Medical gallery of Blausen Medical 2014". WikiJournal of Medicine 1 (2). https://doi.org/10.15347/wjm/2014. 010. ISSN 2002-4436. CC BY 3.0.)

esophagitis, esophageal and stomach ulcers, and risk for esophageal cancer if chronic GERD and esophagitis are not treated.[20] The more common GI side effects of GERD and esophagitis can predispose elderly patients to dysphagia, as well as increase risk of dehydration, electrolyte imbalance, and malnourishment. Hence, it is vital to identify any gastroesophageal symptoms in patients with osteoporosis early in the illness in order to prevent dysphagia. Some preventive measures include avoiding alcohol, tobacco, and other products known to worsen GERD; modifying diet to reduce acid; and remaining upright or elevating the head of bed and avoiding lying flat after intake of a bisphosphonate, which needs to be taken on an empty stomach 30 minutes before any other food or medications. There may be a role for acid suppressive agents recommended by a physician.[21] In addition, dysphagia may occur in those with severe kyphosis from direct mechanical obstruction of the esophagus due to severe spinal deformity.[22,23]

PREVENTION—MODIFIABLE VERSUS NONMODIFIABLE

Fracture risk assessment tools have been created to derive a 10-year predicted fracture probability for patients.[7] Two such tools, the QFracture and FRAX, were endorsed for use in the United Kingdom.[24] The FRAX, a 10-year fracture probability model, is the most used tool globally.[25] It accounts for mortality and is useful at a population level, but it has notable limitations on an individual level because it often underestimates the short-term risk of fracture due to the high risk of death within 10 years without a fracture, causing the fracture probability to be lower than the fracture risk in older patients (risk assumes that the patients will survive to 10 years).[7]

Many fragility fractures occur in the vertebra or following a fall, as a result an assessment of fall risks is critical, and leading osteoporosis societies are promoting the benefit of fall prevention.[7] Performing a medication review to assess agents that pose a risk to bone health and increase risk of falls versus agents that promote bone strength is key during examinations of those who are at higher risk of fracture.[7] PPIs increase the risk of fracture by decreasing the acid-dependent absorption of calcium carbonate. PPIs decrease the acidity in the stomach and thus decrease the absorption of calcium, which leads to an increased fracture risk.[26] Anticonvulsants impair vitamin D absorption and vitamin D deficiency leads to increased fractures.[7] Similarly, antiandrogens in men and antiestrogens in women are known to have a significant adverse impact on bone density and increase the risk of fractures.[7] Many chemotherapy treatment regimens significantly negatively affect bone density, which increases the risk of fractures.[7] Antiserotonergic antidepressants have been suggested to negatively affect bone density, but this has not been proved.[26] If osteoporosis or high fracture risk is detected in a younger adult, they should be evaluated for multiple myeloma, and similarly those with anemia should be worked up for multiple myeloma.[7] All patients with increased risk of fracture need to be encouraged for smoking cessation and limited alcohol intake, which further reduce BMD.[7]

Weight-bearing exercises are beneficial for fracture prevention and falls and may even improve bone density.[7] Supplementation with calcium and vitamin D have been shown to reduce the risk of fracture. Some controversy surrounds the use of calcium supplementation in those with adequate dietary intake of calcium, and expert societies recommend estimating dietary intake of calcium through asking the patient about their intake of oily fish and dairy products or through the use of online dietary calcium calculators.[7] Although adequate calcium consumption can limit the amount of calcium supplementation needed, vitamin D intake from sun exposure and diet is rarely adequate, and supplementation is therefore almost always necessary, especially in the older adult.[7] To determine if vitamin D intake is adequate, measurement of serum levels of cholecalciferol is recommended.[7]

TREATMENT

Bisphosphonates, such as alendronate, are the mainstay of osteoporosis treatment. Other treatment alternatives are listed in **Table 1**, with each class of medication reducing vertebral and/or nonvertebral fractures, including hip fractures.[7] For patients with renal impairment, the only approved agent is denosumab.[7] Unfortunately, denosumab has a small increased risk of infections, including case reports of endocarditis, which should be monitored closely.[7] It is uncertain what the optimum duration for treatment with bone-sparing medications is; however, bisphosphonates have been found capable of maintaining bone density for at least 2 years after treatment withdrawal based on markers of bone turnover, fracture rates, and BMD.[27] Unfortunately, the bone-maintaining effects of other medications seem to wear off soon after the

Table 1
Pharmacotherapy options for osteoporosis

Medication Class	Dosing Route and Frequency	Reduces Fracture Risk in	Potential Adverse Effects
Bisphosphonates • Alendronate • Ibandronate • Risedronate • Zoledronate	As a class, can be oral or intravenous and dosed daily, weekly, monthly or, annually	Hip, nonvertebra and vertebra	Oropharyngeal reflux, musculoskeletal complaints, flulike symptoms, osteonecrosis of jaw, atypical femur fractures
Selective estrogen receptor modulators • Raloxifene	Oral, daily	Vertebra	Leg cramps, hot flashes (vasomotor symptoms), deep venous thrombosis
Parathyroid hormone peptides • Teriparatide	Subcutaneous, daily	Nonvertebra and vertebra	Nausea, headache, arthralgia, hypercalcemia, hypotension
Calcitonin	Intranasal spray or subcutaneous injection	Vertebra	Rhinitis, epistaxis, allergy
Rank L inhibitor • Denosumab	Subcutaneous every 6 mo	Hip, nonvertebra and vertebra	Eczema, nausea, osteonecrosis of jaw, atypical femur fractures
Sclerostin inhibitor/ monoclonal antibody • Romosozumab	Subcutaneous, monthly	Nonvertebra, vertebra	Headache, risk for MI
Hormone replacement therapy • Estrogen	Oral, daily	For osteoporosis prevention only	Increased thromboembolic risk, risk for MI/stroke, breast cancer

Data from "Correction: In the Clinic—Osteoporosis." Annals of Internal Medicine, vol. 167, no. 7, 2017, p. 528., https://doi.org/10.7326/l17-0539.; and Kerschan-Schindl, K. (2020, April). Romosozumab: A novel bone anabolic treatment option for osteoporosis? Retrieved January 02, 2021.

medications are discontinued, such as raloxifene and denosumab.[7] A key complication of bisphosphonate therapy is osteonecrosis of the jaw and atypical femoral fractures.[7] Although these complications are rare, it has been found that a treatment "holiday" (temporarily stopping the drug) can avoid these complications, with a "holiday" typically scheduled after 3 years of treatment with parenteral zoledronate or after 5 years of treatment with oral bisphosphonates.[27]

Patients with a history of vertebral fractures, high risk of fractures, osteoporotic BMD, or any new fractures should be continued on treatment with either the same or an alternative therapy.[7] Many older patients fall into these groups, and it has been shown that the benefits of ongoing therapy outweigh the small risks of the rare complications such as atypical femoral fractures or osteonecrosis of the jaw.[7] If patients are already receiving treatment, have adequate adherence and have had vitamin D and calcium repletion, and a new fragility fracture still occurs, a BMD reassessment should take place, regardless of if treatment has been occurring for 3 to 5 years or less.[7] These patients should have a fall risk assessment, and alternative therapies should be considered if BMD has failed to improve and a fracture has occurred despite therapy.[7] Some patients may also benefit from monitoring markers of bone turnover such as N-telopeptide or serum carboxy-terminal collagen cross-links, and these markers should also be monitored over any treatment holidays, to guarantee that bone turnover is suppressed in these at-risk patients.[7]

> CASE: Unfortunately, about a week after discharge, while at skilled rehab and trying to get to the bathroom unassisted at night, Martha fell again and was found to have a hip fracture. DEXA scan showed a T-Score of 3.5. She was a poor surgical candidate, and thus a non-surgical treatment modality was chosen. On follow up appointment she was found to have extreme pain in her lower back and, upon repeat examination was noted to have a vertebral compression fracture which was noted to be refractory to oral pain control. Kyphoplasty was performed due to her severity of pain and provided optimal relief.

Fragility fractures are defined as fractures sustained when a person falls from a standing height or less without the significant force of a trauma, such as a car accident. Our skeletons should withstand such a fall without developing a fracture, unless there is an underlying reason the bones are weak and fragile, such as from osteoporosis. Hip fractures acquired via tripping or other such falls are classified as fragility fractures and are considered a manifestation of osteoporosis requiring empirical treatment. Therefore, further evaluation and management of osteoporosis is suggested for those with hip fractures regardless of the mechanism of the fall. DEXA scan may be used to establish baseline bone density or to monitor prognosis of treatment and less as a diagnostic tool.

The primary goal of surgical management is to restore function and optimize pain control, and therefore, surgery may not be the treatment of choice for all fractures.[28] Determination of hip fracture and preinjury ambulatory status can help determine the best treatment options, including method of surgical repair if surgery is a possibility. Different surgical options including arthroplasty (total vs hemi) and open reduction and internal fixation remain dependent on type and location of fracture.[29] Fracture types are described as displaced versus nondisplaced, and anatomic locations of the break are defined as intracapsular—femoral head and neck—versus extracapsular—intertrochanteric and subtrochanteric. Nonsurgical and conservative management is reserved for patients who report mild pain, remain bedridden with advanced dementia, have nondisplaced trochanteric fractures, shortened life expectancy, or patients deemed high mortality risk and thereby too unstable for surgery.[30]

The pain from vertebral compression fractures can be managed conservatively with opioid and nonopioid pain management or via the interventional procedures, vertebroplasty and kyphoplasty. These procedures are considered primarily in circumstances when pain control has been refractory to oral analgesia. In addition to management of refractory pain in vertebral compression fractures, they are also recommended for reversal of spinal deformity and height loss and improved function under Britain's National Institute for Health and Care Excellence guidelines.[30] They can be used for pathologic fractures as well. In kyphoplasty, a balloon is inflated within the vertebral body to reshape its deformity and create potential space before allowing bone cement in that space, thereby stabilizing the structure and restoring spinal height. On the other hand, vertebroplasty is considered less invasive, using a smaller gauge needle and with no balloon used but similarly injecting bone cement or a polymerizing agent to offer similar outcomes. In a randomized controlled trial of 300 patients, averaging over 2 years, improved outcomes were seen in the kyphoplasty group versus nonsurgical, standard care group with greater improvement in back pain remaining statistically significant at all time points.[31]

For Martha, we may have engaged her about goals of care in the clinic or on admission to the hospital. Effective communication about the challenges and burdens of osteoporosis and fracture risks is vital. An open and candid conversation about disease awareness and prognosis, eliciting perception of disease and establishing goals is the way to provide appropriate and excellent care to our patients. Unfortunately, our patient's cluster of symptoms and multiple hospitalizations reflect multimorbidity impacting her life expectancy. Ensuring proper social support and network to stabilize remaining in the community and prevent unnecessary hospital admissions which may be burdensome to the patient is crucial.

SURVEILLANCE AND MANAGEMENT

Based on the International Society for Clinical Densitometry guidelines, a follow-up DEXA of hip and spine after 2 years of initiating therapy for osteoporosis is recommended, with less frequent monitoring thereafter. There is no consensus on the optimal frequency of monitoring.[32] In addition, bone turn-over markers such as fasting urinary N-telopeptide or serum carboxy-terminal collagen crosslinks are not recommended for measurement, except for special circumstances where malabsorption of antiresorptive medications may be an issue.[32]

Furthermore, fall prevention in the older adult population is critical to health safety in women with or without osteoporosis. In addition, it is vital to focus on fall prevention for those at risk of osteoporosis including with the utilization of complete geriatric assessment, home safety evaluation, hip protectors, education on regular exercise, and healthy diet.

FUTURE LITERATURE

It is widely known that genetic makeup may affect manifestations of disease, such as osteoporosis. Thus, further research is underway to understand the relationship between gene and bone-forming cells, in the hopes for engineering targeted and effective therapy.[33–40]

CLINICS CARE POINTS

- Osteoporosis is weakening/thinning of bone and is defined by a fracture that occurred following a fall from standing height (fragility fracture); without a fragility fracture a DEXA scan is used to diagnose osteoporosis (T score of -2.5 or less) or osteopenia (T score of -1.0 to -2.5)

- Female gender is a large risk factor for developing osteoporosis; across ethnic and racial groups, more women experience (osteoporotic) fractures than the combined number of women who experience breast cancer, myocardial infarction, and coronary death in 1 year.

- Historically, osteoporosis is underdiagnosed and undertreated, especially in patients older than 75 years, for whom treatment is both most beneficial and most cost-effective.

- Frailty has been defined as a clinical condition that results from aging-related changes and degeneration in patients' psychological, physical, and social functioning, thus leading to increased vulnerability. As people age, frailty begins to play a larger role in their health.

Frailty has been studied in efforts to understand the factors contributing to a rapid decline in health status that ultimately led toward death. Importantly, studies suggest an association between osteoporosis and frailty.

- Fundamentally, it is understood the frailer a person is, the more likely they are to fall and have an osteoporotic fracture and the higher their risk is of having a fracture in the future.

- Many fragility fractures occur in the vertebra or following a fall; as a result an assessment of fall risks is critical, and leading osteoporosis societies are promoting the benefit of fall prevention.

- Just as the risk for osteoporosis increases at menopause with the reduction in circulating estrogens, another important risk factor for osteoporotic fracture is the therapeutic reduction in serum endogenous estrogen levels secondary to breast cancer treatment.

- Bisphosphonates, such as alendronate, are the mainstay of osteoporosis treatment. Other treatment alternatives include denosumab, selective estrogen receptor modulators, and parathyroid hormone peptides. Each of these medications reduces vertebral fracture risk and some even reduce the risk of nonvertebral fractures and hip fractures.

- For patients with renal impairment, the only approved agent is denosumab. Unfortunately, denosumab has a small increased risk of infections, including case reports of endocarditis, which should be monitored closely.

- It is uncertain what the optimum duration for treatment with bone-sparing medications is; however, bisphosphonates have been found capable of maintaining bone density for at least 2 years after treatment withdrawal based on markers of bone turnover, fracture rates, and BMD.

- Hip fractures are generally classified as fragility fractures and are deemed to be a manifestation of osteoporosis.

- Further diagnosis and treatment of osteoporosis is suggested for patients with hip fracture regardless of the mechanism of the fall.

- The mainstay of long-term therapy for osteoporosis remains as bisphosphonate therapy. Thus, it is imperative to be aware of bisphosphonates' several adverse effects profile, including osteonecrosis of the jaw, atypical bone fractures, atrial fibrillation, and more commonly, a milieu of GI sideeffects including, but not limited to, esophagitis, GERD, ulcers, and long-term esophageal cancer.

DISCLOSURE

The authors have nothing to disclose with no potential conflicts of interest.

REFERENCES

1. Silva BC, Leslie WD, Resch H, et al. Trabecular bone score: a noninvasive analytical method based upon the DXA image. J Bone Miner Res 2014;29(3):518–30.

2. Li G, et al. An overview of osteoporosis and frailty in the elderly. BMC Musculoskelet Disord 2017;18(1). https://doi.org/10.1186/s12891-017-1403-x.

3. US Preventive Services Task Force. Screening for osteoporosis to prevent fractures: US preventive services task force recommendation statement. J Am Med Assoc 2018;319(24):2521–31.

4. Rosen CJ. Pathogenesis of osteoporosis. Best Pract Res Clin Endocrinol Metab 2000;14(2):181–93.

5. Musculoskeletal conditions affect millions. (n.d.).. Available at: https://www.who.int/news/item/27-10-2003-musculoskeletal-conditions-affect-millions. Accessed: January 1, 2021.

6. Cauley JA. Defining ethnic and racial differences in osteoporosis and fragility fractures. Clin Orthopaedics Relat Res 2011;469(7):1891–9.

7. Coughlan T, Dockery F. Osteoporosis and fracture risk in older people. Clin Med 2014;14(2):187–91.

8. Staff, Science X. "Study reveals disparities in osteoporosis treatment by sex and race/ethnicity." Medical Xpress - Medical Research Advances and Health News, Medical Xpress, Available at: medicalxpress.com/news/2019-03-reveals-disparities-osteoporosis-treatment-sex.html, Accessed March 6, 2019

9. Hadji P. Cancer treatment-Induced bone loss in women with breast cancer. Bone-KEy Rep 2015;4. https://doi.org/10.1038/bonekey.2015.60.

10. Akram M, et al. Awareness and current knowledge of breast cancer. Biological research. Biomed Cent 2017.

11. "Bone health and osteoporosis." breast cancer now, Accessed May 10, 2019,Available at: breastcancernow.org/information-support/facing-breast-cancer/going-through-treatment-breast-cancer/side-effects/bone-health-osteoporosis.

12. Bartosch P, et al. "Progression of frailty and prevalence of osteoporosis in a community cohort of older women—a 10-year longitudinal study. Osteoporos Int 2018;29(10):2191–9.

13. Sanguineti A. Osteoporosis: good bone gone bad. Elder Care 2018. Available at: https://pogoe.org/productid/21780.

14. KY;, T. (n.d.). Proton pump inhibitors and fracture risk: a review of Current Evidence and mechanisms Involved. Available at: https://pubmed.ncbi.nlm.nih.gov/31060319/. Accessed January 01, 2021.

15. Trémollieres FA, et al. "Osteoporosis management in patients with breast cancer: EMAS position statement." Maturitas, Elsevier. Available at: www.sciencedirect.com/science/article/pii/S0378512216302572. Accessed October 6, 2016.

16. Raisz L. Pathogenesis of osteoporosis: concepts, conflicts, and prospects. 2005. Available at: https://www.ncbi.nlm.nih.gov/pmc/articles/PMC1297264/. Accessed January 01, 2021.

17. Lott A, et al. Admitting service affects cost and length of stay of hip fracture patients. Geriatr Orthopaedic Surg Rehabil 2018. SAGE Publications.

18. Bari MD, et al. Thoracic kyphosis and ventilatory dysfunction in unselected older persons: an epidemiological study in Dicomano, Italy. J Am Geriatr Soc 2004; 52(6):909–15.

19. Lorbergs AL, et al. Severity of kyphosis and decline in lung function: the Framingham study. J Gerontol Ser A 2016. https://doi.org/10.1093/gerona/glw124.

20. M;Salari P;Abdollahi. "Long term bisphosphonate use in osteoporotic patients; a step forward, two steps back. J Pharm Pharmaceutical Sci : a Publication of the Canadian Society for Pharmaceutical Sciences, Societe Canadienne Des Sciences Pharmaceutiques, U.S. National Library of Medicine.

21. Momentum. "Osteoporosis, the voice and swallowing disorders: what women should know." Baylor college of medicine blog network. Available at: bcm.edu/2016/06/07/osteoporosis-the-voice-and-swallowing-disorders-what-women-should-know/. Accessed October 7, 2016.

22. Blechacz B, Gajic O. Severe kyphosis. N Engl J Med 2008;358(24):e28.

23. Goyal N, et al. Kyphosis, a rare cause of dysphagia. Age Ageing 2005;34(5): 521–2.

24. Rabar S, Lau R, O'Flynn N, et al. Risk assessment of fragility fractures: summary of NICE guidance. BMJ 2012;345:e3698.

25. Kanis JA, Oden A, Johnell O, et al. The use of clinical risk factors enhances the performance of BMD in the prediction of hip and osteoporotic fractures in men and women. Osteoporos Int 2007;18:1033–46.

26. Gates BJ, Sonnett TE, Duvall CA, et al. Review of osteoporosis pharmacotherapy for geriatric patients. Am J Geriatr Pharmacother 2009;7:293–323.

27. Compston J, Bowring C, Cooper A, et al. Diagnosis and management of osteoporosis in postmenopausal women and older men in the UK: National Osteoporosis Guideline Group (NOGG) update 2013. Maturitas 2013;75:392–6.

28. Mears SC. Classification and surgical approaches to hip fractures for nonsurgeons. Clin Geriatr Med 2014;30(2):229–41.

29. Freitag MH, Magaziner J. Post-operative considerations in hip fracture management. Curr Rheumatol Rep 2006;8(1):55–62.

30. MA;, Lyon LJ;Nevins. "Nontreatment of hip fractures in senile patients." JAMA, U.S. National Library of medicine.

31. Clarke BI. Balloon kyphoplasty for the treatment of Acute vertebral compression fractures: 2-year results from a randomized trial. Yearb Endocrinol 2011;2011: 231–3.

32. Home. ISCD, Accessed December 14, 2020, Available at: iscd.org/.

33. Urban K. New study identifies causative genes in osteoporosis." University of Michigan. Available at: labblog.uofmhealth.org/body-work/new-study-identifies-causative-genes-osteoporosis. Accessed March 22, 2019.

34. Kerschan-Schindl K. Romosozumab: a novel bone anabolic treatment option for osteoporosis?. 2020. Available at: https://www.ncbi.nlm.nih.gov/pmc/articles/PMC7098919/. . Accessed January 02, 2021.

35. Kessenich CR. Osteoporosis and African-American women. Women's Health Issues 2000;10(6):300–4.

36. Wysham KD, et al. Sex differences in frailty and its association with low bone mineral density in rheumatoid arthritis. Bone Rep 2020;12:100284.

37. Quinn KL, et al. Association between palliative care and healthcare outcomes among adults with terminal non-cancer illness: population based Matched cohort study. BMJ 2020;m2257.

38. Mosti MP;Kaehler N;Stunes AK, et al; "Maximal strength training in postmenopausal women with osteoporosis or osteopenia." J Strength Condition Res, U.S. National Library of medicine.

39. Shanb A, Youssef E. The impact of adding weight-bearing exercise versus non-weight bearing programs to the medical treatment of elderly patients with osteoporosis. J Fam Commun Med 2014;21(3):176.

40. M Lorentzon. "Treating osteoporosis to prevent fractures: current concepts and future developments." J Intern Med, U.S. National Library of medicine.

UNITED STATES POSTAL SERVICE®

Statement of Ownership, Management, and Circulation
(All Periodicals Publications Except Requester Publications)

1. Publication Title	2. Publication Number	3. Filing Date
CLINICS IN GERIATRIC MEDICINE	000 – 704	9/18/2021

4. Issue Frequency	5. Number of Issues Published Annually	6. Annual Subscription Price
FEB, MAY, AUG, NOV	4	$295.00

7. Complete Mailing Address of Known Office of Publication (Not printer) (Street, city, county, state, and ZIP+4®)

ELSEVIER INC.
230 Park Avenue, Suite 800
New York, NY 10169

Contact Person
Malathi Samayan

Telephone (Include area code)
91-44-4299-4507

8. Complete Mailing Address of Headquarters or General Business Office of Publisher (Not printer)

ELSEVIER INC.
230 Park Avenue, Suite 800
New York, NY 10169

9. Full Names and Complete Mailing Addresses of Publisher, Editor, and Managing Editor (Do not leave blank)

Publisher (Name and complete mailing address)

DOLORES MELONI, ELSEVIER INC.
1600 JOHN F KENNEDY BLVD. SUITE 1800
PHILADELPHIA, PA 19103-2899

Editor (Name and complete mailing address)

KATERINA HEIDHAUSEN, ELSEVIER INC.
1600 JOHN F KENNEDY BLVD. SUITE 1800
PHILADELPHIA, PA 19103-2899

Managing Editor (Name and complete mailing address)

PATRICK MANLEY, ELSEVIER INC.
1600 JOHN F KENNEDY BLVD. SUITE 1800
PHILADELPHIA, PA 19103-2899

10. Owner (Do not leave blank. If the publication is owned by a corporation, give the name and address of the corporation immediately followed by the names and addresses of all stockholders owning or holding 1 percent or more of the total amount of stock. If not owned by a corporation, give the names and addresses of the individual owners. If owned by a partnership or other unincorporated firm, give its name and address as well as those of each individual owner. If the publication is published by a nonprofit organization, give its name and address.)

Full Name	Complete Mailing Address
WHOLLY OWNED SUBSIDIARY OF REED/ELSEVIER, US HOLDINGS	1600 JOHN F KENNEDY BLVD. SUITE 1800 PHILADELPHIA PA 19103-2899

11. Known Bondholders, Mortgagees, and Other Security Holders Owning or Holding 1 Percent or More of Total Amount of Bonds, Mortgages, or Other Securities. If none, check box ▶ ☐ None

Full Name	Complete Mailing Address
N/A	

12. Tax Status (For completion by nonprofit organizations authorized to mail at nonprofit rates) (Check one)
The purpose, function, and nonprofit status of this organization and the exempt status for federal income tax purposes:
☒ Has Not Changed During Preceding 12 Months
☐ Has Changed During Preceding 12 Months (Publisher must submit explanation of change with this statement)

PS Form **3526**, July 2014 (Page 1 of 4 (see instructions page 4)) PSN 7530-01-000-9631 PRIVACY NOTICE: See our privacy policy on www.usps.com

13. Publication Title	14. Issue Date for Circulation Data Below
CLINICS IN GERIATRIC MEDICINE	MAY 2021

15. Extent and Nature of Circulation			Average No. Copies Each Issue During Preceding 12 Months	No. Copies of Single Issue Published Nearest to Filing Date
a. Total Number of Copies (Net press run)			143	122
b. Paid Circulation (By Mail and Outside the Mail)	(1)	Mailed Outside-County Paid Subscriptions Stated on PS Form 3541 (Include paid distribution above nominal rate, advertiser's proof copies, and exchange copies)	69	65
	(2)	Mailed In-County Paid Subscriptions Stated on PS Form 3541 (Include paid distribution above nominal rate, advertiser's proof copies, and exchange copies)	0	0
	(3)	Paid Distribution Outside the Mails Including Sales Through Dealers and Carriers, Street Vendors, Counter Sales, and Other Paid Distribution Outside USPS®	31	29
	(4)	Paid Distribution by Other Classes of Mail Through the USPS (e.g. First-Class Mail®)	0	0
c. Total Paid Distribution (Sum of 15b (1), (2), (3), and (4))		▶	100	94
d. Free or Nominal Rate Distribution (By Mail and Outside the Mail)	(1)	Free or Nominal Rate Outside-County Copies Included on PS Form 3541	29	11
	(2)	Free or Nominal Rate In-County Copies Included on PS Form 3541	0	0
	(3)	Free or Nominal Rate Copies Mailed at Other Classes Through the USPS (e.g. First-Class Mail)	0	0
	(4)	Free or Nominal Rate Distribution Outside the Mail (Carriers or other means)	0	0
e. Total Free or Nominal Rate Distribution (Sum of 15d (1), (2), (3) and (4))		▶	29	11
f. Total Distribution (Sum of 15c and 15e)		▶	129	105
g. Copies not Distributed (See Instructions to Publishers #4 (page #3))		▶	14	17
h. Total (Sum of 15f and g)		▶	143	122
i. Percent Paid (15c divided by 15f times 100)			77.51%	89.52%

* If you are claiming electronic copies, go to line 16 on page 3. If you are not claiming electronic copies, skip to line 17 on page 3.

16. Electronic Copy Circulation		Average No. Copies Each Issue During Preceding 12 Months	No. Copies of Single Issue Published Nearest to Filing Date
a. Paid Electronic Copies	▶		
b. Total Paid Print Copies (Line 15c) + Paid Electronic Copies (Line 16a)	▶		
c. Total Print Distribution (Line 15f) + Paid Electronic Copies (Line 16a)	▶		
d. Percent Paid (Both Print & Electronic Copies) (16b divided by 16c × 100)	▶		

☒ I certify that 50% of all my distributed copies (electronic and print) are paid above a nominal price.

17. Publication of Statement of Ownership

☒ If the publication is a general publication, publication of this statement is required. Will be printed ☐ Publication not required.

in the NOVEMBER 2021 issue of this publication.

18. Signature and Title of Editor, Publisher, Business Manager, or Owner

Malathi Samayan - Distribution Controller

Malathi Samayan

Date 9/18/2021

I certify that all information furnished on this form is true and complete. I understand that anyone who furnishes false or misleading information on this form or who omits material or information requested on the form may be subject to criminal sanctions (including fines and imprisonment) and/or civil sanctions (including civil penalties).

PS Form **3526**, July 2014 (Page 3 of 4) PRIVACY NOTICE: See our privacy policy on www.usps.com

Moving?

Make sure your subscription moves with you!

To notify us of your new address, find your **Clinics Account Number** (located on your mailing label above your name), and contact customer service at:

Email: journalscustomerservice-usa@elsevier.com

800-654-2452 (subscribers in the U.S. & Canada)
314-447-8871 (subscribers outside of the U.S. & Canada)

Fax number: 314-447-8029

**Elsevier Health Sciences Division
Subscription Customer Service
3251 Riverport Lane
Maryland Heights, MO 63043**

*To ensure uninterrupted delivery of your subscription, please notify us at least 4 weeks in advance of move.

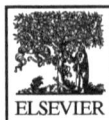

ELSEVIER

www.ingramcontent.com/pod-product-compliance
Lightning Source LLC
Chambersburg PA
CBHW050124240326
41458CB00122B/1332